THE EFFECTS OF STRESS AND POLLUTION ON MARINE ANIMALS

THE EFFECTS OF STRESS AND POLLUTION ON MARINE ANIMALS

*B. L. Bayne, D. A. Brown, K. Burns,
D. R. Dixon, A. Ivanovici, D. R. Livingstone,
D. M. Lowe, M. N. Moore,
A. R. D. Stebbing, and J. Widdows*

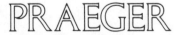

PRAEGER

PRAEGER SPECIAL STUDIES • PRAEGER SCIENTIFIC

New York • Philadelphia • Eastbourne, UK
Toronto • Hong Kong • Tokyo • Sydney

Library of Congress Cataloging in Publication Data

Main entry under title:

The effects of stress and pollution on marine animals.

      Bibliography: p.
      Includes index.
      1. Marine fauna—Effect of water pollution on.
2. Marine fauna—Physiology.   3. Stress (Physiology)
I. Bayne, B. L. (Brian Leicester)
QL121.E34   1985   591.5'2636   84-18145
ISBN 0-03-057019-0 (alk. paper)

Published in 1985 by Praeger Publishers
CBS Educational and Professional Publishing
a Division of CBS Inc.
521 Fifth Avenue, New York, NY 10175 USA
© 1985 by Praeger Publishers

56789 052 987654321

Printed in the United States of America
on acid-free paper

List of Contributors

Dr. B. L. Bayne
Institute for Marine Environmental
  Research
Prospect Place, The Hoe
Plymouth PL1 3DH, England

Dr. D. A. Brown
Southern California Coastal Water
  Research Project
646 W. Pacific Coast Highway
Long Beach, California 90806
U.S.A.

Dr. K. Burns
International Laboratory of Marine
  Radioactivity
Musee Oceanographique
Monaco-Ville, Monaco

Dr. D. R. Dixon
Institute for Marine Environmental
  Research
Prospect Place, The Hoe
Plymouth PL1 3DH, England

Dr. A. M. Ivanovici
Australian National Parks and
  Wildlife Service
PO Box 636
Canberra City A.C.T.
Australia 2601

Dr. D. R. Livingstone
Institute for Marine Environmental
  Research
Prospect Place, The Hoe
Plymouth PL1 3DH, England

Mr. D. M. Lowe
Institute for Marine Environmental
  Research
Prospect Place, The Hoe
Plymouth PL1 3DH, England

Dr. M. N. Moore
Institute for Marine Environmental
  Research
Prospect Place, The Hoe
Plymouth PL1 3DH, England

Dr. A. R. D. Stebbing
Institute for Marine Environmental
  Research
Prospect Place, The Hoe
Plymouth PL1 3DH, England

Dr. J. Widdows
Institute for Marine Environmental
  Research
Prospect Place, The Hoe
Plymouth PL1 3DH, England

Preface

The desire to write this manual arose gradually over a period of years during which the authors were working, both together and independently, in attempts to elucidate some of the physiological, cytological and biochemical responses of sessile marine invertebrates to potentially polluting compounds in the natural environment. Our joint aim was to arrive at measures of these responses that drew upon a fundamental understanding of the processes involved whilst at the same time providing straightforward indicators that could be used in programmes to monitor the effects of pollution. In our earliest discussions we realised that we could not attempt to be comprehensive, either in the methods to be discussed, or in the target species around which our text would be built. The result, inevitably, is a sub-sample of the many processes involved in animals' responses to pollutant stresses, and the primary focus of the manual is on marine bivalves, particularly the common mussel. Having said this, however, we consider that the processes discussed cover a wide range in the repertory of most marine invertebrates as they respond and adjust to the demands of a contaminated environment; and whereas the emphasis on a single group of organisms is particularly relevant to programmes such as Mussel Watch, much of what we say has a much wider potential application amongst both invertebrate and vertebrate phylla.

Although the authors share a common interest, we vary in geographical allegiance. Some of us have worked together for many years at the Institute for Marine Environmental Research in Plymouth, U.K. (Brian Bayne, Dave Dixon, Dave Livingstone, David Lowe, Mike Moore, Tony Stebbing and John Widdows) where a research programme is designed to link studies at the biochemical, cytochemical, cytological and physiological levels into an integrated understanding of toxicological response in marine invertebrates. Kathy Burns first worked on invertebrate responses to hydrocarbons at the Woods Hole Oceanographic Institution in the U.S. and more recently in Monaco. Angela Ivanovici is currently with the Australian National Parks and Wildlife Service but first worked on the energy charge ratio for her doctorate in Melbourne. Dave Brown also first encountered biological polluting effects during his doctorate in Vancouver and has since continued and developed his interest in responses to metals and to organic compounds in California.

In writing this manual, and in attempting to maintain an up-to-date text during a rather long gestation period, we have tried to ensure that the product is, primarily, a useful practical account of a wide variety of techniques covering different levels in the hierarchy of biological response. However, we considered it necessary also to present some of the scientific background to the procedures described, in order that their generality might be appreciated and independently assessed. Most of the techniques have been evaluated both in the laboratory and, importantly, in the natural environment, on individuals exposed to different levels of contamination. In this lengthy process of initial formulation of a physiological or biochemical measurement, through experimentation in the laboratory and eventual testing in the field, one other common aim has been to simplify the required procedures and so to make the technique as widely available and practical as possible.

Our hope, then, is that this manual will serve as a useful starting point for many programmes designed to measure the biological effects of environmental stress factors, including pollution. In this way, by a wide and informed testing of these (and other) procedures, we anticipate significant improvements in our ability to monitor the quality of the natural environment in terms of biological as well as chemical criteria.

B. L. Bayne
Plymouth, 1984

Contents

General Introduction

The observation that organisms are adapted to the environment lies at the foundation of biology. The evolutionary and ecological framework to this observation attributes to the organism a suite of adaptive responses (biochemical, physiological, behavioural) which together enable it to survive and to reproduce within a particular set of environmental conditions. These conditions are seldom constant, however, even for a single individual; there is considerable variability in both the biotic and the abiotic factors experienced by most free-living organisms. The adaptability of the organism may therefore be defined by its capacity to adjust its physiology to operate with optimal efficiency in a variable environment.

It is the role of physiological ecology (and related sub-disciplines of ecology) to understand the adaptive capability of animals and plants. A major contribution of physiology to ecology in recent years has been to provide a set of ideas that allows knowledge of the physiological flexibility of an organism to be related to the demands of the environment. The result of adaptive change by the organism is seen as new functional and structural states that lead to a greater efficiency of performance, and greater fitness for survival in the environment. Three related concepts comprise this contemporary paradigm of functional adaptability in animals.

Kinne (1964) considered the time course of adaptive responses to changes in temperature and salinity and distinguished between the immediate response, the stabilisation of the response and the new steady state of performance. The immediate response to an environmental change occurs over a time span of seconds to hours and often involves over-shoot or under-shoot phenomena in altered rates of physiological or other processes. During the stabilisation of the response, the functional process gradually stabilises over a period of hours to days and eventually achieves the new steady state.

The phenomenon of altered steady states of physiological and biochemical processes in response to environmental change is termed acclimation (when the response is to a change in one environmental variable, usually imposed in a laboratory experiment) or acclimatisation (when the response is to a change in more than one variable, as usually encountered in nature). These concepts were originally explored by Bullock (1955), Prosser (1958) and Precht (1958) and have since been reviewed many times; for more recent reviews see Hazel and Prosser (1974) and Newell (1979). In particular, the classification of the various types of acclimatory response offered by Prosser (1958) has proved useful in studies of the effects of temperature on organisms.

The third related concept is due to Fry (1947) and concerns the relationship between the acclimated condition and the response of the organism to environmental extremes. Fry distinguished between the zone of tolerance, encompassing the range of environmental conditions that could be tolerated indefinitely by the organism, and the zone of resistance, including those conditions tolerable for certain limited periods only. Alderdice (1976) has recently demonstrated the equivalence between the ideas of Fry and those of Prosser and Precht.

Working within this conceptual framework, it becomes possible to characterise, in a quantitative manner, the effects on animals of particular changes in the environment. The response to the environmental stimulus is fully adaptive if the new steady-state condition is quantitatively similar to the numerical value of the physiological variable prior to the environmental change. Under such circumstances acclimation or acclimatisation is said to be complete, and no lasting change in the functional state of the animal can be deduced. However, if the new physiological steady-state is measurably different from its former value, the effect of the stimulus can be recorded as a change in functional state.

An alteration in the functional state or condition of an animal may represent an improvement to the organism's fitness or well-being; the individual may now be better able to compete with others, to escape predators or to grow and reproduce. Equally, a change may represent a deterioration in well-being, rendering the individual less fit. For a full interpretation of the effect(s) of the environmental change, therefore, one must not only assess the resulting change in the organism's physiology, but also judge whether the performance of the organism has been made more or less adaptive (Bayne, 1984).

These ideas were considered by Brett (1958) in his attempt to quantify the damaging effects of environmental changes on fish. He defined "stress" as "a state produced by an environmental or other factor which extends the adaptive responses of an animal beyond the normal range, or which disturbs the normal functioning to such an extent . . . that the chances of survival are significantly reduced". Brett therefore identified a state of stress as the result of the animal's evolved adaptive capability being stretched to the point where damaging effects on fitness result. In more recent usage, however (see Bayne, 1984) the term stress is used to refer to the environmental stimulus (rather than to the physiological state that represents the response) which, by exceeding a threshold value, disturbs normal animal function. When used in this way there is an equivalence with the term as applied to ecosystems (Odum, 1967; Ulanowicz, 1978).

One of the aims of this manual is to illustrate some of these ideas in the context of the effects of environmental deterioration on estuarine and marine invertebrates. Some categories of environmental deterioration may be called pollution, which is the discharge, by man, of substances or energy into the environment such as to create a hazard to its living resources. Studies of pollution in natural ecosystems have many aspects, physical, chemical and biological. The physical aspects include the distribution of potential pollutants (or contaminants) within the ecosystem, and the chemical aspects include the levels and chemical forms of contaminant found within both the biotic and the abiotic components of the ecosystem. However, it is a recognition of the biological effects of contamination (if any) that defines the true significance of the physical and chemical data. No complete assessment of pollution is possible without some understanding of these biological effects. Pollution therefore represents an environmental stress whose effects on organisms can be measured within the framework of ideas just discussed. It is our hope that this manual will help in the making of biological assessments of the environmental impact of pollution.

There is also a wider application for these ideas and for these techniques, however. Not all the potential stress factors in the environment are the result of man's activities. No habitat is totally benign. In seeking to understand the ecology of any species, attention must be directed to the variety of functional processes that sets limits to the adaptability of individuals. The use of experimental procedures that measure the effects of environmental changes within the normal experience of an animal will help in understanding the animal's distribution in nature and its limits of tolerance to natural change, and in providing a quantitative indicator of ecological fitness. These measures may also facilitate the management of stocks of animals in aquaculture, by giving expression to animal well-being.

In this manual, therefore, we shall discuss various procedures for assessing the condition or well-being of estuarine and marine invertebrates, with the wider needs of marine ecology, as well as those of pollution studies, in mind.

In discussing this topic of the adaptation of animals to environmental change, a distinction must be made between general and specific responses to stress. The concept of general stress response was developed by Selye (1950), from work with mammals. He describes a general stress syndrome that is characteristic of the body's response to a variety of environmental insults. In mammals this syndrome includes hormonal, metabolic and cytological symptoms which constitute the general response to the environmental change. The concept is equally applicable to aquatic invertebrates; the components of the "stress syndrome" may vary between species, but the observation that a species (or a higher taxonomic grouping) has a common, general, response to a variety of potentially damaging environmental conditions is probably universal (Pickering, 1981). Much of this manual is devoted to discussing aspects of the general response to such conditions in certain marine invertebrates and to suggesting ways in which the relevant symptoms can be observed and measured.

It is also necessary to recognise that animals respond in specific ways to particular types of pollutant or other stress. For example, a change in the salinity of the medium may induce in aquatic invertebrates certain responses that result in the regulation of cell volume; these responses may be entirely specific to salinity (or, strictly, to osmotic) changes. This observation becomes particularly important in pollution research, where the use of general stress indicators may identify a deterioration in an animal's well-being without being able to suggest the causative factor. When such an observation can be amplified by a specific indication of the type of pollutant involved (metals, petroleum hydrocarbons, etc.) the usefulness of the information for environmental management is greatly enhanced.

Progress in the task of identifying specific responses to known pollutants is helped by the knowledge that most organisms have evolved some means of detoxifying anthropogenic contaminants. Often the detoxifying mechanism has an inducible component; i.e. the animal has the capacity to increase its efficiency at detoxifying a particular contaminant, up to a maximum level. When exposure to the contaminant exceeds the maximum capacity in the detoxifying system, toxic effects result and the organism suffers a deterioration in condition. The identification of the detoxifying mechanism, and the determination of its maximum capacity, provides a means of defining specific pollutant effects and also suggests the quantitative relationship between the concentration of contaminant in the body (the dose) and the biological effect (the response). We devote some sections of this manual to the description of certain detoxifying processes and procedures for their measurement.

Three categories of measurement for assessing the effects of environmental changes on animals can therefore be recognised:

1. The components of the general response to stress.
2. The specific effects of individual contaminants.
3. The change in fitness that results from these responses to environmental stimuli.

These three aspects are all discussed further, together with details of relevant procedures, in this manual.

One other problem remains, namely, the choice of biological material. Of course, in many studies this choice will be made on considerations other than the suitability of the material for registering the effects of environmental deterioration. In other areas, however, and particularly in pollution studies, a choice based on considerations of suitability can be made. This problem has received the attention of many working groups concerned with recommending practices for pollution assessment (McIntyre and Pearce, 1980). In this manual we concentrate our attention mostly on estuarine invertebrates, largely because this is the main field of expertise of the authors, although much of what is discussed could apply to other types of animals, including fish.

The use of sessile invertebrates in environmental quality assessments has much to recommend it. They are unable to escape from environmental deterioration and must either adjust to the change or succumb. Organisms that live in estuaries, which are naturally testing environments, often possess wide physiological tolerance to stress; that is, the boundary between the lethal and the sub-lethal condition, or—in Fry's (1947) terminology—the area of the zone resistance, may be great. This allows for the easier recognition of states of stress, through the measurement of altered physiological or biochemical steady-states, than in other species where the individual's zone of tolerance may be narrow. It is the difference between a eurytopic (wide tolerance to environmental change) and a stenotopic (narrow tolerance) species; the former category, which includes estuarine molluscs, worms and crustaceans, is more suited for environmental quality assessment.

One other consideration is worth mentioning here. Sessile invertebrates, such as bivalve molluscs and some worms, are mostly "primitive" in a taxonomic sense, and whereas certain cellular and metabolic detoxification systems exist in these species, they have not evolved to the degree of efficiency found in more "advanced" species. This has the effect that exposure to certain contaminants will result in a measurable effect on the detoxification system, although, because of the low level of efficiency, general toxic effects will also be felt. Such an organism can therefore provide a general indicator of environmental impact, through measurements of the general response to stress, as well as affording specific indications of the causative agent.

PART **I**

THE SCIENTIFIC
BACKGROUND

1

Physiological Measurements

Physiological responses have three important attributes in providing an assessment of an individual's condition (or health): (1) they represent an integration of the many cellular and biochemical processes that can alter in response to changes in the environment, (2) they represent non-specific (general) responses to the sum of environmental stimuli which are complementary to more specific responses at the biochemical level and (3) they are capable of reflecting deterioration in the environment before effects manifest themselves in the population or the community.

In this chapter the discussion will be limited to those measurements that have been found to be useful in quantifying an organism's physiological condition (i.e. state variables such as body condition index and O:N ratio), its performance (i.e. rate variables such as growth rate) and the efficiency with which the animal functions (such as growth efficiency), in response to environmental stress and pollution. For such responses to be considered useful measures of an animal's condition and therefore suitable for inclusion in this manual, they should fulfill most of the following criteria:

1. To reflect a quantitative or predictable relationship with the stressor or pollutant.
2. To have ecological significance and be shown, or convincingly argued, to be related to an adverse or damaging effect on the growth, reproduction or survival of the individual, the population and ultimately the well-being of the community.

3

3. To be sensitive to stress and pollution and to have a large scope for response throughout the range from optimal to lethal conditions.
4. To have a response time that reflects an integrated steady-state condition that does not alter significantly with short-term fluctuations in the environment (e.g. tidal and diurnal fluctuations).
5. To be measurable with precision and with a high signal-to-noise ratio; i.e. the effect (signal) must be easily detectable above the natural variability (noise).
6. To be easily measured in the laboratory and field under ambient conditions, without the use of very expensive equipment, complicated procedures or high running costs.

With these considerations in mind, it is possible to propose four relevant physiological responses. Although these responses have been developed and evaluated in field monitoring programmes using the common mussel (*Mytilus edulis*) as the indicator species, the fundamental concepts and many of the procedures are immediately applicable to other species. The four physiological stress indices discussed in detail in this section are:

1. Scope for growth—a measure of the energy status of an organism.
2. Growth efficiency—the efficiency with which an individual converts food into body tissues.
3. Oxygen and nitrogen ratio—a measure of the balance between catabolic processes.
4. Body condition indices—indicative of alterations in the nutritional status of the animal.

All the physiological stress indices, except body condition indices, are derived from integrations of basic biological processes, and these are described and discussed under the first index, the scope for growth. A comprehensive knowledge of the test organism's response to a wide range of intrinsic factors (such as size, age, reproduction and nutritional state) and extrinsic factors (such as temperature, salinity, ration, dissolved oxygen, suspended particulates and pollutants) is important at all stages of a monitoring programme (planning, measurement and interpretation of results). But a detailed review of the factors affecting each physiological response (e.g. respiration, feeding, etc.) will not be included in this chapter; instead discussion will be limited to the factors affecting the integrated stress indices themselves.

SCOPE FOR GROWTH

Production of matter (growth and reproduction) is a fundamental property of all living organisms and one that is necessary if a population is to persist in a given environment. The amount of production represents the difference between an individual's or a population's intake and output of matter or energy, and this will vary under different environmental conditions. Alterations in the amount of matter or energy incorporated into growth and reproduction can be described by the balanced energy equation of Winberg (1960):

$$C - F = A = R + U + P \tag{1}$$

or

$$P = A - (R + U) \tag{2}$$

where C = food energy consumed, F = energy lost as faeces, A = energy absorbed from the food, R = energy respired, U = energy excreted and P = energy incorporated into somatic growth and gamete production.

Each component on the right-hand side of Eq. (2) is a physiological process that can be readily measured and converted into energy equivalents (Joules per hour). The energy budget thus provides a means of integrating these basic physiological processes (feeding, food absorption, respiration and excretion) in an index of the energy available for growth and reproduction. This has been termed the "scope for growth" by Warren and Davis (1967) because it is not measured directly but rather is derived by subtraction of energy respired and excreted from the energy absorbed from the food. The advantages provided by this energy budget approach are (1) sensitivity, i.e. when a direct measure of growth may be unable to detect immediately the more subtle effects of an environmental change and (2) an understanding of the bioenergetics of production or an assessment of the energy status of the individual and the various components of growth under different environmental conditions. The direct measurement of growth and production is difficult in many species, especially bivalve molluscs, because a large proportion of the total production can be lost in the form of gametes (either in a single complete release or by gradual spawning) and because the measurement of tissue somatic growth or weight change is impracticable on individuals due to the presence of a shell.

Scope for growth is a useful stress index because it is an integration of the whole organism's response to the total environmental stimulus including both natural and anthropogenic stressors. The growth potential is an indicator of the animal's physiological condition from optimal through sublethal to lethal conditions (Widdows, 1978b). For example, the scope for growth can range from positive values when there is energy available for growth and production of gametes, to negative values when the animal is severely stressed and utilising its body reserves for maintenance metabolism.

Table 1-1 lists many of the studies that have determined "scope for growth" of aquatic organisms. Warren and Davis (1967) were the first to use scope for growth as a method of examining the bioenergetics of production in fish in response to environmental change (e.g. temperature). The use of this index for assessing the physiological condition of mussels in laboratory stress experiments has since been described by Widdows and Bayne (1971), Bayne (1975) and Widdows (1978b). More recently, scope for growth has been measured for animals in the field in response to natural environmental stressors (Bayne and Widdows, 1978) and pollution (Bayne et al., 1979; Widdows et al., 1981b). In addition, Gilfillan (1975) and Gilfillan et al. (1976) have shown that scope for growth (estimated in terms of carbon flux rather than energy units) declined in three bivalve species (*Mytilus edulis*, *Modiolus demissus* and *Mya arenaria*) as a result of exposure to oil.

When the scope for growth has been measured under natural conditions, it has proved to be an accurate predictor of total production (i.e. observed rates of growth and estimated gamete production; Bayne et al., 1979). Even when certain simplifying assumptions are made in the measurement of growth potential, agreement between prediction and field observation is good (Gilfillan and Vandermeulen, 1978; Bayne and Worrall, 1980).

Physiological Components of the Energy Equation

In the following sections is has been necessary to consider the main physiological components of the energy equation as discrete biological processes, but it must be emphasised that any change in a component should be interpreted in the context of the energy equation (or other physiological integrations, e.g. O : N ratio) and not as an isolated response.

A decline in growth rate, for example, can arise from a reduction in energy intake and/or an increase in energy output. A

TABLE 1-1. Summary of Some Studies in Which the Scope for Growth of Marine Invertebrates Has Been Determined

Independent variables	Species	References	Comments
Temperature	*Mytilus edulis*	Widdows & Bayne (1971)	
	Mytilus edulis	Bayne et al. (1975, 1978)	
	Mytilus edulis	Widdows (1978b)	
	Thais lapillus	Stickle (unpublished data)	
Salinity	*Thais lapillus*	Stickle (unpublished data)	
	Mytilus edulis	Widdows (unpublished data)	
Ration	*Mytilus edulis*	Thompson & Bayne (1974)	
	Mytilus edulis	Bayne et al. (1975, 1978)	
	Mytilus edulis	Widdows (1978b)	
	Aulacomya ater	Griffiths & King (1979)	
Body size	*Mytilus edulis*	Thompson & Bayne (1974)	
	Mytilus edulis	Widdows (1978b)	
	Aulacomya ater	Griffiths & King (1979)	
	Perna viridis	Shafee (1979)	
Seasonal cycle	*Mytilus edulis*	Widdows (1978b)	
	Mytilus edulis	Bayne & Widdows (1978)	Field study
	Crassostrea virginica	Dame (1972)	Field study
	Cerastoderma edule	Newell (1977)	Field study
Petroleum hydrocarbons	*Mytilus edulis*	Gilfillan (1975)	
	Mytilus edulis	Widdows et al. (1982)	
	Modiolus demissus	Gilfillan (1975)	
	Acartia tonsa	Gilfillan et al. (unpublished data)	Large enclosure

(continued)

TABLE 1-1. *(Continued)*

Independent variables	Species	References	Comments
Environmental stress and pollution	*Mytilus edulis*	Bayne et al. (1979)	Population differences
	Mytilus edulis	Widdows et al. (1981a)	Pollution gradient
	Mytilus edulis	Widdows et al. (1981b)	Pollution gradient
	Mya arenaria	Gilfillan et al. (1977)	Oil spill
	Calanus hyperboreus	Gilfillan et al. (unpublished data)	Underwater oil seep

reduction in energy intake may be caused by any one or a combination of the following:

1. Reduced feeding rates.
2. Reduced food availability.
3. Reduced efficiency of digestion and absorption of food material.

An increase in energy output or loss may be caused by

1. Increased respiration rate.
2. Increased excretion rate.

A change in any one component can therefore have an important influence on the energy equation and ultimately the scope for growth. However, when changes in these physiological processes are measured in isolation their interpretation is often difficult. In many cases an individual physiological response does not bear a simple quantitative relationship with stress. For example, an increase in respiration rate, and therefore in energy loss, can represent an adaptive response when it is associated with a higher level of feeding activity. Under these circumstances, the increase in food energy intake more than compensates for the increase in respired energy loss and the organism improves its growth rate. In contrast, an increase in metabolic rate resulting from contamination by petroleum hydrocarbons, because it is concomitant with a reduction in feeding rate, causes a lowering of growth rate and this is considered a stress response.

The measurement and interpretation of a physiological response should also be made with due consideration of the effects of extrinsic and intrinsic factors. *Extrinsic factors* that can affect the functioning of marine and estuarine organisms include natural environmental stressors (temperature, salinity, dissolved oxygen, the quality and quantity of suspended particulates, aerial exposure, light intensity and current speed) and anthropogenic stressors (metals, petroleum hydrocarbons and halogenated hydrocarbons and radionuclides). All relevant extrinsic factors should be measured in the normal course of a monitoring programme. There is often sufficient information available, mainly from laboratory studies, to assess the extent to which a particular environmental variable affects the performance of an organism.

In many cases the organism has the ability to compensate for changes in environmental conditions, within defined limits, and this enables certain rates and processes to be maintained relatively independent of alterations in the environment. The capacity of a species to adapt to the normal range of environmental variables, such as temperature, salinity, suspended particulates and pO_2, is likely to be an important consideration in the choice of an indicator organism for an environmental monitoring programme. The mussel, *M. edulis*, is a good example of an organism that is capable of maintaining many of its biological processes relatively independent of the normal fluctuations in natural environmental variables, whilst at the same time remaining responsive to environmental contaminants and natural environmental stressors deviating from the normal range of tolerance. As a result, the level of "noise" or variability in the physiological response is reduced and the "signal-to-noise ratio" increased.

The major *intrinsic causes* of variability include size, age, seasonality related to the cycling of reproductive processes and the effects of nutritional status (i.e. the quantity and quality of body energy reserves).

Body size: The rates of most physiological processes are dependent on individual body size (reviewed by Bayne et al., 1976a, 1976b). The effects of size are traditionally removed from physiological measurements by application of the allometric model relating the rate of the process (Y) to body mass (X):

$$Y = aX^b$$

where a and b are the intercept and the slope of the regression line, respectively. If the sample size is sufficiently large, regression techniques allow an estimate of size-related variance. Regression of physiological responses against body size enables populations of different size ranges to be compared. An alternative and simplified approach is to remove the effect of size by measuring the response of standard-sized animals from a population that has been transplanted to various sites for a period of time (see Chapter 7).

Age: The effect of age on the physiological responses of marine organisms is unknown; this is an area that requires further research but at present there is no evidence to suggest that it is an important consideration.

Reproductive condition: Seasonal variability related to the cycling of reproductive processes is often considerable in marine organisms. Therefore, physiological measurements should be carried out regularly over a seasonal cycle and combined with cytological assessments of the reproductive condition of the animal. Alternatively, measurements may be confined to a particular phase in the reproductive cycle or to one particular season when all organisms are known to be in a similar gametogenic stage. These matters are considered in more detail later.

Nutritional status: Nutritional status, defined as the quantity and quality of body energy reserves, varies seasonally with the reproductive cycle and the availability of food. Its effects on individual physiological responses therefore cannot be considered in isolation from these other two factors.

Respiration

Respiration represents a measure of that part of the food intake (or of available body reserves) which is required to provide energy to support life processes. Energy losses by respiration can be expressed in terms of oxygen utilisation, carbon dioxide liberation or heat production. The direct calorimetric measurement of energy loss in the form of heat resulting from biochemical oxidations and various motor activities is generally regarded as impracticable for routine use on small animals. A much more convenient measure is that of the rate of oxygen consumption, which can subsequently be converted into energy equivalents.

Aerobic and Anaerobic Metabolism. Energy metabolism can be divided into aerobic and anaerobic forms, with the majority of marine organisms obtaining energy from the aerobic oxidation of carbohydrates, lipids and proteins. However, some invertebrates are adapted to withstand periods of reduced oxygen supply, either as a result of inhabiting low oxygen environments or as a result of temporary isolation from the oxic environment, e.g. by shell closure in bivalve molluscs. Under such circumstances anaerobic metabolic pathways are utilised and carbohydrates form the main source of energy (for review, see De Zwaan, 1977). The energy requirement of organisms under hypoxic or anoxic conditions can be calculated, at least in part, from the accumulation of end-products of anaerobiosis (De Zwaan and Wijsman, 1976; Widdows et al., 1979a). The low anaerobic rate of energy consumption and extent to which anaerobiosis is utilised by the majority of marine organisms means that anaerobiosis does not represent a significant energy loss when compared with aerobic metabolic losses. The anaerobic contribution to the energy budget will not be considered further.

Rate of Oxygen Consumption

A review of the extensive literature on the rate of oxygen consumption by marine organisms will not be attempted here because many researchers have measured oxygen consumption as an isolated biological response, ignoring the fact that respiration is covariant with other biological functions, such as behavioural responses, feeding activity and nutrition. Therefore, in many studies it is difficult to interpret the significance of an alteration in the rate of oxygen consumption. For example, the literature concerning the effects of petroleum hydrocarbons on the respiration rate of aquatic organisms provides conflicting evidence (Johnson, 1977), both enhanced and depressed rates of respiration having been reported. But when behavioural responses and respiration are measured simultaneously, it is apparent that the direct effect of hydrocarbons is to enhance oxygen consumption and that the observed decrease in respiration is largely the result of suppression of activity and partial closure or isolation or organisms when exposed to higher hydrocarbon concentrations. It is therefore important that individual physiological responses, such as respiration, are not considered in isolation from other biological functions which act as covariants.

Terminology and Methodology. Several different levels of metabolism can be estimated, depending on the conditions under which respiration is measured. The three most commonly used terms for these levels are standard (= resting), routine and active (Fry, 1947, 1971). The standard metabolic rate is defined as the minimum energy requirement for the maintenance of all essential functions within an inactive animal. It is either determined at zero activity or extrapolated to zero activity from determinations at various levels of induced activity. Active metabolism is the level of oxygen consumption under conditions of maximum activity. The amount of energy available for external work has been termed the "scope for activity" by Fry (1947) and represents the difference between active (maximum) and standard (minimum) metabolism. Routine metabolism is at an intermediate level between active and standard metabolism and represents the rate of oxygen uptake by an animal whose activity is spontaneous and reflects the metabolic rate under natural conditions.

All these terms were originally adopted in fish physiology (Fry, 1947, 1971; Brett, 1965) and have since been applied to metabolic rates of invertebrates (Newell, 1979; Bayne et al., 1976b). In the context of environmental studies and biological effects monitoring, the routine level of metabolism is of most interest. To provide a realistic estimate of the routine rate of oxygen consumption, and ultimately respiratory energy loss in relation to different environmental conditions, it is important to maintain the animal and measure its respiration under conditions as similar as possible to the environment to which it is acclimatized. It is easier to meet this requirement with species such as sessile suspension-feeding organisms that must passively experience the varying conditions in the water mass, than with animals exhibiting a foraging or predatory feeding activity which is usually suppressed in a respirometer.

Correct methodology is extremely important in the measurement of respiration. Winberg (1960), Beamish and Dickie (1967) and Crisp (1971) have reviewed the methodology and identified the precautions to be observed; consequently only the main features and limitations of the various methods will be reviewed in this chapter. Methods for measuring oxygen consumption can be divided into three general categories:

1. Sealed container. This is probably the most common method and involves determining a change in oxygen content in a sealed chamber over a period of time. The closed system is simple to set up, but not all the conditions remain constant; oxygen decreases, carbon dioxide and excretory products increase and a suspension feeder will reduce the particulate concentration

throughout the course of the experiment. Since these factors can affect respiration it is important to flush the respiration chamber at regular intervals, before the factors reach levels that affect the rate of oxygen uptake.

2. Continuous flow system. In this system, oxygen consumption is calculated from the difference in oxygen content between the inflow and outflow at a known flow rate. The advantage of this method is the constancy of conditions, but with low rates of oxygen consumption and consequent small differences in oxygen content between inflow and outflow there is some loss of accuracy.

3. Manometric method. This is generally used when measuring the respiration rate of smaller organisms (Gilson, 1963; Davies, 1966; Lawton and Richards, 1970). It has the advantage that ambient oxygen and carbon dioxide levels are held constant by the replacement of oxygen consumed and absorption of carbon dioxide produced. But it has the disadvantage of not being able to flush the respiration chamber without considerable disturbance, and the method often requires agitation of the chamber to facilitate gaseous exchange.

A flow-through respirometer that is sealed for a limited period of time is recommended as the most suitable method for use in a monitoring programme; the procedures are outlined in detail in Chapter 7.

Energy Losses by Respiration

Oxygen consumption is an important physiological measurement, especially in the context of the energy equation, because it represents a measure of the energy required to support and sustain life. The rate of energy dissipation in metabolism can be obtained from the rate of oxygen consumption by using a factor originally known as the "oxycalorific coefficient" (Ivlev, 1934; Winberg, 1971; Crisp, 1971). However, it should be noted that the calorie as the fundamental unit of energy has now been replaced by the Joule (1 cal = 4.184 J). Table 1-2 gives the oxycalorific coefficients and Joule equivalents for converting oxygen uptake into energy from the three main components of food. It is fortunate that, when the different types of food source are fully oxidised, the variation in energy equivalent for a given oxygen consumption is minimal. Therefore, a single oxycalorific coefficient of 4.86 cal ml^{-1} oxygen (or 20.33 J ml^{-1} oxygen) can be used to convert oxygen consumption to energy equivalents (Crisp, 1971). Energy loss in respiration

TABLE 1-2. Oxycalorific Values of Different Energy Sources (at n.t.p.)

Component	cal ml^{-1} oxygen	J ml^{-1} oxygen
Carbohydrate	5.05	21.13
Fat	4.69	19.62
Protein	4.73	19.79
Approximate mean	4.86	20.33

is therefore calculated from the respiration rate in ml O_2 g^{-1} dry mass h^{-1}, multiplied by 20.33 J ml^{-1} O_2.

Feeding and Digestion

Measurements of feeding and digestion processes provide estimates of the amount of food or energy intake, and of that part of the consumed energy which is absorbed and utilised by the animal and not rejected as faeces. This forms an important component of the energy equation and one that is generally sensitive to stress and pollution. The quantitative measurement of food consumption by animals in laboratory studies is regarded as relatively straightforward, but to make the same measurements of animals that are free in their natural habitat is usually very difficult.

The nature of the feeding mechanism is determined largely by the habitat and the food available to a particular organism. The form and function of the digestive tract are also dependent on the types of food utilised and the organism's feeding mechanism. Suspension feeders, and especially filter feeding bivalve molluscs, have a feeding process that can be measured in the field under near ambient conditions. The discussion of feeding rate measurements in this section will be limited to the suspension feeding of bivalves, again with particular reference to *M. edulis*. For a detailed review of the filtration mechanism, feeding and digestion in *Mytilus* see Bayne et al. (1976b).

Clearance Rate

The rate of suspension feeding is usually measured in terms of clearance rate, which is defined as the volume of water cleared of particles per unit time. In bivalves, the gills filter and remove from the ventilation current all suspended particles greater than 2–5 μm in diameter with 100% retention efficiency (Vahl, 1972; Jorgensen, 1975; Bayne et al., 1977; Møhlenberg and Riisgard, 1978) and even retain particles of 1 μm diameter with ca. 50% efficiency. If clearance rate is based on the filtering of particles greater than approximately 4 μm in diameter (i.e. particle retention efficiency is 100%), then clearance rate is equal to the ventilation (or pumping) rate.

Clearance rates can be measured either in static or in flow-through systems (reviewed by Bayne et al., 1976b). In the static system, which is the simpler method, the bivalve is confined in an appropriate volume of water containing a suspension of suitable particles (usually unicellular algae), and the filtration results in an exponential decline in the particle concentration. The theoretical basis of the method is discussed by Coughlan (1969), who points out that the different forms of the exponential relationship which have been used by various workers are essentially the same. The flow-through system, however, offers many advantages over the static system: steady-state conditions can be maintained over relatively long periods of time without disturbance to the animal (e.g. the amount of particulate matter available to the animal does not decline), there is no reduction in pO_2 or accumulation of ammonia and other excretory products and it is possible to detect periods of non-activity. Clearance rate is determined in a flow-through system by expressing the particle concentration in the water before and after the animal in relation to flow rate. The flow-through method is preferred and is described in detail in Chapter 7.

The degree to which clearance rate is maintained at a steady-state under constant experimental conditions is largely dependent upon the species being studied. In many intertidal bivalves, of which M. edulis is a good example, pumping rate or clearance rate is maintained at a constant level over considerable periods of time (Bayne et al., 1977; Brand and Taylor, 1974). In contrast, subtidal bivalves like Arctica islandica show a very intermittent pattern of pumping activity (Brand and Taylor, 1974). The feature of essentially continuous feeding represents an important consideration when selecting an experimental animal suitable for measurement of physiological stress indices such as the scope for growth, because the feeding rate can be easily determined without the need to establish an average daily feeding rate from constant measurement and integration of feeding over several hours.

Filtration Rate and Absorption Efficiency

The filtration rate, defined as the quantity of particulate material filtered out of the water per hour, is obtained by multiplying the clearance rate (litre h^{-1}) by the particle concentration (mg litre^{-1}). The filtration rate (mg h^{-1}) is then converted to energy equivalents by multiplying by the energy content of the particulate organic material.

A large and variable proportion of the particulate organic matter (POM) is refractory and not utilised as an energy substrate by heterotrophic organisms. The proportion of POM in the total seston and the proportion of utilisable food will vary with season and physical environmental factors (e.g. substratum, wave action, tidal movements). At one extreme, oceanic waters have a low total seston concentration of ca. 0.5 mg litre^{-1}, of which ca. 65% is POM and only 40% is utilisable (e.g. Shetland Islands; Widdows et al., 1981a). Towards the other extreme, estuarine and brackish waters have a higher total seston (especially in autumn and winter when there are high freshwater inputs and sediment resuspension), e.g. 40 mg litre^{-1}, of which 12% is POM and 5% is utilisable as food (Widdows et al., 1979b). These environmental differences in the proportion of utilisable organic matter in the seston will be reflected in the efficiency with which organic material is absorbed by the animal.

A suspension feeding bivalve, such as *Mytilus*, filters all particles greater than a minimum diameter from the ventilation current and transports them, via the mouth, to the stomach and digestive gland for digestion and absorption. The efficiency with which food material is absorbed by the digestive system can be determined in several ways (reviewed by Calow and Fletcher, 1972):

1. Gravimetric method. The ratio of the food absorbed into the organism to the total amount of food ingested, i.e. $(C-F)/C$, is measured either in terms of dry ash-free weights or, preferably, as units of energy. The difficulty with this method is that the amount of food ingested and faeces egested must be determined over an interval of time sufficiently long to be representative of a steady state.

2. Radiotracer method. Food absorption is estimated by measuring the difference between the amount of isotope ingested and egested by the animals. However this technique also requires the quantitative collection of faeces and the complete removal of non-absorbed isotope from the gut.

3. Indicator method. This technique involves measuring the increase in concentration of an inert, non-absorbed substance as it passes through the gut. The non-absorbed substance may either be part of the food, e.g. ash (Conover, 1966), or be added by the experimenter, e.g. chromic oxide (McGinnis and Kasting, 1964). The advantage of this method is that food ingested and faeces egested do not have to be collected quantitatively. However, it is based on two assumptions: that only the organic fraction in the food is significantly affected by the digestive processes, and that there are minimal losses of metabolic secretions, e.g. mucus, and excretory products into the faeces. Such losses will result in an underestimate of absorbtion efficiency.

4. Dual-radiotracer technique. The use of two isotopes (^{14}C and ^{51}Cr) together not only enables a distinction to be made between faecal material derived from food and that derived from metabolic secretions, but also facilitates estimation of assimilation efficiencies from small samples of faeces only (Calow and Fletcher, 1972). This new technique is a combination of the radiotracer and indicator methods and involves measuring the ratio of an absorbed (e.g. ^{14}C) to a non-absorbed (e.g. ^{51}Cr) indicator in samples of both food and faeces.

Although the dual-radiotracer technique is recognised as an improvement on other procedures it is not suitable for routine use with many organisms, including suspension feeders, as would be envisaged in a monitoring programme. Therefore, for reasons of practicality, simplicity and cost, the ratio method of Conover (1966) is to be recommended. The Conover ratio is based on the proportion of ash-free material (i.e. organic) in the food and the faeces:

$$\text{Absorption efficiency} = \frac{F - E}{(1 - E)F} \times 100$$

where F = ash-free dry weight:dry weight ratio in the food, and E = ash-free dry weight:dry weight ratio in the faeces. This ratio method is particularly suitable for suspension feeders where there is usually a high proportion of inorganic matter in the food ingested (30–90%) to act as a non-absorbed indicator.

Factors Determining Absorption Efficiency

The efficiency with which food is absorbed can be altered by environmental factors, the type and condition of the food, and the physiological condition of the animal, but the main factor is the amount of food available, or the ration level.

Many organisms show an inverse relationship between absorption efficiency and total amount of food consumed. In the case of M. edulis, this relationship can largely be explained by the functional response of the feeding and digestive system to increasing concentrations of suspended particulates (Widdows et al., 1979b). At very low particle concentrations, all the material filtered from the ventilation current by the gills is ingested through the mouth and transported via the stomach to the digestive gland for digestion. Following food absorption, the material that remains is passed to the intestine and rejected as "glandular faeces" (Van Weel, 1961; Thompson and Bayne, 1972). As the particle concentration increases, the digestive gland is unable to digest and absorb all the food material entering the stomach. The excess material, after by-passing the digestive gland, is transported through the gut undigested and is rejected as "intestinal faeces" (Van Weel, 1961). The absorption efficiency therefore declines as the ingestion rate and the proportion of intestinal faeces increases with increasing particle concentration. At these particle concentrations it is possible to distinguish between the two components of the faeces (Thompson and Bayne, 1972).

At a particle concentration of approximately 5 mg litre^{-1} a threshold is reached (Widdows et al., 1979b), above which further material filtered by the gills cannot be ingested and is carried away from the mouth by rejection tracts on the labial palps and deposited as pseudofaeces (Foster-Smith, 1975a, 1975b). Bernard (1974) suggested that the main function of labial palps was to reduce mass volume prior to ingestion and to reject excess material, but more recent studies by Kiorboe et al. (1980) and Kiorboe and Møhlenberg (1981) indicate that M. edulis, as well as other bivalve species, exhibit a degree of particle selection and this appears to be related to the size of the labial palps.

At progressively higher particle concentrations, increasing amounts of excess material are rejected in the form of a slow but continuous stream of pseudofaeces, produced along the ventral side of the septum dividing the inhalent from the exhalent siphon. At particle concentrations where both faeces and pseudofaeces are produced, it can be difficult to distinguish between them, and the Conover ratio is then based on the ash-free dry weight:dry weight ratio of the combined faeces and pseudofaeces. Kiorboe et al. (1980) and Kiorboe and Møhlenberg (1981) have stated that the "Conover ratio is valid only when the particle selection efficiency of the

bivalve is known or when there is no pseudofaeces production."
This assumption, however, is incorrect if both faeces and
pseudofaeces are collected and used to determine E in the Conover
ratio. Under these circumstances absorption efficiency is related to
the total material filtered rather than to material ingested (Bayne
and Widdows, 1978).

Nitrogen Excretion

A small proportion of the total energy absorbed by an animal is
excreted as metabolic waste products via the kidneys or across the
body surface. The energy lost as excreta therefore forms a negative
component of the basic energy equation.

Nitrogenous excretory products are derived from the catabolism of proteins, by way of amino acids which may be trans-
aminated and deaminated, and also nucleic acids. The amount of
nitrogenous waste is determined by the utilisation of protein for
energy and by the rate of breakdown and turnover of body cell
constituents.

No organism limits its nitrogen excretion to one product, but
it is well established that aquatic invertebrates commonly excrete
much of their nitrogen in the form of ammonia. $M.$ $edulis$ is an
example of such an ammonotelic animal, excreting at least
80-90% of the total nitrogen as ammonia, approximately 5-10%
as amino-N (Bayne and Scullard, 1977; Livingstone et al., 1979)
and 5% as urea (Bayne, 1973a). The proportions of nitrogenous
excretory products may vary with season and as a result of
environmental stress.

Ammonia is highly toxic and must therefore be excreted
rapidly from the body. This presents no difficulty to aquatic
animals with permeable surfaces, but in bivalves and other invertebrates that can isolate themselves from their environment, valve
closure may result in a build up of ammonia in the mantle cavity
and body tissues which in turn inhibits further NH_4 production.

The rate of ammonia excretion can be incorporated into the
energy equation following conversion into energy equivalents
(1 mg NH_4-N is equivalent to 24.87 J; Elliot and Davidson, 1975).

Factors Affecting the Scope for Growth

A review of the intrinsic and extrinsic factors affecting scope for
growth can serve (1) to illustrate the response of each physiological

component of the energy equation to a particular variable; (2) to provide the understanding necessary to interpret the response of scope for growth over a wide range of conditions; and (3) to demonstrate the sensitivity and utility of the scope for growth as a measure of an organism's physiological condition.

Intrinsic Factors

Body Size

Figure 1-1 illustrates the increase of all components of the energy equation (respiration, feeding, absorption and excretion) with increase in body mass of *M. edulis* (Widdows, 1978a, 1978b). The slope or weight exponent of the regression line, describing a particular rate as a function of body size, is normally less than 1 (ranging from 0.4 to 0.8), indicating that the weight-specific rate (i.e. rate per unit mass) declines with increasing body size.

Reproductive Condition

The reproductive condition of the animal can alter the physiological performance of *Mytilus*. When the mantle tissue contains mature gametes the respiration rate is ca. 33% higher than at other times of the year when the animal is in a state of early gametogenic development (Fig. 1-2). This increased energy requirement during the period of gamete maturation is normally concomitant with a slight increase in the clearance rate of *Mytilus* and as a result the scope for growth is usually maintained, given that ration conditions are similar.

Extrinsic Factors (Natural Environmental Stressors)

Temperature

Littoral and estuarine organisms live in an environment that subjects them to changing ambient temperatures over tidal, diel (short-term) and seasonal (long-term) cycles. Despite being poikilotherms, *Mytilus* and other littoral invertebrates are capable of temperature acclimation which results in many of their physiological rates being maintained relatively independent of temperature (Bayne et al., 1976b). Both respiration and clearance

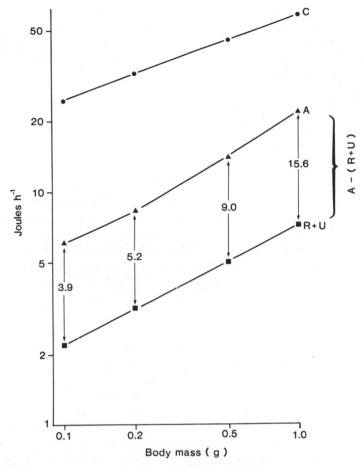

FIG. 1-1. Effect of body size of *M. edulis* on scope for growth and components of the energy equation (*C*, energy consumed; *A*, energy absorbed; *R*, energy respired; *U*, energy excreted). Ration level = 1.4 mg algal cells litre^{-1}. (From Widdows, 1978b.)

rates of *M. edulis* show a marked degree of temperature independence (Q_{10} 1 to 1.6) after a period of adaptation (approximately 2 weeks) to changes in both constant temperature and fluctuating temperature regimes (Widdows, 1976). *Mytilus edulis* acclimates to temperatures between 5 and 20°C (Fig. 1-3), and consequently within this range the importance of temperature as a factor determining the respiration, feeding rates and ultimately scope for growth is reduced (Widdows, 1978b). Above 20°C there is a breakdown in temperature compensation mechanisms (Fig. 1-3)

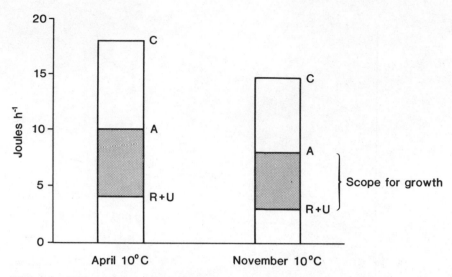

FIG. 1-2. Effect of reproductive condition of *M. edulis* on scope for growth and components of the energy equation. April (period of gamete maturation); November (period of gametogenic quiescence). Body mass = 0.5 g. Ration level = 0.56 mg algal cells litre^{-1}. (From Widdows, 1978b.)

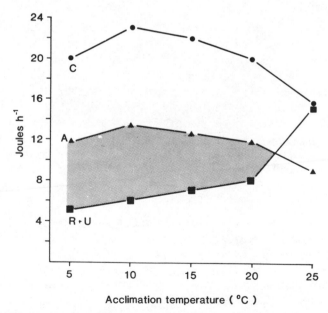

FIG. 1-3. Effect of acclimation temperature on scope for growth and components of energy balance of *M. edulis*. Body mass = 1 g. Ration level = 0.56 mg algal cells litre^{-1} (From Widdows, 1978.)

22

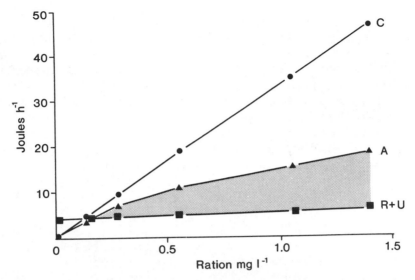

FIG. 1-4. Effect of ration (mg algal cells litre^{-1}) on scope for growth and components of energy balance of *M. edulis*. Body mass = 1 g. Temperature = 10°C. (From Widdows, 1978b.)

demonstrated in terms of an increase in respiration rate (R) and a decline in clearance rate (C), and at 25°C and above this results in a negative scope for growth. Under these conditions an animal can only maintain itself by utilising nutrient reserves in the body as a source of energy. Such a physiologically determined maximal limit of thermal tolerance is comparable with an ecologically derived estimate of 26.7°C, based on the mean summer seawater temperature at the southern distribution limit for *M. edulis* in North America (Wells and Gray, 1960).

Food Concentration

The quantity and quality of particulate food varies seasonally and differs markedly in different environments. The relationship between the scope for growth for *M. edulis* and ration level, expressed as mg particulate food material per litre, is illustrated in Fig. 1-4 (Widdows, 1978b). At low food concentrations the energy consumed (C) and absorbed (A) is less than the energy lost through respiration (R) and excretion (U). This results in a negative scope for growth, which signifies the utilisation of body energy reserves by a severely stressed animal. As the food concentration increases there is a level, known as the maintenance ration, at which the energy absorbed by the animal equals the energy lost and there is neither body weight gain nor weight loss. At concentrations above the maintenance ration, scope for growth is positive and energy is available for somatic growth and/or reproduction. There is a gradual increase in scope for growth with increasing food concentration until a plateau representing maximum growth rate is reached. The main factor limiting scope for growth at the higher food concentration is the rate of energy absorption from the food. In response to increasing food concentration, the rate of energy consumption (C) is simply proportional to the ration level, the absorption efficiency declines and the resultant, the rate of energy absorption (A), increases more gradually than C. A similar relationship between scope for growth and ration has been recorded in the ribbed mussel *Aulacomya ater* by Griffiths and King (1979). At the very high concentrations of suspended particulates found in some estuaries, the scope for growth of *M. edulis* is reduced as a result of a combination of lower clearance rates, lower absorption efficiency and the higher concentration of suspended silt which lowers the proportion of organic material in the seston filtered (Bayne and Widdows, 1978; Widdows et al., 1979b).

Dissolved Oxygen

Mussels inhabit a variety of coastal and estuarine environments that may be subjected to fluctuations in oxygen tension (pO_2); for example, lagoons and enclosed areas of brackish water, muddy shores of estuaries, salt marshes and areas exposed to organic pollution. Mussels have been shown to be capable of some regulation of their physiological processes under hypoxic conditions (Bayne, 1971; Bayne and Livingstone, 1977), so that the relationships between ventilation (clearance rate), respiration rate and ultimately scope for growth, and oxygen tension take the form shown in Fig. 1-5. Consequently, scope for growth as well as the other basic physiological rates, are maintained relatively independent of oxygen tension within the "normal environmental range" and down to approximately 1×10^4 Pa (80 mmHg or 50% oxgygen saturation). As a result, oxygen tension, like other environmental variables, becomes a significant factor determining respiration, ventilation rate and scope for growth only when the limit of the animal's adaptive capacity is exceeded.

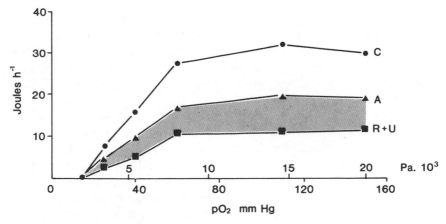

FIG. 1-5. Effect of dissolved oxygen on scope for growth and components of energy balance of *M. edulis*. (From Bayne, 1971, 1975).

Salinity

Mytilus edulis and many other estuarine organisms are capable of adaptation to fluctuating salinities from 35°/oo to at least 20°/oo (sinusoidal salinity cycle of 12 hours). All components of the energy equation are held relatively independent of salinity changes within this range (Fig. 1-6A). In response to salinity changes below 20°/oo, respiration, clearance rate and scope for growth decline (Stickle and Sabourin, 1979; Shumway and Youngson, 1979; Widdows, unpublished data). The degree of adaptation to reduced salinities improves following a period of acclimation to constant conditions. Figure 1-6B demonstrates that at 15°/oo partial acclimation to the salinity occurs. Recent evidence, however, suggests that different populations of *Mytilus* can show marked differences in capacity to acclimate to salinity changes. Mussels subjected to melt water from glaciers along the coast of Alaska are able to compensate for wide fluctuations in salinity (Stickle and Sabourin, 1979), whereas mussels from Long Island Sound show more limited salinity adaptation (R. I. E. Newell, personal communication).

Aerial Exposure

Bivalve molluscs in the littoral environment experience periods of exposure to air, the duration of which depends on their distribution

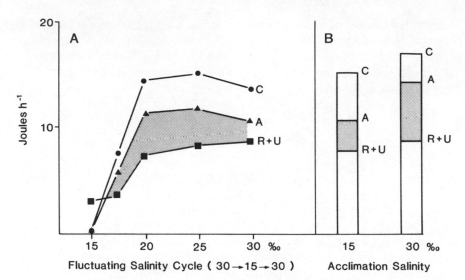

FIG. 1-6. Effect of salinity on scope for growth and components of the energy balance of *M. edulis*. A. Response to fluctuating salinities between 30 and 15⁰/₀₀. B. Acclimated response to 30 and 15⁰/₀₀. (Widdows, unpublished data.)

on the shore and on the form of the tidal cycle. The effect of air exposure on the various physiological components of scope for growth is illustrated in Fig. 1-7. During exposure, although due to the cessation of feeding there is no energy consumption from food, there is some energy loss through respiration and excretion $(R + U)$. The degree of energy utilisation varies depending on the species (Widdows et al., 1979a). *Mytilus edulis*, for example, maintains closed valves when exposed to air and thereby reduces its oxygen consumption to approximately 10% of the aquatic rate. Under these circumstances anaerobiosis occurs, but the calculated energy utilisation associated with anaerobic metabolism is only ca. 12% of the total energy utilisation in water. Following reimmersion, the resumption of filter feeding leads to a continuation of food consumption and absorption at a rate similar to that prior to air exposure. The respiration and excretion rates, however, are enhanced and gradually return to a steady state within one to three hours of reimmersion. This decline in oxygen consumption is referred to as the payment of an oxygen debt built up during air exposure.

It is therefore important, when using *Mytilus* as an indicator organism, to allow the animal at least one hour to recover from any extended period of aerial exposure. After this time has elapsed, the temporary disturbances in feeding, respiration and excretion rates—and consequently in the scope for growth—will have disappeared, and the measured rates will then more closely reflect the steady-state condition of the animal.

Field Application of Scope for Growth Measurements

Comparison between Populations

There are now a number of studies where the concept of scope for growth has been used to compare different bivalve populations. Initial studies investigated the seasonal variation in the individual physiological components of the energy equation, including scope for growth, of mussels inhabiting two different environments (Lynher—estuarine; Cattewater—power station effluent). Figure 1-8 shows that differences between the scope for growth of the two populations of mussels were measurable and particularly evident as low and negative values for mussels from

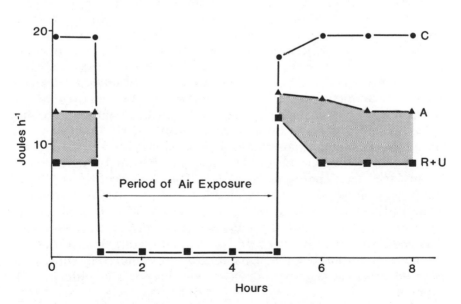

FIG. 1-7. Effect of aerial exposure on scope for growth and components of energy balance of *M. edulis*. (From Widdows et al., 1979b; Widdows, unpublished data.)

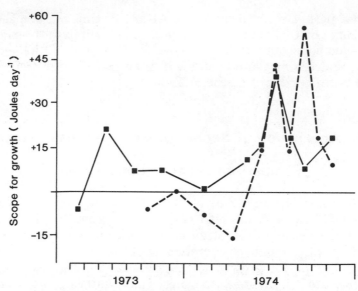

FIG. 1-8. Seasonal changes on the scope for growth of *Mytilus edulis* (1 g dry mass) from two populations: Lynher River (■) and Cattewater power station (•). (Redrawn from Bayne and Widdows, 1978.)

the Cattewater during a period of elevated temperature in the winter of 1973–74 (Bayne and Widdows, 1978).

A simulation model of the growth of *Mytilus*, based on the physiological components of the energy equation, provided growth curves that could then be compared with observed growth rates for mussels from the Lynher, estimated by the traditional methods of size–class analysis. When both types of curve are plotted in terms of body weight gain (Fig. 1-9), and weight loss due to spawning is also incorporated into the simulation model, there is good agreement between the predicted growth curve and the maximum and minimum observed growth curves (Bayne and Radford, unpublished data; Bayne et al., 1979). Therefore, scope for growth can provide a reliable estimate of the growth potential of mussels from different populations or sites in a monitoring programme.

More recently, mussel populations around Sullom Voe in the Shetlands were measured as part of a monitoring programme. A comparison between the scope for growth of mussels from five sites formed part of a baseline study (Widdows et al., 1981a) and showed significant population differences (October 1978, Fig. 1-10). The two populations most isolated from "human activities" within the Sullom Voe region had the highest scope for growth.

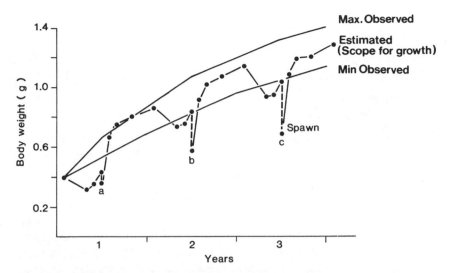

FIG. 1-9. Growth curves for *M. edulis* from the Lynher population. Estimated growth curve based on scope for growth measurements starting with an assumed dry tissue mass of 0.4 g at the beginning of year 1; a, b and c are predicted periods of mass loss due to spawning. Minimum and maximum observed growth curves are also shown, as calculated from monthly sampling for year class and length-mass analysis. (Redrawn from Bayne et al., 1979.)

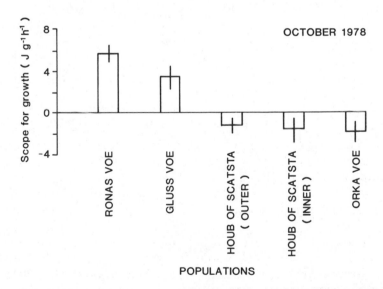

FIG. 1-10. A comparison between the scope for growth of *M. edulis* from five sites in the vicinity of Sullom Voe Oil Terminal. Ronas Voe and Gluss Voe populations are the most isolated from "human activities" in the Sullom Voe region. (From Widdows et al., 1981a.)

Anthropogenic Stressors

Scope for growth has been related to toxicant levels in both field and laboratory studies using crustacea and bivalve molluscs.

Laboratory Studies

To date, scope for growth has been measured in the laboratory only in response to petroleum hydrocarbons. Gilfillan (1975) showed that exposure to progressively greater concentrations of seawater extracts of crude oil from 0.12 mg litre^{-1} to 6 mg litre^{-1} reduced scope for growth in *M. edulis* and *Modiolus demissus*. In a more recent study by Widdows et al. (1982), mussels chronically exposed for 5 months to an environmentally realistic concentration of petroleum hydrocarbons (e.g. 30μg litre^{-1} total hydrocarbons derived from the water-accommodated fraction of North Sea crude oil) showed a significant reduction in scope for growth. This effect was primarily a function of a reduced clearance rate and elevated respiration and excretion rates in hydrocarbon-exposed mussels (Fig.1-11*A*). In a review by Anderson (1977), it was concluded that there was little agreement between sublethal responses of marine organisms and the level of hydrocarbon contamination in the tissues. However, Widdows et al. (1982) recorded a negative correlation ($r = -0.9$) between scope for growth and aromatic hydrocarbon concentration in the tissues of *Mytilus* (Fig. 1-11*B*). A similar relationship was recorded in *Mya arenaria* exposed to an oil spill (Gilfillan et al., 1977; see below). In a laboratory study, Edwards (1978) exposed a shrimp (*Crangon crangon*) to progressively increased levels of water soluble fraction (WSF) of North Sea Oil at 10, 15 and 20°C. At each temperature, scope for growth was reduced with increasing WSF content; the reduction in scope for growth was greatest at 20°C.

The use of large experimental enclosures represents an intermediate stage between laboratory and field studies. Researchers at the Graduate School of Oceanography, Rhode Island, have found that 3 weeks exposure to 250 ppb oil greatly reduced the scope for growth in the copepod *Acartia tonsa* (Gilfillan, unpublished data, and cited by Bayne et al., 1980a).

Field Studies

A number of field monitoring programmes have determined physiological components of the energy equation and calculated

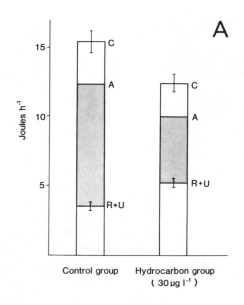

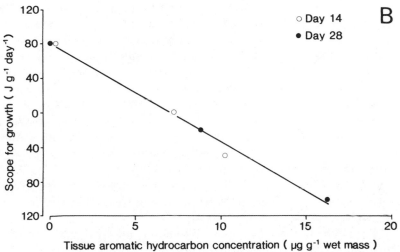

FIG. 1–11. *A.* Effects of 100 days exposure to 30 μg petroleum hydrocarbons litre^{-1} (water accommodated fraction of North Sea crude oil) on scope for growth of *M. edulis.* (From Widdows et al., 1982.) *B.* Relationship between scope for growth of *M. edulis* and tissue aromatic hydrocarbon concentration. Correlation coefficient $r = -0.9$. (From Widdows et al., 1982.)

scope for growth as a physiological stress index. Although it is recognised that a cause–effect relationship is difficult to establish in environmental studies because of the number of factors that could influence the biological responses, in most cases there is good evidence to link a decline in the physiological condition of a population (e.g. scope for growth) with causative agent(s), e.g. anthropogenic stressors, by virtue of other natural stressors remaining relatively constant. In a pollution monitoring programme it is important for the experimenter to select transplant sites with the aim of minimising the effects of local variations in natural environmental stressors, e.g. temperature, salinity and suspended particulates. This may, for example, involve placing the transplanted mussels away from a freshwater input or an area with elevated concentrations of suspended particulates.

An example of a combined chemical and biological effects monitoring programme involving the transplantation of mussels along a pollution gradient was carried out by Widdows et al. (1981b). Mussels were transplanted to sites along a pollution gradient in Narragansett Bay. After one month, they were sampled for chemical analysis of body tissues (concentrations of metals and hydrocarbons) and measurement of physiological stress indices including scope for growth. Figure 1-12 summarises the results and demonstrates the decline in scope for growth with increasing concentration of contaminants within the water and tissues. In this study the natural environmental stressors most likely to affect the physiological condition of an animal, such as temperature, salinity, dissolved oxygen and total seston concentration, all remained relatively constant along the length of Narragansett Bay. Consequently there was good evidence to suggest that the reduction in condition of mussels transplanted to the northern region of the bay was caused by anthropogenic stressors rather than natural environmental variables.

In a similar field study of soft-shell clams (*Mya arenaria*) from three different oil spill sites in Maine, Gilfillan et al. (1976) have shown that scope for growth (measured in terms of carbon flux) correlated with elevated body burdens of hydrocarbons, particularly aromatic hydrocarbons (Table 1-3). In a further study, increased scope for growth in *Mya* correlated with increased somatic growth (Gilfillan and Vandermeulen, 1978). An investigation of the effects of an underwater oil seep on scope for growth in *Calanus hyperboreus* from Baffin Bay (Gilfillan unpublished data, and cited by Bayne et al., 1980a) found that copepods in the seep area exhibited greatly reduced feeding rates, respiration rates in

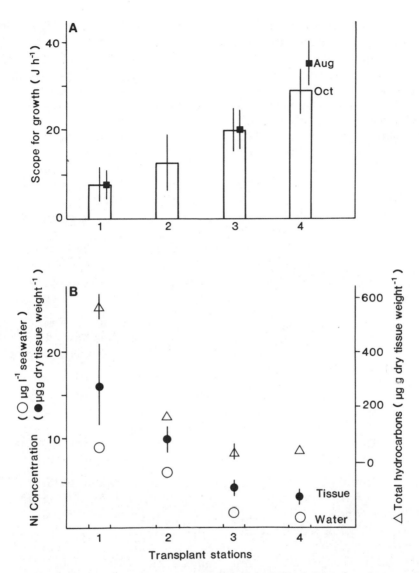

FIG. 1-12. Relationship between scope for growth of *M. edulis* and environmental pollution. A. Scope for growth of mussels transplanted to four stations along a pollution gradient in Narragansett Bay (measurements carried out in August and October 1977). B. Pollution gradient described in terms of total hydrocarbon concentration in the mussel body tissues (△), the Ni concentration in the water (○) and in the mussel body tissues (•) at four transplant stations in Narragansett Bay. (Redrawn from Widdows et al., 1981a.)

TABLE 1–3. Scope for Growth and Tissue Aromatic Concentrations of *Mya arenaria* from Sites around Casco Bay, Maine

Location	Scope for Growth*	Tissue aromatic fraction ($\mu g\ g^{-1}$ wet tissue wt)
Prince Point	130.2	1.1
Falmouth B	119.7	1.8
Chandler Cove	81.27	1.0
Falmouth A	64.6	2.1
Mussel Cove B	45.9	2.0
Long Cove	43.4	2.7
Chebeague Spit	36.9	2.6
Mussel Cove A	18.5	2.6
	Correlation coeff. $r = -0.78$	

From Gilfillan et al. (1977).
*C flux in mg C gained per 100 mg animal from Aug 1974 to Feb 1975.

the seep area were higher than in nearby areas and the scope for growth was greatly reduced as a result. All studies have therefore demonstrated a significant negative correlation between scope for growth and oil pollution.

GROWTH EFFICIENCY

An additional physiological stress index can be calculated from the energy equation in order to provide further information on an animal's condition. The scope for growth as a proportion of the absorbed ration represents net growth efficiency (K_2; Ivlev, 1961) and is a measure of the efficiency with which food is converted into body tissues (Paloheimo and Dickie, 1965, 1966a, 1966b; Thompson and Bayne, 1974; Widdows, 1978b):

$$K_2 = \frac{A - (R + U)}{A}$$

where A = absorbed energy, R = respired energy and U = excreted energy. A reduction in K_2 is therefore indicative of a stressed condition since a greater proportion of the energy absorbed from the food is being used to maintain the animal, and consequently a smaller proportion is available for growth.

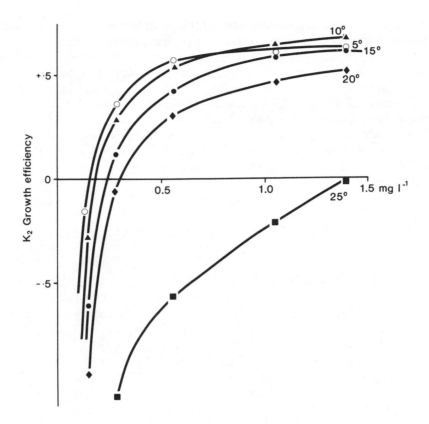

FIG. 1-13. Effect of acclimation temperature on the relationship between growth efficiency (K_2) of *M. edulis* (1 g dry mass) and ration. (From Widdows, 1978b.)

TABLE 1-4. Calculated Growth Efficiencies for *Mytilus edulis* transplanted along a pollution gradient in Narragansett Bay

Transplant station	K_2 net growth efficiency (%)	Ni concentration tissues ($\mu g\ g^{-1}$ dry wt)	Total hydro-carbons in tissues ($\mu g\ g^{-1}$ dry wt)
1. Sabin Point	64	3.6	40
2. Conimicut Point	47	4.4	40
3. Conanicut Island	32	10	160
4. E. R. L. Narragansett	30	16	560

From Widdows et al. (1981b).

Figure 1-13 illustrates the effect of both ration and temperature on growth efficiency. Like scope for growth, the zero value for K_2 represents the maintenance ration and negative values indicate that the animal is utilising body reserves in order to survive.

In a field study, K_2 growth efficiencies were calculated for mussels transplanted along a pollution gradient in Narragansett Bay (Widdows et al., 1981b). An increase in pollution, measured in terms of tissue concentrations of contaminants, resulted in a reduction in the net growth efficiency (Table 1-4).

OXYGEN TO NITROGEN RATIO

A general response by an organism to stress is the utilisation of nutrient reserves to meet a metabolic requirement that may have been enhanced above normal values. In some instances this can be measured in terms of a depletion of carbohydrate, protein and lipid stores, but generally these changes in chemical composition occur only in response to conditions of extreme stress (Bayne and Thompson, 1970). An alternative approach, and one that is often more responsive to stress, is to determine alterations in the balance between the catabolism of carbohydrate, protein and lipid substrates.

The ratio between oxygen consumed and nitrogen excreted (O:N, calculated in atomic equivalents) provides an index of the relative utilisation of protein in energy metabolism (Corner and Cowey, 1968; Bayne et al., 1976d; Widdows, 1978b). A high rate of protein relative to carbohydrate and lipid catabolism results in a low O:N ratio, which is generally indicative of a stressed condition. A high O:N value therefore indicates a predominance of lipid and/or carbohydrate catabolism over protein degradation. The theoretical minimum value for O:N, with uniquely protein catabolism, is approximately 7 (Mayzaud, 1973).

Measurement of the O:N ratio is based on data for the rate of oxygen consumption and the rate of ammonia excretion, both of which are determined as components of the energy equation or scope for growth. The O:N ratio has been documented for planktonic crustacea (Conover, 1978) and benthic molluscs (Bayne, 1975; Bayne et al., 1976d). There are likely to be interspecific and intraspecific differences in the O:N value for a healthy animal, depending upon trophic level and the nature of the food and nutrient reserves. The interpretation of O:N should therefore be based on relative changes rather than on absolute values.

For *M. edulis*, perhaps one of the most documented species, a value of above 50 is representative of a healthy mussel, whereas a value of 30 or below is generally indicative of a stressed animal with a relatively high protein catabolism.

Factors Affecting the O:N Ratio

Intrinsic Factors

Seasonal/Gametogenic Cycle

In *M. edulis* the rate of oxygen consumed to nitrogen excreted varies seasonally as a result of reproductive and nutrient storage cycles (Bayne et al., 1976d; Widdows, 1978b). Consequently, any alteration in O:N due to environmental stress and pollution will be superimposed on the annual cycle and has to be interpreted in the light of the reproductive/storage cycle. The main feature of the seasonal variation in O:N is the marked decline during and immediately after the spawning period (Fig.1-14); the time of this will vary from population to population depending upon both intrinsic and extrinsic factors. This seasonal picture reflects the poor condition of the animals at a time when the mantle is under-going tissue autolysis, reorganisation and regeneration following spawning. For most of the year, however, the O:N ratio for healthy mussels is approximately 50, with brief periods of elevated O:N when nutrient reserves are high and the animals are in a state of gametogenic quiescence. Therefore, during the period after spawn-ing when animals are naturally stressed and the low O:N ratio is not responsive to additional stressors, e.g. ration (Fig.1-14), the ratio of oxygen consumed to nitrogen excreted does not provide a suitable index of the effects of environmental stress and pollution.

Extrinsic Factors

Ration

Ration, or food availability, is an important factor determining the O:N ratio of *Mytilus* (Fig.1-14). Starvation and very low ration

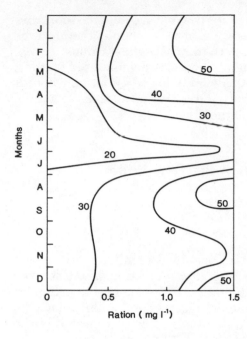

FIG. 1-14. Isopleths of O:N ratio of *M. edulis* (1 g dry mass) as a function of season and ration. (Redrawn from Widdows, 1978b.)

levels result in low O:N values of approximately 20, which generally increase to 50 at a higher food concentration. The decline in O:N is a consequence of a small reduction in metabolic rate and/or an increase in the rate of ammonia excretion. The effects of starvation on the O:N ratio have been recorded for *M. edulis* (Bayne, 1973a, 1973b; Bayne and Scullard, 1977; Widdows, 1978b) and for *Donax vittatus* (Ansell and Sivadas, 1973). Furthermore, Gabbott and Bayne (1973) have demonstrated that during starvation, when *M. edulis* has a low O:N ratio, a significant fraction of body protein is lost. An O:N ratio of approximately 25-30 appears to correspond to the maintenance ration with the exception of the spawning period when the ratio is extremely low at all ration levels (Fig. 1-14).

Temperature

The relationship between temperature and O:N (Fig. 1-15) is similar to that for scope for growth (Widdows, 1978b). *M. edulis* shows a significant decline in O:N above 20°C and this is indicative of a stress condition.

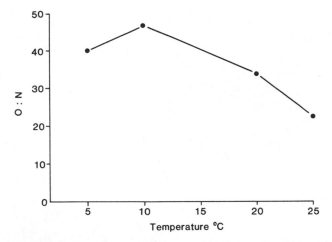

FIG. 1-15. Effect of acclimation temperature on the O : N ratio of *M. edulis.* (From Widdows, 1978b.)

Anthropogenic Stressors

The field application of O:N has been demonstrated in a monitoring programme in Narragansett Bay (Widdows et al., 1981b). Mussels transplanted along a pollution gradient in August showed a decline in O:N from 75 to 30 with increasing environmental contamination (Fig. 1-16). However, when repeated in October no environmentally induced effects were discernible, because all animals had relatively low O:N ratios following spawning in the autumn. This confirms the possible limitation of the O:N ratio at certain times of year and also emphasises the need to measure stress indices outside of the spawning period.

Little detailed information is available on the effect of other extrinsic factors, although the ratio is known to respond in a manner consistent with the concept of reduced O:N values with increasing stress, e.g. exposure to air and reduced salinities.

BODY CONDITION INDEX

A condition index of long standing in studies of commercially important shellfish is the proportion of the internal shell volume which is occupied by the body tissues (Baird, 1958, 1966). Baird

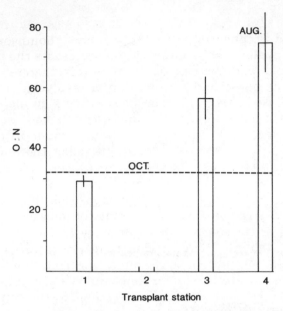

FIG. 1-16. O : N ratios of *M. edulis* transplanted to four stations along a pollution gradient in Narragansett Bay. Station 1 at Sabin Point was the most polluted site. Effect of pollution on O : N was discernible in August but not in October. (From Widdows et al., 1981b.)

(1958) determined the condition index of mussels and oysters as follows:

$$\frac{\text{Weight or volume of wet flesh}}{\text{Shell cavity volume}} \times 100$$

An alternative index based on dry weight instead of wet tissue weight avoids the very considerable difficulties involved in standardising the method of removing and measuring wet tissue. Furthermore, wet tissues can contain variable amounts of water, which can obscure fluctuations in condition (Shaw et al., 1967). Walne (1970) therefore recommended the following dry meat condition index:

$$\frac{\text{Dry tissue weight (g)}}{\text{Shell cavity volume (ml)}} \times 1{,}000$$

The condition index is a simple index that reflects long-term changes in the nutrient state of bivalve molluscs and has mainly been used to demonstrate seasonal changes in samples from natural populations (Walne, 1970; Gabbott and Walker, 1971; Gee et al., 1977) and from hatchery and laboratory populations (Gabbott and Stephenson, 1974; Bayne and Thompson, 1970) of mussels and oysters. The nutrient state represents the total tissue glycogen, lipid and protein content and is therefore a useful measure of the physiological condition of bivalves.

An increase in the condition index reflects an increase in the organic constituents associated with growth and is dependent upon the balance between food availability, rates of feeding and rates of catabolism. A reduction in the index therefore reflects either periods of stress involving utilisation of reserves or spawning.

Changes in the biochemical composition have also been measured to determine the nutrient state of mussels and oysters. Much of the work on seasonal changes in metabolic stores has been reviewed by Gabbott (1976). Changes in the total quantities of glycogen, lipid and protein were found to correlate with those of condition index (Walne, 1970; Gabbott and Walker, 1971; Gabbott and Stephenson, 1974), although alterations in the concentration and distribution of the three storage materials were controlled primarily by the demands of gametogenesis.

The advantage of the body condition index is that it is a simple measurement to carry out and requires only basic laboratory equipment; the disadvantages are its insensitivity and relatively low signal-to-noise ratio. Therefore, significant changes in the condition index are only likely to be measurable after long-term (months/years) exposure.

Factors Affecting the Body Condition Index

Season

There is a marked seasonal cycle in the body condition index of bivalves, the form of which will largely depend upon the spawning cycle and food availability. A typical seasonal pattern for *M. edulis* is illustrated in Fig. 1-17. In the spring, usually March/April, there is a rapid decline in condition index associated with spawning, followed by an increase in condition as tissue reserves are built up. There may be a second spawning in the autumn in some populations (see Fig. 1-20) (Gee et al., 1977), and if the available food is significantly below the maintenance ration during the winter there may be a gradual fall in condition between November and February.

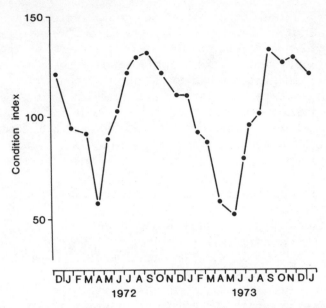

FIG. 1-17. Annual cycle of condition index for sublittoral *M. edulis* (65 mm) in the Conwy estuary. (Redrawn from Dare and Edwards, 1975.)

Ration

The condition index has been shown to respond to ration when measured over a period of several months. For example, Bayne and Thompson (1970) recorded a decline in the condition index of unfed mussels compared with fed mussels when maintained in a laboratory for 80 days, and there was a concomitant loss of carbohydrate and protein reserves. Gabbott and Stephenson (1974) demonstrated a similar effect in *Ostrea edulis* (Fig. 1-18). The condition index therefore reveals the utilisation of body reserves under conditions of nutritive stress, but it is less likely to record a change if tissue growth is accompanied by a proportional amount of shell growth.

Height on the Shore

Baird (1966) has demonstrated that the body condition index for *M. edulis* decreases as the period of exposure to air increases with the height on the shore (Fig. 1-19). This inverse relationship is presumably a result of the reduction in time spent feeding and the consequent low tissue growth rate by mussels higher on the shore.

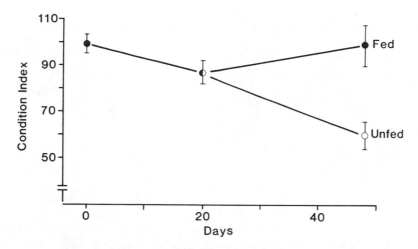

FIG. 1-18. Effect of ration (fed and unfed) on the condition index of *Ostrea edulis*. (From Gabbott and Stephenson, 1974.)

Environmental Stress and Pollution

The body condition index has not been applied in an environmental monitoring context, but there are examples where mussel populations have been compared over two or more annual cycles (Dare and Edwards, 1975; Gee et al., 1977). Two mussel populations in southwest England (Gee et al., 1977) demonstrated population differences, the extent of which varied from year to year (Fig. 1-20).

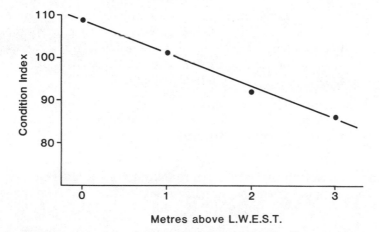

FIG. 1-19. Effect of tidal level (metres above low water extreme spring tides) on the condition index of *M. edulis*. (From Baird, 1966.)

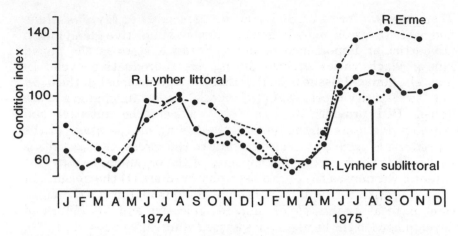

FIG. 1-20. Effect of different estuarine environments on the monthly values for condition index of *M. edulis*. River Lynher littoral site (solid lines); River Lynher sublittoral site (dotted lines); River Erme site (dashed line). (Redrawn from Gee et al., 1977.)

In the autumn (1974) the Lynher population had a lower condition index than the Erme population due to an autumn spawning. The following year, after the spring spawning period, there was a rapid improvement in condition in both populations but the Lynher population was significantly lower in condition index than the Erme population throughout the summer and autumn. Without additional information on the physiological, cytological and biochemical stress responses, together with detailed environmental data, it is difficult to relate these differences to environmental quality, but the recorded differences in condition index do appear to correlate with the degree of pollution at these two sites (Lowe and Moore, 1978, and unpublished observations).

Body Component Index

The changes in nutrient state are reflected also in the relative size of various tissues in the organism. Relative size can be expressed as a body component index (BCI), which is defined as follows:

$$BCI = \frac{\text{dry weight of a tissue}}{\text{total dry weight of flesh}}$$

There are two forms of BCI that are applicable to *Mytilus edulis* and other bivalves, namely gonad index and digestive gland index. Of particular importance in mussels and oysters is the gonad index, which varies greatly during the reproductive cycle. In mussels, gonadal tissue is distributed throughout most of the body but the majority is present in the mantle. Following changes in the gonad, BCI provides an index that reflects the nutritive and reproductive state of the animal. Depending on the stage of the reproductive cycle and the magnitude of the stress, changes ensue that reduce the reproductive capacity of the organism to different extents. Responses that have been observed are (1) the absence of spawning with a gradual recession of the gonadal mass, (2) reduction of total quantities of gametes released and (3) failure of development in the larvae from stressed adults (Bayne et al., 1978).

A similar BCI is that describing the relative size of the digestive gland. This tissue forms a major nutrient store and plays an important role in regulating nutrient distribution to other body tissues. In response to stress (e.g. nutritive and temperature), the energy reserves from the digestive gland are the first to be mobilised (Thompson, 1972; Widdows, 1972) and the relative size declines.

2

Cytological and Cytochemical
Measurements

Investigation of specific aspects of cellular functions offer a means
of developing rapid and sensitive indicators of adaptive responses
to environmental alterations. It should be possible to observe
structural-functional alterations in individual cells or groups of
cells at an early stage of a stress response, before an integrated
cellular alteration would manifest itself at the level of whole-
animal physiological processes. Some of these cellular responses
may be generalised, whereas others are likely to be specific to a
particular type of stressor. Considerations such as these have led
to many cytological (or "histopathological") investigations of
stress responses in marine invertebrates.

When cells are stressed they undergo a series of often irreversible biochemical and cellular changes, which manifest themselves
as alterations in the animal's physiology. Histology and cytology
offer approaches and techniques for studying changes in the structure of tissues and their composite cells, thus giving indications of
the degree of stress and of the adaptive capability of the organism.

It is useful in investigations of tissue and cellular responses
to stress to start with tissues that are presumptive indicators of
the adaptive capability and general condition of the animal concerned. The four main functional categories that attract most
attention in stress studies are the processes of reproduction,
respiration, digestion and excretion. If the stressor affects feeding
and digestion then the animal may die of starvation; if respiration
is affected then anoxia may ensue; while a loss or decline in
reproductive capability can affect the fitness of the population.

Although many classical treatises deal with human and veterinary (including fish) histology and pathology, by comparison few deal with invertebrate animals and only a small proportion of these with marine invertebrates. This lack of established literature on invertebrate pathology causes certain problems to the pathologist with regard to such basic matters as classification and terminology of the disease condition (Stewart, 1976). This dilemma was discussed by Sparks (1972) in his excellent book on invertebrate pathology. Sinderman (1970) reviewed studies of the principal diseases of marine fish and shellfish. One aspect of fish pathology which has received particular attention is parasitology; three useful books on this subject are those by Reickenback-Klinke and Elkan (1965), Van Duijn (1967) and Mawdesley-Thomas (1974).

In recent years, the awareness of marine pollution has led to many investigations of the cytological effects of pollutants—e.g. surfactants (Abel and Skidmore, 1975; Schmid and Mann, 1961) and metals (Skidmore and Tovell, 1972)—on fish gills. Fish have proved to be good indicators in this respect as the thickness of the gill filaments increases after exposure of the contaminants, which in turn affects oxygen transport efficiency. This parameter has been used as a measure of pollutant effect by Hughes and Perry (1976). Another factor that has received particular attention is neoplasia in fishes; however, correlating the incidence of neoplasia with environmental pollutant levels is difficult and the majority of cases tend to be circumstantial (Wellings et al., 1976; Mearns and Sherwood, 1976). Attention has turned in recent years from fish to bivalves (particularly oysters, clams and mussels) and their associated cytological changes induced by environmental stressors. These animals have certain advantages over fish for use in toxicological studies; fish are expensive and prone to secondary stressors (such as handling and infection by fungi or bacteria) whereas bivalves are sessile, plentiful, inexpensive and relatively easy to maintain in the laboratory.

Oysters, clams and mussels are commercially valuable, and this has been a contributing reason for their scientific investigation. However, these organisms can also concentrate a variety of chlorinated hydrocarbons (Risebrough et al., 1976), aromatic hydrocarbons (Di Salvo et al., 1975; Fossato and Canzonier, 1976) and metal ions (Friedrich and Filice, 1976; Philips, 1979; Simpson, 1979; Lowe and Moore, 1979) within their tissues, and therefore they represent good indicators of xenobiotic bioaccumulation. In view of this, Goldberg (1975) proposed that mussels should be used on a world-wide basis as indicators of environmental pollution. Bayne (1976) elaborated this proposal and suggested that mussels could also be used to measure the biological effects of observed pollution load, thus reflecting the ecological consequences of environmental contamination.

Mussels have been exposed to a variety of experimental stressors, and there is a wealth of literature on effects induced by starvation (Gabbott and Bayne, 1973; Bayne, 1973a), oxygen tension (Bayne, 1975; Coleman, 1973), salinity gradients (Bayne, 1973a; Bayne, 1975) and temperature fluctuations (Bayne, 1973a; Read and Cummings, 1967; Wallis, 1975). Much of this work has had a biochemical or physiological orientation, although some recent investigations have adopted a multivariate and multi-disciplinary approach which has enabled the correlation of cytological observation with functional parameters. For instance, cytological quantitation using microstereology has been applied to the combined effects of salinity, temperature and feeding regimes on the development of gametes and the role of mantle reserve tissues in glycogen utilisation (Bayne et al., 1978). Langton (1975) has also used cytological parameters in describing the cyclical activity of the digestive tubule epithelium in *Mytilus edulis*. Other applications of cytological assessment of the cellular responses to stress in mussels include the effects of injections of anthracene and various steroids on digestive cells (Moore et al., 1978a, 1978b), digestive tubule degeneration in response to starvation (Thompson et al.,1974), digestive cell responses to temperature, exposure and nutritional extremes (Thompson et al., 1978) and gill damage induced by elevated temperature (Gonzalez and Yevich, 1976). In addition, regression of reproductive tissues in response to combinations of thermal, osmotic and nutritional stressors has been described in *M. edulis* (Bayne et al., 1978). A tissue response involving the occlusion of the vascular haemolymph system of *M. edulis* by granular blood cells has been shown to be associated with sites of chronic environmental pollution (Lowe and Moore, 1979). However, the stressor that induces this condition has not been specifically identified; this is also the case with a neoplastic haemocytic disorder, not unlike certain mammalian leukaemias, which occurs in a population of mussels exposed to discharges of aromatic hydrocarbons (Lowe and Moore, 1978). Similar presumptive neoplastic conditions have also been reported in oysters and mussels from polluted areas in the United States (Farley, 1969; Farley and Sparks, 1970; Mix, 1976).

The effects of ionizing radiation on the digestive and reproductive systems in oysters have been described by Mix and Sparks (1970, 1971a, 1971b) and Mix (1972). These effects included

haemocytic infiltration, loss of digestive tubule epithelial cells, abscesses and mitotic inhibition in response to a range of dose levels of gamma radiation. Investigations of tissue regeneration following a short period of irradiation have revealed cellular division and repopulation of the digestive tubule epithelium with normally functioning cells (Mix and Sparks, 1971b; Trenholm and Mix, 1978).

Clearly, then, cytology offers an approach whereby the biological effects of stress and environmental pollution can be measured in terms of the adaptive capability of the animal and the cellular changes associated with these adaptive processes. It is obviously necessary to have a thorough knowledge of the cells in their normal functional state in order to detect alterations from the norm. The most positive indication of cell injury is the condition of the nucleus, while the commonest change associated with cell death is pyknosis, in which the nucleus shrinks and becomes very dense. The nuclei of dead or dying cells may also fragment (karyorrhexis) or even dissolve (karyolysis).

Although the nucleus is a good indicator of cell injury and death, cytoplasmic changes also accompany these conditions. Many of these are best realised only at ultrastructural levels of resolution where cellular injury can induce dramatic alterations in the endoplasmic reticulum, with swelling and rupture of other membranous systems such as mitochondria, which additionally show loss of cristae, as well as general cytoplasmic disorganisation. Damage to the lysosomal system is often apparent at both the light microscopic and ultrastructural levels where it involves the loss of integrity of the lysosomal membranes, resulting in "leaky" lysosomes which can thus release their hydrolytic enzymes into the cytosol. Light microscopy can also be used to demonstrate reductions in the intensity of staining for glycogen and lipids which can accompany cell death. Moreover, changes such as swelling of the cells can occur while at the same time the cytoplasm becomes granular and eventually diminishes, thus giving rise to a dense, opaque acidophilic mass.

Cell death is, however, not the only measurable response to stress; many cells adapt to the stressor in characteristic ways, such as increased secretion of mucus or muscular hypertrophy. It is only when this adaptive capability is exceeded that cell death occurs.

It is perhaps pertinent at this point to mention post mortem degeneration. These are changes, not unlike those already described, that occur in cells after death; if tissues are not rapidly

fixed for examination the changes could be misconstrued to indicate cellular manifestations of stress or even terminal pathology.

The methodologies of histology and cytology can therefore provide the means to determine manifest alterations in an animal's physiology and general health. A sound knowledge of the normal histology and cytology of the animal permits the formulation of stress indices based on alterations from the norm in the cells and tissues. While it may be possible to derive indices from subjective estimations of tissue changes and intuitive reasoning, it is obviously better to rely on objective measurements of alterations in structure. Some tissue changes, such as those induced by parasitism or neoplasia, need little or no quantitation; however, alterations in reproductive or digestive cycles can be fully determined only by objective quantitation. During the course of several years of both field and experimental investigations of the marine mussel *M. edulis*, a number of stress indices have been derived at the histological and cytological levels. These are described in detail later in this chapter.

So far we have concentrated mainly on the morphological alterations that can be induced by stressors; however, it has become increasingly clear that there is a fundamental unity between the structural organisation of cellular components and their physiological functions. The subcellular organelles are endowed with unique functional properties which are an integration of their molecular structure and biochemical functions. Cytochemistry provides a connecting link between descriptive morphology and biochemistry, allowing us to look at cellular biochemistry in relation to the structural matrix. This offers an integrated approach to problems involving alterations in both cellular structure and biochemistry, such as pathological changes induced by environmental stressors. Two such systems that have been employed for this purpose are lysosomal integrity involving the latency of the hydrolytic enzymes within the lysosome, and the stimulation or induction of the microsomal marker enzyme NADPH-neotetrazolium reductase which is believed to be linked with mixed-function oxidase (MFO) systems. The first of these two systems involves an apparently generalised response to a wide range of physical, chemical and biological stressors, while the second is a fairly specific response to certain types of organic xenobiotics.

These two systems are discussed in detail later in this chapter and serve as examples of the use of specific cytochemical tests as markers of functional morphological entities, i.e. lysosomes and

smooth endoplasmic reticulum, respectively. Both of these systems are present, to a greater or lesser extent, in all cell types ranging from the fungi to vertebrates, so these types of cytochemical tests should be applicable on a fairly widespread basis. Many other histo- or cytochemical reactions have been used to identify and quantify specific cellular components. These include, for instance, succinate dehydrogenase and NAD-dependent isocitrate dehydrogenase for mitochondria, 5'-nucleotidase for plasma membrane, and nucleoside diphosphatase and glucose-6-phosphatase for smooth endoplasmic reticulum (Hardonk and Koudstaal, 1976). Non-enzymic components such as DNA can be identified and measured in tissue sections using the Feulgen reaction and microdensitometry, while many metals such as copper, zinc, lead, mercury and iron can also be localised in specific cellular sites (Pearse, 1972). With the application of cytochemistry at the ultrastructural level, more detailed information can be obtained about the structural relationships of many enzyme systems (Pearse, 1972).

The use of this type of methodology, associated where necessary with biochemistry, subcellular fractionation and cytological techniques in order to check the validity of specific localisation, should provide rapid and sensitive indicators of responses to altered environmental conditions. They are particularly promising in investigations of responses to stress in invertebrates, where cells are seldom organised into highly specific organ systems and where many tissues consist of a number of very different cell types, thus making biochemical interpretation difficult in some instances. Other advantages of using cytochemical techniques are that they permit the use of very small samples of tissue and, through the use of unfixed hexane-frozen cryostat sections, avoid problems associated with the homogenisation of tissues.

HISTOPATHOLOGICAL CONDITIONS

Granulocytomas

Granulocytomas—so called because their dominant cell type is the granular haemoctye, or granulocyte—are non-neoplastic inflammatory responses to a range of environmental pollutants. This condition was first described by Lowe and Moore (1979) in the digestive gland and mantle tissue of *M. edulis*. It is quite distinct from haemocytic responses to invading tissue parasites which are composed of macrophages and hyaline haemocytes. The granulocytes that dominate granulocytomas exhibit coagulation of the cytoplasmic granules (Fig. 2-1). This condition originates in the haemolymph vessels from which it spreads, overcoming encapsulation responses, to invade the surrounding connective tissue where it induces atrophy and autolysis of the digestive tubule epithelial cells. In a survey of nine populations of mussels, there appeared to be a good correlation between the incidence of granulocytomas and the levels of anthropogenic stress (Fig. 2-2) (Lowe and Moore, 1979; and unpublished data). In view of the degenerative effects on the digestive cell this condition is thought to be indicative of a general loss of condition.

Haemopoetic Neoplasms

There are, as yet, no established criteria on which invertebrate neoplasia can be diagnosed. However, Pauley (1969), in his review of molluscan neoplasia, suggested that the infiltration, invasion or replacement of normal cells by actively mitotic, atypical cells is an indication of a potentially neoplastic condition. Suspect neoplasms in marine invertebrates that fulfil Pauley's criteria have been described in a number of bivalves including *Ostrea lurida* (Mix, 1975, 1976), *Granostrea virginica* and *Crassostrea gigas* (Farley, 1969a) and *M. edulis* (Farley, 1969b; Lowe and Moore, 1978; Mix et al., 1979). In mussels, this condition was characterised by the infiltration and replacement of the adipogranular tissue (Froutin, 1937) by enlarged, mitotically active, haemocyte-like cells (Fig. 2-3). These abnormal cells, which were rich in cytoplasmic RNA and had significantly higher DNA values than normal haemocytes (Lowe and Moore, 1978), were observed to be associated with degeneration of the digestive cells (Fig. 2-3, C and D). The replacement of the adipogranular tissue would ultimately lead to a loss of glycogen and protein storage capacity with the possible cessation or loss of gametogenic capability. Similarly, the degeneration of the digestive cells would gradually lead to a loss of intracellular digestive capability and, ultimately, probable starvation.

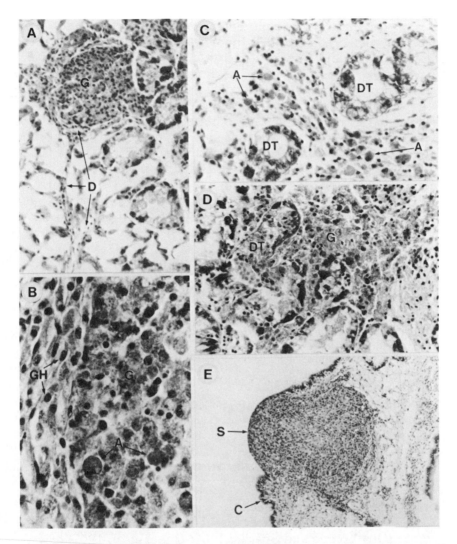

FIG. 2-1. *A.* Section of the digestive gland of *Mytilus edulis* showing a small granulocytoma (G) within a dilated haemolymph duct (HD) (×320). *B.* Section of a granulocytoma (G) showing amorphous bodies (A) and a surrounding layer of fusiform granulocytes (GH) (×800). *C.* Section showing granulocytoma cells, with asociated amorphous bodies (A), invading the digestive gland tissues between the digestive tubules (T) (×500). *D.* Section showing the breakdown of the digestive tubules, adjacent to invading granulocytoma cells (G), resulting in a loss of cellular integrity (×320). *E.* Section showing metaplastic changes in the epidermal cells of the digestive gland from ciliated columnar (C) to simple squamous (S) (×125).

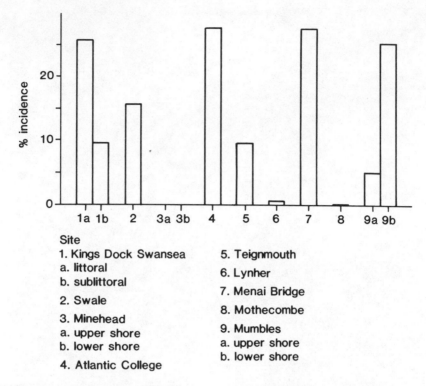

FIG. 2-2. Incidence of granulocytomas in mussels from 12 sites in England and Wales.

Haemocytic Infiltration of Tissues

Localised increases in blood cells or haemocytes can be induced by a variety of factors including parasitism, injury such as shell damage (Des Voigne and Sparks, 1968; Bubel et al. 1977) or even the natural process of tissue resorption following spawning (Bayne et al., 1978). These increases may involve either a single type or several classes of haemocyte. However, it is not always apparent whether these localized increases involve the promotion of additional blood cells, or represent a redeployment of the existing complement of haemocytes. Increases in haemocyte numbers in response to elevated temperature have been demonstrated in *Crassostrea virginica* by Feng (1965) who postulated that as haemocytes participate in nutritional processes their numbers may fluctuate depending on whether or not the animals are feeding. Thompson et al. (1978), working with *Mytilus californianus*,

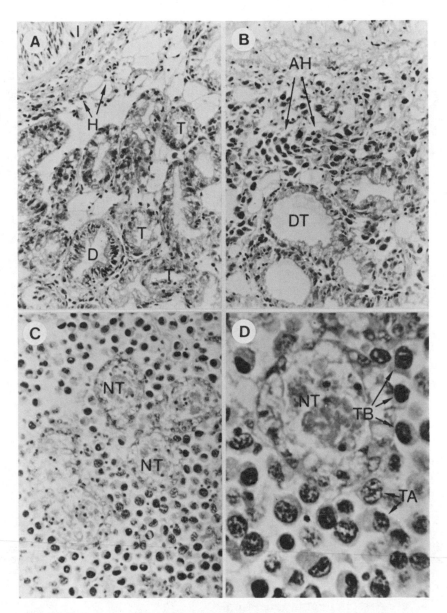

FIG. 2-3.　*A.*　Section through normal digestive gland tissues of *M. edulis* showing digestive tubules (T), ducts (D) and hemocytes (H) in connective tissues underlying the intestine (I) (×312). *B.*　Section as in *A* showing degenerating digestive tubules (DT) and infiltration of the connective tissue underlying the intestine by enlarged atypical hemocytes (AH) (×312). *C.*　Section showing severe infiltration of connective tissues by atypical hemocytes with associated necrotic digestive tubules (NT) (×312). *D.*　Section showing necrotic digestive tubule (NT) with infiltrating type A (TA) and type B (TB) atypical hemocytes (×788).

showed that the change from a starved condition to high food ration did not induce an increase in haemocyte numbers, and neither did a combination of increased ration and increased temperature; however, exposure to the atmosphere at elevated temperature led to an immediate increase which returned to baseline once the animals were immersed. Clearly, the numbers of haemocytic responses are usually focal and of a transient nature. Moreover, in those situations where haemocyte numbers generally remain within natural limits, always bearing in mind the natural variability, no loss of condition can be inferred. When haemocytes exceed natural limits and the cells are evident in very large numbers throughout the connective tissue matrix, this is taken to be a manifestation of a stress response and is classified as indicative of loss of condition.

Parasitic Infestation

The presence of parasites in animal tissues does not necessarily indicate a stressful condition, one example being *Mytilicola intestinalis* in *M. edulis* (Moore et al., 1978c); however, the larvae of digenetic trematodes can induce castration, sex reversal or inhibition of gametogenesis (Smyth, 1966), which could be significant at the population level. Investigations of oysters have indicated that the number of parasites per animal actually increases when the host is subjected to various types of crude oil (Barszcz et al., 1978), suggesting that contaminant-induced stress may incapacitate the hosts' cellular defence mechanisms. The use of parasitism as an index of stress can only be considered sound if the parasite has an effect that is known to be detrimental to the host. However, there are indications that an otherwise benign parasite can be detrimental if the host organism is stressed. Such a synergism is believed to have been responsible for mortalities in mussels parasitised with *M. intestinalis* during an exceptionally hot summer when black-body temperatures rose to 28–37°C (Davey, personal communication).

Alterations in Reproductive Cycles

The reproductive cycles of many marine molluscs are well documented and are generally interpreted in the form of a series of nominal stages, which range from stage 0, or neuter state, to a stage 6 representing the spawning process (Chipperfield, 1953; Lubet, 1957). Such a technique does not readily lend itself to investigations of cause and biological effect, because the method by which the stages are derived is based on subjective estimates while the scale of events is too unrefined to describe the dynamic aspects of the reproductive process. Microstereology has been used, therefore, to describe the cellular processes leading up to and including spawning in mussels; Bayne et al. (1978) showed that stressed mussels produce fewer and smaller eggs than unstressed animals. The technique has also been used to demonstrate different reproductive cycles in mussels from various parts of Great Britain (Lowe et al., 1982), as well as differences induced by the effects of local environments. A comparison of three different mussel populations in southwestern England revealed that each population had its own distinct cycle. The three populations came from very different habitats; these were exposed open coast (Whitsand), outer estuarine (Mothecombe) and inner estuarine (Lynher River). The reproductive cycles of these populations were quantitatively described in terms of the cellular composition of the mantle tissues in which the gametes develop (Figs. 2-4, 2-5, 2-6). Nutritional reserves for gametogenesis and maintenance metabolism are stored in the adipogranular cells (Froutin, 1937; Lubet, 1959), which are rich in proteins, lipids and carbohydrates (glycogen), and in the vesicular connective tissue cells (Lubet, 1979) where carbohydrate (glycogen) is also stored. As these reserves decline, as indicated by a decrease in the volume fractions of the two cell types, gamete development takes place until at full maturation both the adipogranular cell and vesicular connective tissue cell volume fractions are minimal. Mussels from both the Mothecombe and Whitsand populations exhibited a well-synchronised reproductive cycle (Figs. 2-4, 2-5), whereas those from the Lynher population showed a considerable degree of variation (Fig. 2-6); nevertheless, the overall trends remained the same. The reasons for this difference in synchrony are not immediately apparent.

Differences among the three populations became apparent following stereological investigation of the composition of the mantle connective tissue storage cell system. The ratios of the volume fractions of vesicular connective tissue cells to adipogranular cells showed that in mussels from both the Mothecombe and the Lynher populations, the adipogranular cells dominated for a considerable part of the year (Figs. 2-4, 2-6), while in mussels from Whitsand the vesicular cells were always dominant (Fig. 2-5).

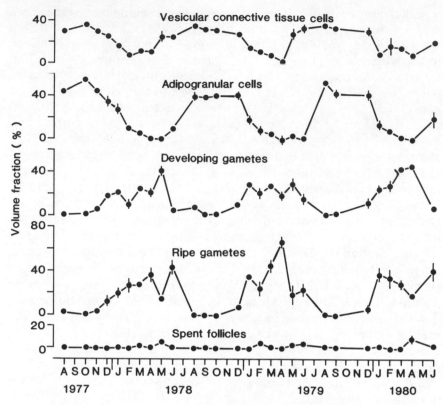

FIG. 2-4. Volume fractions (means ± standard errors) of mantle tissue from Mothecombe mussels.

The reason for this dominance of the vesicular cells in the latter population is not known; however, it may well be a feature of exposed or open coast populations of mussels which are subject to lower temperatures than those from estuarine populations. In addition, the estuarine mussels probably have greater availability of food throughout the year than those from open coast situations.

Loss of Synchrony in Digestive Tubules

Digestion in bivalves has been shown to occur at two sites: extracellular digestion is brought about by the action of the crystalline style in the stomach, whilst intracellular digestion occurs in the digestive cells of the digestive diverticula. In *Crassostrea*

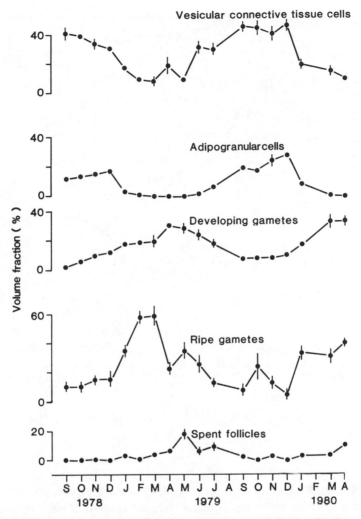

FIG. 2-5. Volume fractions (means ± standard errors) of mantle tissue from Whitsand mussels.

virginica, C. gigas and *Ostrea edulis* it has been shown that the crystalline style dissolves and reforms during every tidal cycle (Morton, 1971; Bernhard, 1973; Langton and Gabbot, 1974). However, it has also been shown in *Cardium edule* and *M. edulis* that phasing of the digestive cells is linked not to the tidal cycle but to the influx of food (Owen, 1972; Langton, 1975). Of course, in the case of littoral animals the presence of food is dependent on the tidal cycle (Morton, 1977).

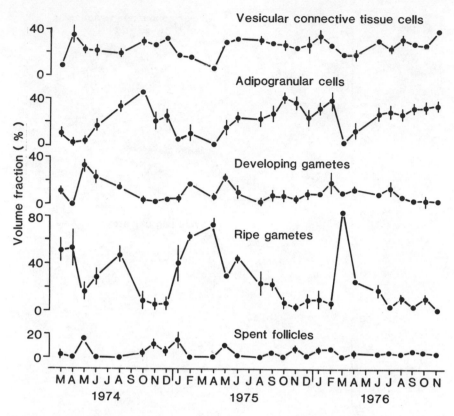

FIG. 2-6. Volume fractions (means ± standard errors) of mantle tissue from Lynher mussels.

The principal phases in the digestive cells of molluscs have been characterised as absorption, digestion, fragmentation, excretion and reconstitution (Owen, 1966; Langton, 1975; Bayne et al., 1976b) (Fig. 2-7). In some species these phases are synchronised so that at any one time all digestive cells are in the same phase (Langton, 1975), although this is by no means true of all bivalves. Langton (1975) has shown that in mussels all the various phases of the digestive cells can be found any time during the tidal cycle.

Several stressors have been shown to upset the digestive rhythm in mussels; these include spawning, which induces structural alterations in the digestive cells resulting in autolytic changes (Bayne et al., 1978), and starvation (Thompson et al., 1974) which results in structural alterations correlated with a decline in digestive gland index (Chapter 8). Elevated temperature

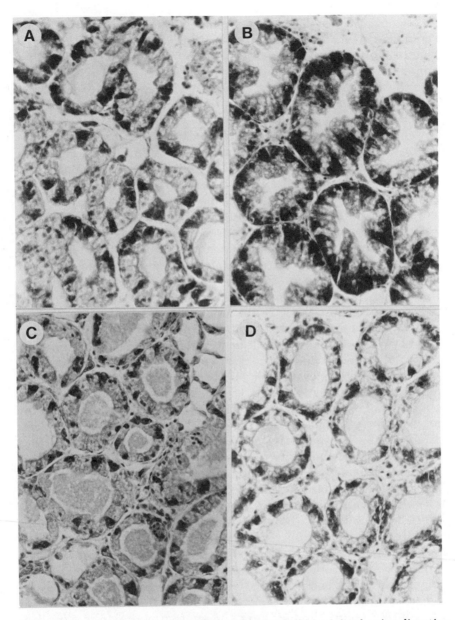

FIG. 2-7. *A.* Section through the digestive gland of *M. edulis* showing digestive tubules with digestive cells in the holding phase. The dark-staining cells are basiphil cells. *B.* Section as in *A* showing digestive cells in the absorption phase. *C.* Section as in *A* showing digestive cells in the fragmentation phase. *D.* Section as in *A* showing digestive cells in the reconstitution phase.

has also been shown to alter tubule structure in *M. californianus* (Thompson et al., 1978), and Moore et al. (1978a, 1978b) reported structural alterations in the digestive cells of mussels in response to injected anthracene and 17β-estradiol.

Routine screening of sections of the digestive diverticula of mussels, from environments of different quality, has indicated that all the tubules emanating from one duct are in the same phase (Lowe, unpublished data). This observation is supported by the findings of Langton (1975) that food is passed into small groups of tubules served by a single duct, therefore indicating that their digestive cells would be active while those not served by that duct might be in a different phase. Mussels from environments that are known to be highly contaminated have been observed to exhibit a greater number of digestive cells in the fragmentation phase (Lowe, unpublished data), and experimental evidence has indicated that changes in the digestive cell phasing can be induced by stress (Widdows et al., 1982). Further evidence indicative of tissue alterations under stress can be found in the work of Bayne et al. (1979) and Moore et al. (1978b) who observed decreased lysosomal stability in the digestive cells with an increasing degree of stress. Bayne et al. (1976a) showed a significant correlation between lysosomal stability and scope for growth. As this increased incidence, or induction, of digestive cell fragmentation and decreased lysosomal stability apparently represents different aspects of the same phenomenon, it might also be expected that a significant increase in the incidence of digestive cells exhibiting fragmentation would be indicative of reduced scope for growth and therefore loss of condition.

The various phases of intracellular digestion in molluscs have previously been quantified by ascribing a nominal stage to each phase. Such a technique has one major drawback, namely that digestion is a highly dynamic process and therefore to attain accurate representation by this method would demand numerous stages. One of the principle differences among the various phases of digestive tubules is the thickness of the tubule epithelial cells. This property has been used to develop a technique to characterise digestive changes in an objective quantitative manner, which takes into account the fact that the system is dynamic. Application of this technique to mussels which had been exposed to the water-accommodated fraction of crude oil (30 μg litre^{-1}) showed that the mean cell height of the digestive tubule epithelium relative to that of the control was significantly reduced (Fig. 2-8), with an associated reduction in mean variance (Lowe et al., 1981; Widdows et al., 1982).

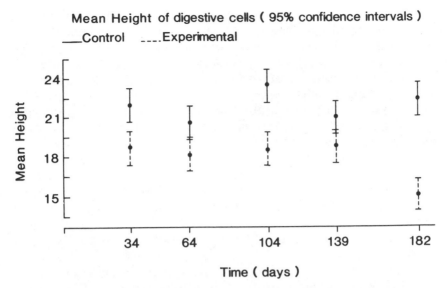

FIG. 2-8.   The effects of aromatic hydrocarbons (30 μg litre^{-1}) in the water-accommodated fraction of North Sea crude oil on digestive tubule epithelial cell depth.

DESTABILISATION OF LYSOSOMES

Mammalian lysosomes are known to be responsive to many types of stressor (see Dingle and Fell, 1969a, 1969b), and lysosomes are an ideal starting point for investigations of generalised cellular stress responses in invertebrates. The gastrodermal cells of coelenterates (Tiffon, 1971; Moore and Stebbing, 1976) and the digestive cells of bivalves and gastropods are especially rich in lysosomes (Summer, 1969; Owen, 1972; Moore and Halton, 1973, 1977; Moore, 1976).

The lysosomal–phagosomal complex forms a vacuolar intracellular digestive system capable of catabolising both endogenous cellular components and exogenous substances which are engulfed by the processes of autophagy and heterophagy, respectively. Autophagy involves the segregation of cytoplasmic components within internal membrane-bound vacuoles, and this process is believed to be central to the normal turnover of these components (Ericsson, 1969). When an organism is stressed, autophagy can function as a physiological survival mechanism (i.e. autodigestion or resorption) or in severe cases it can represent a pathological condition (Ericsson, 1969). The autolysosomes, that are formed during this process are also believed to be more fragile than heterolysosomes, which are involved in heterophagy (Ericsson, 1969). Heterophagy, in contrast, involves the endocytosis (pinocytosis and phagocytosis) of materials, frequently nutritive, from the extracellular environment and their subsequent transport into the lysosomal-vacuolar system, thus providing the means for the intracellular digestion of external substances.

One of the fundamental biochemical properties of lysosomes is the structure-linked latency of many of their hydrolytic degradative enzymes which is a direct consequence of the impermeability of the lysosomal membrane to many substrates as well as the internal membrane-bound nature of many of the enzymes which renders them inactive (Fig. 2-9). However, the membrane stability or fragility of the lysosomes can be altered under certain physiological and pathological conditions (Bitensky et al., 1973) which activate and in some instances release the previously bound enzymes (Fig. 2-9).

Some of the lysosomal stress responses investigated in mammals include tissue injuries induced by a wide variety of toxic organic and inorganic chemicals, atomic and ultraviolet radiation,

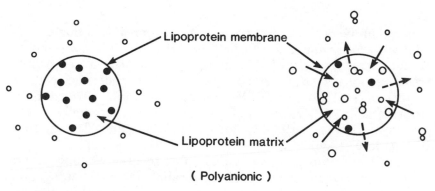

I Lysosome in 'normal' cell   II Lysosome in 'stressed' cell

Lipoprotein membrane

Lipoprotein matrix

(Polyanionic)

o Substrates

● Acid hydrolases (bound or inactive)

O Acid hydrolases (free or active)

FIG. 2-9. Lysosomes in unstressed cells are largely impermeable to many substrates, and the lysosomal hydrolases are inactive or latent. Many stress conditions destabilize the lysosomal membrane, resulting in increased permeability to substrates, activation of previously latent hydrolytic enzymes (reduced latency), disruption of normal lysosomal function and possible release of hydrolases into the cytoplasm where they could cause cytolytic damage.

and photo-sensitisation by visible light; these have been reviewed by Allison (1969) and Slater (1969). In addition, degenerative diseases of bone (Vaes, 1969) and neurons (Holtzman, 1969) and bacterial infections (Allen, 1969) also involve deleterious alterations in lysosomes. These stressors and xenobiotics can in many instances damage or destabilise the integrity of the lysosomal membrane, thus inducing activation and release of previously latent degradative enzymes which initiate catabolism of cellular components and, in severe instances, cell death.

Lysosomes are noted for their sequestration and accumulation of a variety of compounds, including aromatic hydrocarbons, carbon tetrachloride, asbestos, silica, aminoazobenzene derivatives, beryllium, metal powders and viruses (Allison, 1969) as well as the ions of copper, iron, lead, zinc, nickel, tellurium, silver, mercury and plutonium (Koenig, 1963; Rahman and Lindenbaum, 1964; Abraham et al., 1967; Barrett and Dingle, 1967; Scheuer et al., 1967; Vaughan et al., 1967; Verity and Reith, 1967; Slater, 1969; Brun and Brunk, 1970; George et al., 1976; Sternlieb and Goldfischer, 1976; Moore and Stebbing, 1976; Moore, 1977; Moore and Lowe, 1977). Many of these substances are capable of destabilising the lysosomal membrane if the storage capacity is overloaded, with subsequent activation and release of degradative lysosomal enzymes. For an organism, this property of lysosomes could be of considerable environmental consequence through its potential for catabolic disruption of cellular systems (Bayne et al., 1978).

The latency of lysosomal enzymes (lysosomal stability) has therefore been used in both vertebrates and invertebrates as a measure of the condition of the lysosomes in response to a variety of stressors (Allison and Mallucci, 1964; Gahan, 1965; Allison, 1969; Gabrielescu, 1970; Bitensky et al., 1973; Kaw et al., 1975; Moore, 1976; Moore and Stebbing, 1976; Bayne et al., 1976a; Kohli et al., 1977; Matthay et al., 1977; Moore et al., 1978a, 1978b; Bayne et al., 1978; Moore, 1979). Much of the work with invertebrates has been carried out with *M. edulis*, although a number of other bivalves have also been studied as well as the hydroid *Campanularia flexuosa* (Moore and Stebbing, 1976) and the marine snail *Littorina littorea* (Moore et al., 1982).

Lysosomal stability in the digestive cells of *Mytilus* has been found to respond to a range of experimental physical and chemical stressors. These include hyperthermia (Moore, 1976), hypoxia (Moore et al., 1979), starvation, hyposalinity, induced spawning (Bayne et al., 1978), injection of polycyclic aromatic hydrocarbons

(Moore et al., 1978b; Moore, 1979; Bayne et al., 1979) such as 2-methylnaphthalene, 2,3-dimethylnaphthalene, phenanthrene (Table 2-1) and anthracene (Tables 2-2, 2-3) as well as exposure to 12.0 μg litre^{-1} of the water-soluble fraction of crude oil from the Auk field (Moore, 1980a) (Table 2-4; Fig. 2-10, A and B). In all these experiments, lysosomal stability was reduced, indicating that the stressors were inducing functional alterations in the lysosomes and in certain instances structural changes, which were indicative of cytotoxicity (Moore et al., 1978b; Bayne et al., 1978).

The lysosomes of the endodermal cells in the hydroid C. flexuosa are also destabilised by exposing the organism to low levels of copper, cadmium and mercury ions (Stebbing, 1976; Moore and Stebbing, 1976). This organism is highly sensitive to low levels of metal ions, and Stebbing (1976) has developed a bioassay system that employs an index of colonial growth (Chapter 5). Threshold values (Stebbing, 1976) of the response of this index to exposure to copper, cadmium and mercury have been compared with values based on increased activity of lysosomal hexosaminidase as an index of lysosomal fragility (Moore and Stebbing, 1976); these are presented in Table 2-5. Lysosomal deterioration is apparent at lower concentrations of the toxic metals than those which induce an integrated response such as the decline in colonial growth rate (Table 2-5).

Evidence of the value of lysosomal stability as a measure of cellular condition and catabolic potential is provided by significant positive linear correlations between this index and the physiological scope for growth (Bayne et al., 1976a; Bayne et al., 1979), in experimental as well as field investigations. In summary, lysosomal destabilisation induced by environmental stressors results in the activation and release of lysosomal degradative enzymes in both Mytilus and Campanularia, and this appears to be a fairly generalised response. The level of destabilisation in both of these organisms bears a quantitative relationship to the degree of stress (Bayne et al., 1976a; Moore and Stebbing, 1976; Moore et al., 1978b) and governs the intensity of catabolic or degradative effects, as well as the level of pathological change that results. Undoubtedly, degradative damage to functional physiological modules within a cell will eventually have wide-ranging effects on the integration of cellular, tissue and, ultimately, whole-organism physiological processes.

Cytochemical techniques such as the measurement of lysosomal stability can also give insight into the mechanisms of

TABLE 2-1. The Effects of Aromatic Hydrocarbons on the Labilisation Period of Lysosomal Hexosaminidase in the Digestive Cells of *M. edulis* after 24 h

Treatment (100 μl/mussel)		Labilisation period of latent lysosomal hexosaminidase (% of vehicle control, VC; mean ± S.E., $n = 5$)	U-test*
VC I		100.0 ± 5.3	
VC II		97.8 ± 5.4	$P > 0.05$
Naphthalene (10^{-2} M)		108.7 ± 4.4	$P > 0.05$
2-Methylnaphthalene (10^{-2} M)		73.9 ± 8.7	$P < 0.05$
2,3-Dimethylnaphthalene (10^{-2} M)	I	43.5 ± 4.4	$P < 0.01$
	II	52.2 ± 5.2	$P < 0.01$
Phenanthrene (10^{-2} M)		69.6 ± 4.3	$P < 0.01$

*Comparing treatments with VC I.

TABLE 2-2. The Effects after 24 h of Different Levels of Injected Anthracene on the Labilisation Period of Latent Lysosomal Hexosaminidase in the Digestive Cells and Mantle Adipogranular (ADG) Cells of *M. edulis*

Treatment (μg anthracene/mussel)	Primary labilisation period[a] (min; mean ± S.E., $n = 5$)	
	Digestive cells	ADG cells
0 (Vehicle Control)	25 ± 1.0	20 ± 2.0
10	$17 \pm 2.0, P < 0.05$	$6 \pm 1.0, P < 0.01$
25	$17 \pm 2.6, P < 0.05$	$6.3 \pm 1.3, P < 0.01$ ($n = 4$)
50	$15 \pm 1.0, P < 0.01$	$7 \pm 3.4, P < 0.05$
100	$8 \pm 2.0, P < 0.01$	$3 \pm 1.2, P < 0.01$
100[b]	$5 \pm 1.0, P < 0.01$	

[a]Mann-Whitney U-test, comparing treatment with vehicle control.
[b]Replicate experiment.

TABLE 2–3. The Effects of Injected Anthracene (100 μg) over a Period of 168 h on the Labilisation Period of Lysosomal Hexosaminidase in the Digestive Cells of *M. edulis*

Time after injection of anthracene (h)	Primary labilisation period (min; mean ± S.E., $n = 5$)	
	Vehicle control	Experimental* (100 μg)
24	22 ± 1.22	8 ± 2.00, $P < 0.01$
48	22 ± 2.00	8 ± 3.00, $P < 0.05$
96	25 ± 1.01	5 ± 1.01, $P < 0.01$
168	23 ± 2.00	17 ± 3.39, $P > 0.05$

*Mann-Whitney U-test, comparing treatment with vehicle control.

TABLE 2–4. The Effects of Exposure to Water-soluble Fraction of Auk Crude Oil (12.0 μg litre^{-1}) on the Labilisation Period of Latent Lysosomal Hexosaminidase in the Digestive Cells of *M. edulis*

Treatment	Labilisation period of latent lysosomal hexosaminidase (min; mean ± S.E., $n = 10$)	U-test
Control 2 days	21.0 ± 0.7	
Control 7 days	24.0 ± 0.7	
Experimental 7 days	14.0 ± 0.6	$P < 0.001$
Experimental 14 days	15.0 ± 1.2	$P < 0.001$
Control 21 days	21.0 ± 1.9 ($n = 5$)	
Experimental 21 days	14.5 ± 1.4	$P < 0.01$
Experimental 28 days	14.0 ± 2.1	$P < 0.01$
Control 35 days	23.0 ± 0.8	
Experimental 35 days	12.0 ± 0.8	$P < 0.001$
Control 39 days	22.0 ± 1.2 ($n = 5$)	
Experimental 39 days	14.0 ± 1.0 ($n = 5$)	$P < 0.01$

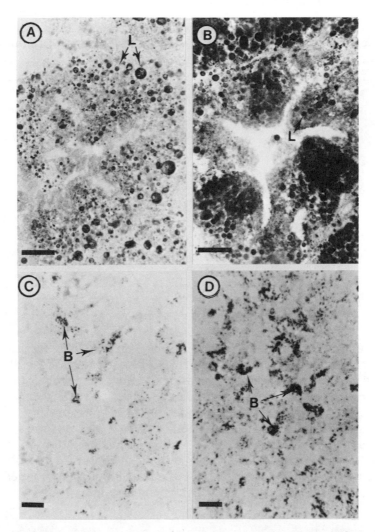

FIG. 2-10. (Scale bar ≡ 20 μm.) *A.* Section through the digestive tubules of *M. edulis*, from the control condition of the Auk crude oil exposure experiment (21 days), following 10 min labilisation (pH 4.5 at 37°C) and showing slight staining reaction for hexosaminidase in lysosomes (L) of the digestive cells. *B.* Section as in *A* of *M. edulis*, exposed for 28 days to the water-soluble fraction of Auk crude oil (12.0 μg litre^{-1}), following 10 min labilisation (pH 4.5 at 37°C) and showing intense staining reaction for hexosaminidase in lysosomes (L) of the digestive cells. *C.* Section through the connective tissue of the digestive gland of *M. edulis*, from the control condition of the Auk crude oil exposure experiment (35 days), showing blood cells (B) stained for NADPH- neotetrazolium reductase activity. *D.* Section as in *C* of *M. edulis*, exposed for 35 days to the water-soluble fraction of Auk crude oil (12.0 μg litre^{-1}), showing increased staining reaction for NADPH-neotetrazolium reductase in the blood cells (B).

69

TABLE 2-5. Growth Rate and Lysosomal Hexosaminidase Cytochemical Threshold Values for Exposure to Copper, Cadmium and
Mercury

Metal	Exposure no.	Threshold for colonial growth (μg litre^{-1})	Threshold for cytochemical index (μg litre^{-1})
CuCl$_2$	1	(2.4)*	1.20
	2	13	1.39
	3	10	1.90
	4	12	1.24
	5	18	—
CdCl$_2$	1	110	40
	2	280	75
HgCl$_2$	1	1.6	—
	2	1.7	0.17

*A different sub-culturing technique was used in this experiment.

cytoxicity, although caution is required in the interpretation of
loss of lysosomal integrity as a primary toxic effect when, in fact,
it may in some instances be a secondary effect. Nevertheless, information can still be obtained which is related to toxic mechanisms
involving changes in the physico-chemical properties of the
lysosomal membranes. In addition, the role of lysosomes in the
accumulation of certain metals and organic xenobiotics is also
important in terms of their role as a detoxication system which
effectively isolates these materials from the cytoplasm unless the
storage capacity of the lysosomes is overloaded.

STIMULATION OF MICROSOMAL
NADPH-NEOTETRAZOLIUM REDUCTASE

Detoxication of foreign compounds is an important survival
mechanism for organisms living in chronically polluted environments. Many organic xenobiotics, including pesticides and
aromatic hydrocarbons, are metabolised by the microsomal (smooth

endoplasmic reticulum) mixed-function oxidases, which require NADPH and oxygen (the biochemical properties of this system are discussed in Chapter 4). A number of the intermediates that can be formed, such as epoxides, are primary carcinogens or mutagens, so the mixed-function oxidases must be viewed as comprising both detoxication and toxication elements (Lee et al., 1977). Many foreign compounds stimulate the proliferation of the smooth endoplasmic reticulum (microsomes) with its associated mixed-function oxidases and NADPH-producing enzymes such as 6-phosphogluconate dehydrogenase and glucose-6-phosphate dehydrogenase (Altman, 1972); some of the possible interactions and effects of environmental chemicals on these systems have been reviewed by Conney and Burns (1972). The use of this phenomenon of induction of mixed-function oxidases by xenobiotics has been proposed by Payne (1977) as a possible method of monitoring the biological effects of petroleum hydrocarbon pollution in marine organisms, although he was able to demonstrate induction only in fish and not in invertebrates.

NADPH-neotetrazolium reductase is believed to be linked with mixed-function oxidases in mammals (Altman, 1972; Hardonk and Koudstaal, 1976) and to represent the NADPH-oxidising activity of the microsomal respiratory chains terminating in cytochrome P-450 (Chayen, 1978; Henderson, 1979). Cytochemically and biochemically determined activity for NADPH-neotetrazolium reductase is stimulated in mammals by phenobarbitol, hexobarbitol and methylcholanthrene, which also induce mixed-function oxidase activity (Koudstaal and Hardonk, 1969, 1972; Altman, 1972; Richards, 1973; Linder and Beyhl, 1978). NADPH-neotetrazolium reductase has also been used as a marker enzyme for smooth endoplasmic reticulum and as a potential indicator for mixed-function oxidase systems in *M. edulis* (Moore 1979; Bayne et al., 1979). This enzyme has been localised in the intestinal epithelial cells and developing oocytes (Moore, 1979); activity determined microdensitometrically has been shown to be stimulated by anthracene (Tables 2-6 and 2-7), dimethylnaphthalene, phenanthrene and phenobarbital (Table 2-8) (Moore, 1979; Bayne et al., 1979), as well as the water-soluble fraction of crude oil (7.7–68 μg litre^{-1}) (Fig. 2-10, *C* and *D*; Table 2-9) (Moore, 1980a; Moore et al., 1980). This enzyme system can therefore be used as a cytochemical index of stimulation of microsomal enzyme activity by aromatic hydrocarbons and phenobarbital.

TABLE 2-6. The Effect of Anthracene on the Staining Intensity of NADPH-Neotetrazolium Reductase in the Blood Cells of *M. edulis* over a Period of 24 h

Treatment	Relative absorbance of NADPH neotetrazolium reductase (% of VCI; mean ± S.E., $n = 5$)	U-test*
VC I	100.0 ± 4.61	
VC II	101.8 ± 3.97	$P > 0.05$
10 μg Anthracene	150.8 ± 13.46	$P < 0.01$
25 μg Anthracene	155.2 ± 2.71	$P < 0.01$
50 μg Anthracene	153.4 ± 8.20	$P < 0.01$
100 μg Anthracene I	179.0 ± 11.93	$P < 0.01$
100 μg Anthracene II	184.0 ± 11.92	$P < 0.01$

*Comparing treatments with VC I.

Studies on mammals also point to the use of NADPH-neotetrazolium reductase as in indicator of the stimulation of the microsomal detoxication system. This enzyme is present in the digestive cells and blood cells of *Mytilus* and responds to phenobarbital and polycyclic aromatic hydrocarbons in the same way as in mammalian cells. This particular response is believed to be specific to certain groups of xenobiotics (Moore et al., 1980) and has been applied to monitoring for pollutant effects induced by oil-derived hydrocarbons (Moore et al., 1982).

TABLE 2-7. The Effect of 100 μg of Anthracene on the Staining Intensity of NADPH-Neotetrazolium Reductase in the Blood Cells of *M. edulis* over a Period of 7 days

Time (days)	Relative absorbance of NADPH-neotetrazolium reductase (arbitrary units of absorbance; mean ± S.E., $n = 5$)		U-test
	Vehicle control	100 μg Anthracene	
1	15.77 ± 1.08	29.01 ± 1.88	$P < 0.01$
2	16.48 ± 0.53	26.21 ± 1.54	$P < 0.01$
4	16.35 ± 1.24	22.51 ± 2.82	$P > 0.05$
7	17.37 ± 1.89	22.16 ± 1.06	$P < 0.05$

TABLE 2–8. The Effects of Phenobarbital and Aromatic Hydrocarbons on NADPH-Neotetrazolium Reductase Activity Determined Microdensitometrically in the Blood Cells of *M. edulis* after 24 h

Treatment (100 µl/mussel)		Relative absorbance (% of vehicle control, VC; mean ± S.E., $n = 5$)	U-test*
VC (Phenobarbital)	I	100.0 ± 8.8	
	II	112.8 ± 4.6	$P > 0.05$
Phenobarbital (0.85×10^{-2} M)	I	156.1 ± 6.9	$P < 0.01$
	II	157.5 ± 5.1	$P < 0.01$
VC (aromatic hydrocarbons	I	100.0 ± 14.5	
	II	105.6 ± 17.9	$P > 0.05$
Naphthalene (10^{-2} M)		75.7 ± 10.5	$P > 0.05$
2-Methylnaphthalene (10^{-2} M)		80.1 ± 16.5	$P > 0.05$
2,3-Dimethylnaphthalene (10^{-2} M)	I	265.0 ± 19.5	$P < 0.01$
	II	252.2 ± 46.7	$P < 0.05$
Phenanthrene (10^{-2} M)		147.7 ± 13.1	$P < 0.01$

*Comparing treatments with VC (phenobarbital) I and VC (aromatic hydrocarbons) I.

TABLE 2–9. The Effects of Exposure to Water-soluble Fraction of Auk Crude Oil (12.0 µg litre^{-1}) on NADPH-Neotetrazolium Reductase in the Blood Cells of *M. edulis*

Treatment		Relative absorbance of NADPH-neotetrazolium reductase (arbitrary units of absorbance; mean ± S.E., $n = 5$)	U-test
Control 7 days	I	18.23 ± 2.00	
	II	16.21 ± 2.13	$P > 0.05^a$
Experimental 7 days	I	33.84 ± 3.05	$P < 0.01$
	II	33.09 ± 2.37	$P < 0.01$
Experimental 14 days	I	32.06 ± 3.23	$P < 0.01$
	II	30.32 ± 3.07	$P < 0.01$
Control 35 days	I	21.30 ± 1.94	
	II	23.94 ± 2.19	$P > 0.05^b$
Experimental 35 days	I	35.63 ± 2.29	$P < 0.01$
	II	42.18 ± 3.91	$P < 0.01$

[a]Comparing treatments with control 7 days I.
[b]Comparing treatments with control 35 days I.

The presence of mixed-function oxidases can facilitate the formation of mutagenic intermediates with the potential for damage to the genome. In this context, neoplastic blood cells have been reported from a number of bivalves including *Mytilus* (Farley, 1969; Farley and Sparks, 1970), and Lowe and Moore (1978) have demonstrated that a native population of mussels with this condition had been exposed to a range of aromatic hydrocarbons. In the case of the individual, somatic mutation is of no ecological consequence unless it results in widespread mortality; however, genetic damage to the developing gametes could have far-reaching effects in relation to their viability and survival.

3

Chromosomal Aberrations

The continuing contamination of the marine environment with chemical and physical agents of known or suspected mutagenic and carcinogenic activity poses an insidious threat to marine life and to those organisms, including man, that are trophically dependent upon it (Beardmore et al., 1980). Samples from polluted marine environments have been shown by standard genetic toxicological methods to cause damage to DNA (e.g. Colombatti et al., 1976; Parry et al., 1976). A variety of marine animals has been shown to accumulate certain classes of pollutants in their tissues (Chipman, 1972; Roberts, 1976; Grimås, 1979), and many of these organisms, including several important food species, are known to have the metabolic capability for transforming various xenobiotics to mutagens (Payne and Martins, 1980). It follows that there is a need for genetic screening of water samples and living material collected from those environments known to be at risk from pollution (IAEA, 1979; Beardmore et al., 1980).

Pollution can act on genetic material in two ways. First, pollutants may exert selective pressure on the genetic structure (allele frequencies) of whole populations by modification of the environment. Discussion of this is beyond the scope of this chapter; there are a number of reports in the literature of this type of genetic adjustment in natural populations of marine animals exposed to pollutants (see Mitton and Koehn, 1975; Nevo et al., 1977, 1978; Battaglia and Beardmore, 1978). Also, using laboratory-grown populations Battaglia et al. (1980) have demonstrated changes in the genetic constitution of the copepod *Tisbe* in response to toxicant exposure.

Second, pollutants are also capable of causing mutation by inflicting damage directly to the DNA molecule within the individual cell nucleus. Since events of this kind occur at random with respect to the environment, they tend to be deleterious, introducing errors into the genetic blue-print which controls the structure and function of the cell. Unless mutations are severely limiting in their action, such as to cause the death of the carrier cell, the altered genome may be transmitted to daughter cells (Fig. 3-1). In

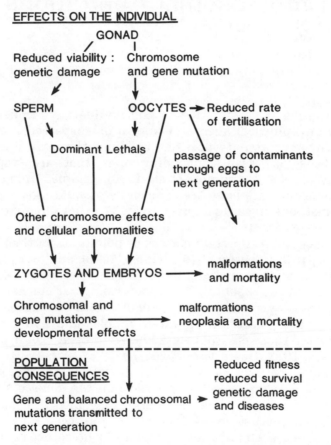

FIG. 3-1. Diagram depicting how pollution effects incurred at one stage in development may not finally be expressed until some later stage, even into the next generation (the example shown here refers to the sensitive reproductive tissues of a marine invertebrate, e.g. tubeworm or mussel). Hence, genetic effects are amongst the more insidious consequences of marine pollution.

the case of somatic cell mutation, this may produce a mosaic individual or possibly lead to neoplasia; mutations in the germ cell line are transmitted through the gametes to the next generation of individuals which, because of their altered genomes, will be at a selective disadvantage compared to their unaffected relatives. Either way the outcome is the same: a reduction in the *fitness* of the affected individuals.

There are two types of mutation, gene mutations and chromosomal mutations; the latter are usually referred to as "aberrations" in order to avoid confusion between the two. Gene mutation is a change at or within a single locus (Drake and Flamm, 1972) that becomes evident only after it gains phenotypic expression. The frequency with which gene mutations occur is relatively low; most estimates of natural mutation rate in germinal tissues fall in the range 1×10^{-7} to 1×10^{-5} per locus per gamete per generation (Beardmore et al., 1980). On the basis that the natural rate of gene mutation (sometimes misleadingly called the spontaneous rate) is extremely low, it has been argued that the effect of any pollutant acting to increase the mutation rate would be compensated for by natural regulatory processes (Cook and Wood, 1976; Berry, 1977). This argument does not apply to the second type of mutation, chromosomal aberration, which involves whole chromosomes, or segments carrying large numbers of genes. In man, the most-studied species, abnormal chromosome complements are found in approximately 7% of all conceptuses (Hook, 1982) and are responsible for congenital abnormalities, reduced fertility, decreased life-span, senility and cancer (Kihlman, 1966; Sutton and Harris, 1972; Carter, 1977; Magee, 1977). While less is known about the natural aberration level in the cells of aquatic organisms, control values are generally reported as being about 1% (e.g. Kligerman, 1979), although in some cases the level could be significantly higher (Fig. 3-2).

Numerical chromosome aberrations fall into two categories: types that involve single chromosome deviations from the normal diploid number (e.g. $2n + 1$, $2n - 1$), which are termed aneuploid (Dixon, 1982), and types involving whole multiples of the haploid condition (n, $3n$, $4n$, etc.), which are collectively described under the heading of haplo/polyploids (Fig. 3-2). For information regarding the features that characterise a chromosome (i.e. chromatids, chromosome arms and centromere), the reader is referred to general texts on cytogenetics (e.g. Swanson, 1957; John and Lewis, 1968), while details of chromosome nomenclature are given by Levan et al. (1964).

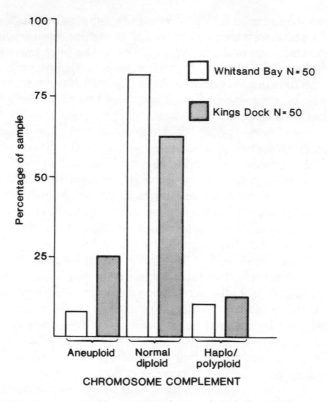

FIG. 3-2. The percentage frequencies of normal and abnormal mussel (*Mytilus edulis*) embryos in samples originating from clean (Whitsand Bay) and polluted (King's Dock) sites.

The other major category of chromosomal aberration includes all those *structural* effects involving one or both chromatids in the chromosome. Primary damage inflicted on a chromosome by a mutagen leads to the formation of a lesion (Bostock and Sumner, 1978, p. 437) which is either repaired or remains as a gap, a chromatid break or a chromosome break, depending upon the extent of the damage and the stage in the cell cycle when the damage occurs (Evans, 1962). Broken ends of chromosomes have a strong mutual attraction which results in the majority of them rejoining either in their original orientation, so that evidence of damage may be demonstrated only by radio or chemical labelling techniques (Bostock and Sumner, 1978), or abnormally so that unscheduled configurations are formed, namely inversions, translocations and duplications. The loss of a piece of chromosome is termed a deletion (Evans, 1962; Kihlman, 1966; Savage, 1975).

Types of chromosomal damage that cannot be seen as changes in chromosome structure but nonetheless involve genic rearrangements, e.g. pericentric inversions, can be made visible by the use of one of the modern chromosome banding techniques (e.g. Salemaa, 1979; Sharma and Sharma, 1980). Failing this, their presence is often indicated by abnormal chromosome pairing during the first division of meiosis (Ahmed and Sparks, 1970). The paper by Savage (1975) provides a detailed classification of induced chromosomal structural changes and is an essential reference for workers in this field.

Brief mention should be made of a third category of chromosomal aberration which is sometimes encountered in mutation studies. This heterogeneous group contains those aberrations resulting from damage to the mitotic spindle that give rise to an abnormal segregation of chromatids at anaphase, e.g. tripolar anaphases (Fig. 3-3). This category also contains all those chromosomal aberrations whose aetiology is not fully understood; these include the pulverised nuclei generally encountered only in radiation studies (Savage, 1975), and the so-called sub-chromatid or "stickiness" phenomena that lead to the formation of pseudo bridges in anaphase nuclei (Evans, 1962; Gregory et al., 1974; Nichols et al., 1977).

Recent expansion of interest in environmental mutagenesis (Auerbach, 1976; Scott et al., 1977), and the recovery of mutagens from the tissues of marine organisms (for references, see above),

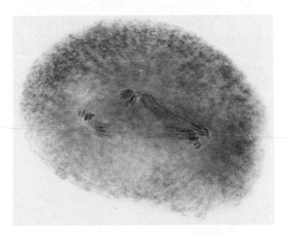

FIG. 3-3. A case of aneuploidy (individual chromosome deviations from the diploid number): tri-polar anaphase in a cell with three centrioles (scale bar ≡ 10 μm).

has led to a search for suitable genetic systems for investigation. Interest has focussed primarily on fish cells because of the importance of this group as food species for man; in particular, because of the ease with which they can be kept in the laboratory, most of this work relates to freshwater species. For the most part, the studies have dealt with radiation effects, usually at high dosage levels; Kligerman (1979) has recently reviewed the literature on aquatic radiation from the point of view of methodology.

Longwell (1976) carried out field-based investigations on the influence of general pollution stress and acute hydrocarbon pollution on the incidence of various developmental abnormalities, including some chromosomal aberrations, in the planktonic eggs and larvae of two marine fish species. Her results, supported by the findings of radiation studies (IAEA, 1979), show that the cells of fish, especially the eggs and early developmental stages, are very sensitive to chromosome damage arising from contact with water-borne mutagens.

Less is known about chromosomal aberrations in the cells of aquatic invertebrates. Using a range of direct- and indirect-acting mutagens, Pesch and co-workers (1980, 1981) have demonstrated that the larvae of the sediment-dwelling polychaete *Neanthes arenaceodentata* can be used as the basis for an extremely sensitive, *in vivo*, assay for measuring chromosomal effects. Recently, Pesch's sister chromatid exchange technique has been successfully applied to the adults and larvae of the mussel *Mytilus edulis* (Dixon and Clarke, 1982; Harrison and Jones, 1982). The level of sensitivity exhibited by the cells of these two marine invertebrates for standard mutagens is comparable to that recognised for mammalian cells.

The cytogenic techniques described in Chapter 9 use the reproductive stages of the marine tubeworm *Pomatoceros triqueter* as a test system for investigating the effects of pollutants on genetic material.

4

Biochemical Measurements

Biochemical indices of stress involve the measurement of molecular components of the cells of tissues or of extracellular fluids such as blood serum. These indices complement other measurements of stress effects at different levels of organisation (physiological, cytological, cytochemical) and, although they are at present in the early stages of development, they will be a necessary part of an effective programme of biological-effects monitoring. For a particular biochemical response to be acceptable as an index of biological effect, it must, like other stress indices, fulfill two important criteria:

1. The measurable change in the biochemical process must result from, or be a response to, a change in the environmental factor. The relationship between the biochemical index and the environmental factor may be quantitative but is more likely to be semi-quantitative or even qualitative. For example, the synthesis of an enzyme may be induced by the presence of a pollutant but may not then be increased by further increases in the concentration of the pollutant. The activity of the enzyme will not then be quantitatively related to the concentration of the pollutant but will be indicative of its presence and of an effect.
2. It must be possible to demonstrate that the change in the biochemical process will have a detrimental effect on growth, reproduction or survival of the organism. For example, it is possible that a change in one biochemical process could be

compensated for by a change in another process such that no decline in biological performance results. A modification to this requirement is the situation where a change in a biochemical process cannot be shown directly (or mechanistically) to affect growth, etc., but may simply be characteristic of a physiological condition which does have this affect, e.g. the taurine:glycine ratio (Jeffries, 1972). Such an index could still be useful, given sufficient background information for interpretation.

The importance of fulfilling the second criterion above cannot be over-emphasised. In the absence of this, the biochemical index cannot be used as a measure of biological effects and becomes simply a means of measuring pollutant levels, rather than their effects, a role that has been suggested for the aryl hydrocarbon hydroxylase system of fish (Penrose, 1978). It is only in the latter context that the existence of a quantitative relationship between the biochemical index and the environmental factor (first criterion above) is important. In the context of biological effects monitoring, the important relationship is that between the biochemical index and the particular measure, usually energetic, of the resulting biological performance of the animal. At least in the case of a *general biochemical index of stress* (see below), it is the quantitative nature of this relationship which will transform the index from a "number" into an operational tool and which will determine and limit its application in environmental monitoring. If the relationship is semi-quantitative, then the application of the biochemical index will be semi-quantitative. Different considerations may apply for *specific biochemical indices of stress* (see below) such as, for example, the production of metallothioneins, where no biological effect occurs (other than the energy cost of protein synthesis) until the detoxification system is saturated with metal (see below). The relationship between the biochemical index and the particular measure of biological performance can therefore be complicated and also may be dependent on the criterion used for the latter. These aspects are discussed in more detail in some of the sections below. The ideal biochemical index of stress is that which is itself a meaningful and acceptable measure of biological performance.

The particular usefulness of biochemical indices is likely to result from a number of features of such responses:

1. Sensitivity to sublethal stress. Responses to an environmental change, at whatever level of cellular organisation, are

fundamentally biochemical. Therefore, biochemical indices should be the most sensitive to environmental change and provide the earliest warning of a decline in animal condition. Two sorts of sensitivity are possible. (1) Sensitivity in "time". This will be the more usual case where in the biological response to a stressor, the change in the biochemical process (registered as the biochemical index) occurs before changes in other processes, including physiological ones. Because a decline in biological performance is likely to be the result of a series of such events, implicit in the use of such sensitive indices is that the decline in biological performance will result only if the particular stressor (environmental condition) is maintained. This, of course, assumes that the biochemical changes are reversible. (2) Sensitivity to the level of the stressor. This sensitivity is conveyed by the fact that a biochemical process responds to, say, a level of pollutant that does not affect other processes being measured, including physiological ones. In practice, therefore, such a biochemical index is only possible if it is also a measure of biological performance which is regarded as having significance in terms of ecological consequence. The usual measures of biological performance would not register a change in the presence of such low levels of stressors.

2. Ease of measurement. Biochemical indices consist of measuring the qualitative or quantitative aspects of biological molecules, usually by enzymatic or chemical means. Such indices, once they have been fully interpreted and understood, often can be reduced to simple assays or tests which lend themselves to automation.

3. Specificity of the response. The possibility of attributing a biological effect to a specific pollutant or type of pollutant, or even to a pollutant as opposed to a natural variable, decreases the higher the level of organisation in the individual that is considered. Therefore, where specific enzymes or enzyme systems are induced by particular pollutants, for example, it may be possible to use such indices or changes to identify the offending stressor in a complex environmental situation. This feature of biochemical indices has led to their categorisation into *general indices of stress* and *specific indices of stress* (e.g. Bayne et al., 1980b).

In terms of the monitoring of biological effects, it is possible to envisage two types of biochemical response which can be termed *primary* and *secondary* responses, and which may show one, two or all of the above features. A *primary response* is one in which the biochemical process responds immediately to an environmental change. Such a response will clearly be sensitive and may or may not be specific. A *secondary response* is one that occurs at a later stage in the biological response as a consequence of other metabolic events. Therefore, it will be no more sensitive than a physiological or a cytological change and, as it does not have a direct functional relationship to the environmental variable, it may not be specific. However, a strong case could exist for the use of such a response by virtue of the ease of its measurement as compared with, for example, a physiological index.

In recent years, research into biochemical responses to pollution has been increasing. The studies have involved many different marine organisms, and all the major groups of pollutants. As a result of a number of workshops and symposia, problems in the application and use of biochemical studies have been identified and various recommendations made for the future areas of research that will be most useful for environmental monitoring purposes (Giam, 1978; I.C.E.S., 1978; Bayne et al., 1980b; Lee et al., 1980; Uthe et al., 1980). Some of these discussions are considered in the sections on the individual biochemical indices and towards the end of this section.

Any molecule is a possible site for a response, but it is likely that certain areas of metabolism, or certain types of molecules, will offer more potential for incorporation into biochemical indices. Low molecular weight compounds such as the substrates and products of intermediary metabolism generally have attracted least attention. The usefulness of such molecules is probably limited by their general nature, rapid turnover (concentrations can change during extraction) and low concentrations within tissues. Exceptions to this, however, include free amino acids, adenosine phosphates and some blood metabolites which appear to be useful as indices of stress. Certain physiological responses involving small molecules have also been suggested as potential areas for the derivation of stress indices. For example, osmotic and ionic regulation by fish and certain invertebrates are vulnerable to polychlorinated hydrocarbons and metals, while the balance between different end-products of nitrogen metabolism may be disturbed by various environmental stressors including metals (see I.C.E.S., 1978).

Macromolecules stored as energy reserves (carbohydrate, lipid, proteins) are probably limited in use, at least in mussels, due to their very marked seasonal variation, although Jeffries (1972) recorded substantial depletion of carbohydrate in clams from an estuary polluted with hydrocarbons. For oysters, Gabbott and Walker (1971) found that measurements of a simple condition index correlated well with measures of glycogen content, and it has been suggested that, for routine monitoring purposes, this could suffice as a crude estimate of nutritional status (Bayne et al., 1980b). Measurements of storage macromolecules are more useful when their utilisation is directly linked to reproductive processes. In such cases, they offer potential as indices of ecological consequence, e.g. the phosphoprotein, vittellogenin, has been suggested as a measure of vittellogenesis and larval development in flounder (I.C.E.S., 1978, suggested from Emmersen and Emmersen, 1976), and the lipid content of the eggs of *Mytilus edulis* has been found to reflect the degree of stress experienced by the adults (Bayne et al., 1978).

The molecules that probably offer the greatest potential for the monitoring of biological effects and have attracted most attention are enzymes and other "functional" proteins such as metallothioneins (e.g. see I.C.E.S., 1978; Bayne et al., 1980b; Lee et al., 1980). Both general and specific enzymes and enzyme systems have been investigated in relation to the major groups of pollutants and aspects of this are considered later in this chapter. Informational molecules have received less attention, with the exception of steroids, but must offer similar potential. Nervous and endocrine function, DNA and RNA changes and steroid metabolism have been recommended as prime candidates for future development (Giam, 1978; I.C.E.S., 1978; Lee et al., 1980). Also recommended for study were immunological responses, reproductive biochemistry, membrane biochemistry and lipid metabolism.

Much ignorance clearly exists with regard to many areas of biochemistry and their interaction with pollutants, and this led Giam (1978) to propose the following for future investigation: (1) Biochemical differences exist between different organisms; selection of species for study should therefore be based either on systematic phylogenetic surveys (one or more species, from different habitats, per phylum) or on field and laboratory observations of pollutant-resistant and pollutant-sensitive species. In the latter case, comparison of the two types might identify the biochemical processes responsible for the resistance to pollution. (2) More information is required on the rates and routes of pollutant accumulation and release by marine organisms and on the bioavailability of food-adsorbed and sediment-adsorbed pollutants (to this we can add inorganic and organic chemical speciation in the water column). (3) Histopathological and ultrastructural studies may provide information about the cellular and subcellular sites and modes of action of the pollutant. (4) Study and identification of specific toxification and detoxification systems are required, together with comparison of the pollutant metabolites and conjugates to the parent compound for toxicity and mutagenicity. (5) Study of the interactions between different pollutants (synergism, antagonism, etc), between pollutants and natural environmental stresses (salinity, temperature, dissolved oxygen) and between pollutants and biological parameters (sex, age, season, nutritional state, etc) are required.

Problems that are likely to be encountered in the application of biochemical studies to biological effects monitoring have been commented on at length by Uthe et al. (1980). Many of these problems can be accommodated by working with a single sentinel species such as *M. edulis* or with several closely related species such as the bivalve molluscs (see Bayne et al., 1980b). Criteria can be established for a sampling strategy that will meet the problems of age and heterogeneous genetic constitution, while, on the basis of detailed biochemical knowledge, interpretation of changes is possible against a background of season, sex and tissue specificity. In addition to being suitable organisms for pollutant surveys because of their bioaccumulating properties (Goldberg et al., 1978), bivalve molluscs, and in particular *M. edulis*, have been the subject of a considerable biochemical research effort over the last ten years. Knowledge of their biochemistry, particularly in relation to seasonal aspects and tissue specificity, has increased and is increasing rapidly. Recent reviews on aspects of their metabolism include: amino acid and protein metabolism (Campbell and Bishop, 1970; Lange, 1972; Schoffeniels and Gilles, 1972; Bayne et al., 1976c), anaerobic and carbohydrate metabolism (Goddard and Martin, 1966; De Zwaan et al., 1976; De Zwaan and Wijsman, 1976; De Zwaan, 1977), energy metabolism in general (Gabbott, 1976), lipid and sterol metabolism (Voogt, 1972), and population genetics (Levinton and Koehn, 1976).

GENERAL INDICATORS OF STRESS

Amino Acids and the Taurine:Glycine Ratio

In comparing populations of the hard clam *Mercenaria mercenaria* from polluted and clean habitats of Narragansett Bay, Rhode

TABLE 4–1. Responses of the Taurine:Glycine Ratio to Stress in Bivalve Molluscs

Species	Tissue	Stressor[a]	Control[b] animals	Stressed[b] animals	Reference
Hard clam, *Mercenaria mercenaria*	gill and mantle	1. hydrocarbons (F) 2. general (L)	2.3–2.9	5.0–6.6 2.5–4.9	Jeffries (1972)
Oyster, *Crassostrea virginica*	haemolymph	1. parasitic infection (F)	0.5–2.0	1.3–9.1	Feng et al. (1970)
Clam, *Protothaca staminea*	gills	1. chlorinated seawater (L)	3.5	4.7–5.7	Roesijadi (1979)
Anadara trapezia	—	1. reduced salinity (L)	0.9	no change	Lee et. al. (1980)
Oyster, *Saccostrea commencialis*	—	1. reduced salinity (L)	2.3	4.5	Lee et. al. (1980)
Oyster, *Crassostrea gigas*	adductor muscle	1. hydrocarbons (F)	0.9	2.3–2.4	Neff (pers. comm.)
Clam, *Macoma inquinata*	adductor muscle, foot and mantle	1. hydrocarbons (F)	0.6	0.9	Roesijadi and Anderson (1979)

T:G ratio

[a]L: laboratory exposures; F: field exposures or field comparisons.
[b]Range of values represents change with time.

87

TABLE 4–2. Responses of the Taurine:Glycine Ratio and the Sum of Threonine and Serine of the Whole Tissues (Less Digestive Gland) of *M. edulis* to Stress

Stressor(s)[b]		T:G ratio[a]		(thr ± ser) (μmol g^{-1} dry wt)[a]		Source
		Control	Experimental	Control	Experimental	
(a)	Increased temperature	1. 1.9–2.4	2.7–3.9	18–28	no change	Bayne et al. (1976c) (T:G ratio) and Livingstone, unpublished data (thr + ser).
		2. 1.8	no change	87	70	Livingstone and Feith, unpublished data
(b)	Starvation	1. 1.9–2.4	no change	18–28	no change	Bayne et al. (1976c) (T:G ratio) and Livingstone, unpublished data (thr + ser).

(c)	Increased temperature and starvation combined	1. No interaction—results as for (a)1			Bayne et al. (1976c) (T:G ratio) and Livingstone, unpublished data (thr + ser).
(d)	Hydrocarbons	1. 1.6–1.1	no change	75–64	69–54	Widdows et al. (1982)
		2. 1.3	no change	87	71	Livingstone and Feith, unpublished data
(e)	Hydrocarbons and increased temperature combined	1. 1.8 [interaction: data from expt. of (a)2 and (d)2]	2.1	no interaction		Livingstone and Feith, unpublished data
(f)	Reduced salinity	1. 2.1	4.2–12.1	60	19	Calculated from Livingstone et al. (1979)

[a]Range of values represents change with time or intensity of stressors.
[b]Laboratory experiments.

TABLE 4–3. Taurine:Glycine Ratio and the Sum of Threonine and Serine of the Whole Tissues (Less Digestive Gland) of Field Populations of *M. edulis*

Population	Environment	T:G ratio[a]	(thr + ser)[a]
Ronas Voe[b]	clean—oceanic	1.1 ± 0.1	115 ± 13
Mothecombe[b]	clean—estuarine	1.6 ± 0.1	114 ± 7
Mumbles[c]	clean—coastal	1.9 ± 0.03	106 ± 8
Teignmouth[c]	domestic sewage	1.9 ± 0.1	99 ± 2
Minehead[c]	domestic sewage	2.0 ± 0.3	50 ± 3
Lynher[c]	hydrocarbons	2.5 ± 0.2	64 ± 4
Houb of Scatsa	peat bed run-off	2.9 ± 0.5	26 ± 4
Atlantic College[c]	industrial effluent	3.0 ± 0.1	27 ± 2
Swansea Dock[c]	hydrocarbons, metals	3.2 ± 0.4	24 ± 3
Swale[c]	paper mill effluent	3.5 ± 0.3	35 ± 3

After Livingstone and Fieth, unpublished data.
[a] Means ± S.E., $n = 5$, (thr + ser) in μmol g^{-1} dry wt.
[b] Collected October 1977.
[c] Collected August 1977.

Island, Jeffries (1972) described a stress syndrome in the polluted stock in terms of a series of morphological, cytological and biochemical observations. Prominent amongst these were changes in the concentrations of the free amino acids of the gill and mantle tissues: the major components, taurine and glycine, respectively increased and decreased in response to environmental or laboratory stress. Jeffries therefore proposed the tissue molar ratio of taurine to glycine (T:G ratio) as a convenient index of stress, an increase in the ratio being characteristic of a decrease in animal condition (Table 4-1). Increases in the T:G ratio have subsequently been demonstrated for several species of bivalve molluscs, including *M. edulis*, in response to a variety of stressors (Tables 4-1, 4-2 and 4-3). However, the increases have been due mainly to decreases in glycine rather than to changes in taurine (e.g. Bayne et al., 1976c; Roesijadi, 1979; Neff, pers. comm.; Roesijadi and Anderson, 1979), while in the case of low salinity stress taurine also decreases (but less than glycine, so the T:G ratio increases) (Livingstone et al., 1979). Increased taurine concentrations have been observed for *M. edulis* but only in comparisons of field populations (Livingstone and Fieth, unpublished data). A few other organisms have been investigated with variable results: in plaice, *Pleuronectes platessa*, the T:G ratio was higher in oil-exposed fish (Neff, pers. comm.); in the gastropod *Pyrazus ebeninus*, the ratio did not change at low salinity (Lee et al., 1980); in shrimp, *Palaemonetes pugio*, alterations in glycine metabolism occurred in response to PCBs (Roesijadi et al., 1976); and in the polychaete *Neanthes arenaceodentata*, glycine decreased at low salinity and a decrease was indicated at reduced oxygen tension (Abati and Reish, 1972).

Smaller changes in other free amino acids have been reported, but no consistent responses have been discernable (Schafer, 1961, 1963; Abati and Reish, 1972; Jeffries, 1972; Sansone et al., 1978; Neff, pers. comm.; Roesijadi and Anderson, 1979). An exception is the sum of threonine and serine (thr + ser) of the tissues of *M. edulis* which decreased in response to salinity, temperature and hydrocarbons (Table 4-2) and is observed to be reduced in stressed field populations (Table 4-3).

The Taurine:Glycine Ratio as an Index of Stress

In bivalve molluscs, the T:G ratio fulfills the first criterion of an index of stress, namely it responds to a number of natural and man-made environmental stressors. It is therefore a general index of stress, although to date no effect of starvation has been recorded. It also fulfills the second criterion in that elevated values are associated with experimental conditions and field environments that lead to a reduction in animal performance. However, the application of the index in biological effects monitoring is at present limited by the lack of information on the function of taurine and glycine in the stressed animal and on the relationship between the index and more fundamental measurements of animal condition. The situation can be summarised as follows:

1. Role of taurine and glycine. Most of the studies have been empirical and have not investigated the fate of taurine and glycine. Only in the case of salinity stress are their roles known: they (and other components of the free amino acid pool) are used as osmotic effectors in the process of *isosmotic intracellular regulation*, the concentrations being decreased (low salinity adaptation) and increased (high salinity adaptation) in order to regulate cell volume (see Bayne et al., 1976c; Bishop, 1976; Livingstone et al., 1979). The response to salinity is therefore different from that of other stressors and is identifiable by the decrease in taurine (low salinity stress).

The function of taurine and glycine in the responses to other stressors is speculative. Taurine is a primary amine rather than an amino acid, viz. $NH_2(CH_2)_2SO_3H$, and the pathways of its synthesis are similar to those of vertebrate systems (Allen and Garrett, 1971; Finney, 1978). It is present in high concentrations in marine invertebrates but is absent from freshwater and terrestrial species, which suggests that its main function is indeed osmoregulatory (Allen and Garrett, 1971). However, taurine is also a key intermediate of sulphur metabolism, and the other functions that have been suggested for it or its derivatives are (Allen and Garrett, 1971): (1) as a regulator of the transmission of nerve impulses; (2) in the maintenance of ion balance in nerve cells; (3) as a regulatory factor in energy release; (4) as a phosphagen (particularly in marine polychaetes), e.g. phophotaurocyamine; and (5) in the production of polysaccharide sulphates. Of these functions, (5) is perhaps the most likely to be relevant to the stress response because of its general nature and because many functions of bivalves depend upon a copious supply of sulphonated polysaccharides. The turnover of taurine is indicated to be slow relative to that of glycine (Baginski and Pierce, 1975, 1977; Livingstone et al., 1979) and this may be a factor in explaining its lack of change in short-term laboratory exposures in contrast to more elevated concentrations in stressed field populations. Glycine is the simplest amino acid, viz. $CH_2(NH_2)COOH$, and is also present in high concentrations in many marine invertebrates (Awapara, 1962). A role as a readily mobilisable source of energy is possible but, although this has been suggested for the free amino acid pool in general, there is as yet little evidence to support it (De Zwaan, 1977; Felbeck, 1980).

2. Relationship between T:G ratio and animal condition. Simultaneous measurements of the T:G ratio and the energetic condition of bivalves have been made in only a few instances, and the results are variable. The T:G ratio increased and condition index decreased in *M. inquinata* exposed to oil-contaminated sediment (Roesijadi and Anderson, 1979). In temperature-stressed *M. edulis*, the T:G ratio increased with increasing total calorie deficit (calculated as scope for growth) but was low in other stress situations where there was a reduced scope for growth (Bayne et al., 1976c; Widdows et al., 1981b). Establishing a relationship between

the T:G ratio and some more-fundamental measure of animal condition or performance will be important if the application of the index is to be made quantitative. A complicating factor in this will be that taurine and glycine have more than one function in bivalve molluscs. Whereas the changes during low salinity adaptation are rapid and are clearly part of a *primary biochemical response* to the stressor, those that result from other stressors probably occur only after several weeks or longer and most likely represent a *secondary biochemical response*. The sensitivity of the T:G ratio as an index of stress is therefore difficult to assess. An index that reflects a primary biochemical response will be more sensitive than one that reflects a secondary response, but in the case of the changes in T:G ratio it is the significance of these (in terms of animal condition) that is unresolved.

There is some evidence of a "dose-response relationship" for the T:G ratio, the index changing more with increased levels of stress (Bayne et al., 1976c), but the information is limited. Changes in taurine and glycine have been observed to be reversible in field populations (Widdows et al., 1981a) and for experimentally induced salinity stress (Livingstone et al., 1979). As with many aspects of bivalve biochemistry, the concentrations of most of the free amino acids (and consequently the T:G ratio) vary seasonally (Fig. 4-1) (see also Zurburg et al., 1979; Zurburg and De Zwaan, 1981). The pattern of change is regular and will need to be established as a base-line for any population studied. In long-term studies of populations of *M. edulis*, differences in T:G ratio have still been apparent despite the seasonal variability (Table 4-4). Changes in T:G ratio have been observed in several tissues (Table 4-1), and any further question of tissue selection will depend on increased knowledge of the functions of taurine and glycine.

Present studies indicate that the T:G ratio can be applied as an indicator of stress to marine bivalve molluscs in general, although the ranges of values will be different for different species. The applicability of the index to other classes and phyla is questionable. Although the results appear encouraging, major biochemical differences exist between marine organisms, e.g. the total concentration of free amino acids in plaice (*P. platessa*) is only 30 mM compared with 200 mM for oyster (*C. virginica*; Neff, pers. comm.); crustaceans are capable of *extracellular anisosmotic regulation*, whereas bivalves largely are not (Bayne et al., 1976b).

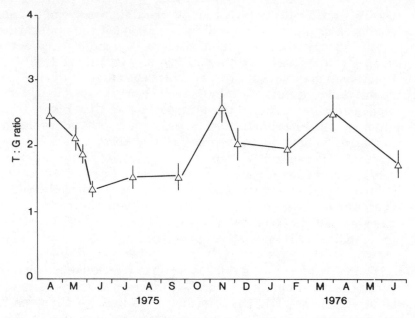

FIG. 4-1. Seasonal variations in the T : G ratio of the whole tissues (less digestive gland) of *M. edulis* (Lynher population). (Livingstone and Fieth, unpublished data.)

However, if the functions of taurine and glycine during the stress response are very general, then it may be that the index will have wide applicability.

Threonine and Serine, and Other Amino Acids, as Indices of Stress

The concentration of threonine plus serine (thr + ser) in the whole tissues of *M. edulis* appears to be a sensitive index of stress. It is more sensitive than the T:G ratio because, when its values are high, it is reduced by levels of stress that have no effect on the T:G ratio, i.e. for increased temperature and hydrocarbons [see Table 4-2, experiments (a)2 and (d)2, respectively]. Also, in the study of field populations, (thr + ser) tended to be either high or very low; only two populations (Lynher, Minehead) showed intermediate values (Table 4-3). This possibly suggests that relatively low levels of stress cause a marked reduction in the concentrations of threonine and serine. A problem arises from the large seasonal

TABLE 4-4. Comparison of the Pooled Data (Recorded over a Number of Years) for the Taurine:Glycine Ratio and the Sum of Threonine and Serine of the Whole Tissues (Less Digestive Gland) of Four Populations of *M. edulis*

Population	Period of time samples collected	T:G[a]	(thr + ser)[a]	Sampling times[b] (%)			
				S	Su	A	W
Ronas Voe	Octover 1977 to May 1980	1.2 ± 0.1 (25)	94 ± 6 (20)	40	0	40	20
Mothecombe	October 1977 to September 1979	1.5 ± 0.1 (37)	89 ± 4 (37)	14	0	57	29
Swansea Dock	August 1977 to June 1979	2.6 ± 0.2 (50)	30 ± 3 (50)	30	30	20	20
Lynher	April 1975 to June 1979	2.7 ± 0.2 (99)	46 ± 3 (88)	34	34	16	16

After Livingstone and Fieth, unpublished data.

[a]Means ± S.E, number of samples in brackets, (thr ± ser) in μmol g^{-1} dry wt.

[b]The samples were collected over a number of years and the sampling times are described in terms of the percentage for each season. S:Spring (March–May); Su:Summer (June–August); A:Autumn (September–November); and W:Winter (December–February).

variation in the concentrations of amino acids (Fig. 4-2) which may make it difficult to use the index at certain times of the year, e.g. see Table 4-2, experiment (a)1. However, as with the T:G ratio, where populations have been studied over a period of time, differences are readily evident despite the seasonal fluctuations (Table 4-4). The functional basis of the index is speculative (except for salinity stress, where the function is the same as for glycine) but a role as an energy supply is a possibility (see Livingstone et al., 1979). As in the case of the T:G ratio, further work is required on matters such as tissue selection and species applicability.

Application of (thr + ser) and the T:G ratio together will strengthen their use in programmes of biological effects monitoring. It is possible to envisage an early change in the former being followed by a change in the latter as environment and animal condition deteriorate. Future studies may identify other components of the free amino acid pool that will be useful in stress monitoring, either as general or specific indices. The composition of the free amino acid pool may well be found to provide not only a "fingerprint" identifying a particular organism (Awapara, 1962), but also a "fingerprint" of its state of health. This concept was approached in the work of Jeffries (1972) in which he also tried to describe changes in the total composition of the free amino acid pool by using ecological diversity indices.

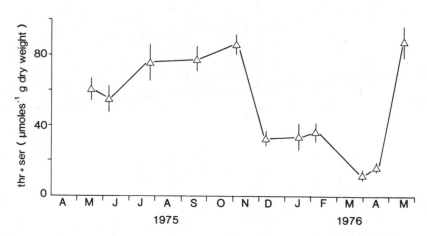

FIG. 4-2. Seasonal variation in the (thr + ser) of the whole tissues (less digestive gland) of *M. edulis* (Lynher population). (Livingstone and Fieth, unpublished data.)

Adenylate Energy Charge

The adenylate system of adenosine triphosphate (ATP), adenosine diphosphate (ADP) amd adenosine monophosphate (AMP) is ubiquitous in living organisms as the system of stoichiometric energy transduction between metabolic sequences. The extent to which such a system may be said to contain potentially available chemical energy is determined by the extent to which its components are not at equilibrium. The adenine nucleotide system contains much chemical energy by virtue of the fact that the ATP/ADP concentration ratio *in vivo* is normally about 10^8 times the value that would exist if ATP were hydrolysed to equilibrium. The *adenylate energy charge* was proposed by Atkinson in the late 1960s (Atkinson and Walton, 1967; Atkinson 1968, 1969) as a means of expressing the energy status of the system; it is given by the relationship

$$\text{Energy charge} = \frac{\text{ATP} + \frac{1}{2}(\text{ADP})}{\text{ATP} + \text{ADP} + \text{AMP}}$$

The energy charge ratio can be calculated from any given set of molar concentrations of ATP, ADP and AMP and has a value in the range of 0 to 1. Atkinson chose to describe the energy status of the adenylate system in terms of mole fractions (this is the stoichiometric parameter corresponding to a concentration ratio) because the interactions of the system with metabolic sequences are stoichiometric, and because mole fractions are linearly related to other properties of chemical interest, e.g. the amount of available energy and the amount of chemical reaction that has occurred. The term $\frac{1}{2}(\text{ADP})$ appears in the numerator because in addition to energy being obtained from both the γ-phosphate bond of ATP (ATP $\rightarrow$ ADP + Pi) and the β-phosphate bond by pyrophosphate cleavage (ATP $\rightarrow$ AMP + PPi), energy can also be obtained from the β-phosphate bond of ADP indirectly through conversion to ATP by the action of the enzyme adenylate kinase (E.C.2.7.4.3) (2 ADP $\rightleftharpoons$ AMP + ATP). Thus two molecules of ADP are equivalent to one of ATP, and the desired effective mole fraction of ATP is the mole fraction of ATP plus half the mole fraction of ADP. In simple terms, the energy charge is therefore a measure to which the ATP-ADP-AMP system is "filled" with high-energy phosphate groups. If all the adenine nucleotide in the cell is ATP, the adenylate system is completely filled and will have an energy charge of 1. At the other extreme, if all the adenine nucleotide is present as AMP, the system is empty of high-energy phosphate groups and has an energy charge of 0. If it is only half-full of high-energy groups, it has an energy charge of 0.5.

In addition to being the energy-coupling system of living systems, ATP, ADP and AMP participate in metabolic regulation through their action as modulators of many key allosteric enzymes. On the basis of such observations and the belief that the universal energy-transducing system (the adenylate system) should serve also as the primary basis of the kinetic correlation of metabolism, Atkinson proposed that energy charge itself should be a major factor in the regulation of pathways that produce and utilise high-energy phosphate groups (for reviews, see Atkinson 1971a, 1971b, 1976, 1977). Experiments in vitro with enzymes from glycolysis and the citrate acid cycle and with the first enzymes in biosynthetic sequences have demonstrated this (Fig. 4-3). Regulatory enzymes from catabolic sequences are maximally active at low values of energy charge, and their activities decrease as the charge nears the value of 1. Regulatory enzymes from biosynthetic sequences show the opposite response; activity is low except at relatively high values of the charge. The metabolic steady state in which ATP production is equal to ATP utilisation is given by the intersection of the two curves, corresponding to an actual energy charge of about 0.85. From these results, obtained in vitro, it appeared that the energy charge in vivo should be strongly stabilised around 0.85, since a decrease in the charge would be counteracted by the resulting increase in the rate of ATP-yielding sequences and decrease in the rate of ATP-consuming sequences, and an increase in charge would lead to the opposite result. This was confirmed by analyses of nucleotide concentrations in vivo and it is now well established that the energy charge values of normally metabolising cells are between 0.75 and 0.95. The ATP-ADP-AMP system thus is poised to run optimally in steady state in which the energy charge is about 0.85 and strongly resists any deviations from it. In case of short-term emergencies, the cell will resist a decrease in energy charge by the removal of AMP through the action of the enzyme adenosine monophosphate deaminase (E.C.3.5.4.6) ($AMP + H_2O = IMP + NH_3$).

Despite the wide application of the energy charge concept, it has been criticised both as an expression of the energy status of cells and as the regulator of the pathways of energy production and utilisation. First Lehninger (1975) mantained that the

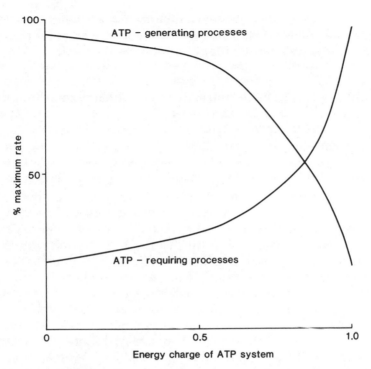

FIG. 4-3. Response of the ATP-generating processes and ATP-utilising reactions to the AEC.

phosphorylation potential—the ratio (ATP)/(ADP)(Pi)—is a more sensitive indicator of the energy status of cells because it includes the concentration of inorganic phosphate, an essential reactant in oxidative and glycolytic phosphorylations. Its value varies from 200 to 800 M^{-1}, depending on metabolic state. Atkinson, however, has pointed out that the phosphorylation potential, unlike energy charge, is not linearly related to the amount of available energy. Second, Purich and Fromm (1972, 1973; see also Atkinson and Fromm, 1977) have demonstrated that the *in vitro* responses of enzymes to energy charge are markedly influenced by other factors including pH, the level of free uncomplexed Mg^{2+}, the total adenylate concentration and the concentration of the other substrates. Fromm concludes that the concept of cellular energy control by energy charge is untenable. Atkinson argues that such objections simply reflect aspects or details of the mechanism yet to be fully understood, and that the case for the ubiquitous regulatory significance of the balance among the concentrations of the adenine nucleotides, which can be most conveniently expressed as the adenylate energy charge, is well established.

Application of Adenylate Energy Charge to Biological Effects Monitoring

The application of adenylate energy charge (AEC) as a biochemical index of sublethal stress has been proposed by Ivanovici (Ivanovici and Wiebe, 1981; Ivanovici, 1980a). They interpret the index in terms of a measure of the metabolic energy that is (potentially) available to the organism at the time of sampling. Three ranges of values of AEC are identified as typical in multicellular organisms and microorganisms in culture (Table 4-5), namely 0.8–0.9 for optimal environmental conditions, 0.7–0.5 for limiting or non-optimal conditions and less that 0.5 for severe conditions. Where examined, organisms with values between 0.7 and 0.5 had slower growth rates and reproduction did not occur; the organisms were viable, however, and on return to normal conditions they resumed all characteristics of their normal, unstressed state. In contrast, if values fell below approximately 0.5, viability was lost, and the organisms did not recover on return to optimal conditions. These findings are summarised in Table 4-6 and represent data from microorganisms (Chapman et al., 1971; Montague and Dawes, 1974; Knowles, 1977, plants (Simmonds and Dumbroff, 1974), invertebrates (Ivanovici, 1977, 1980b; Skjoldal and Bakke, 1978) and vertebrates (Ridge, 1972; Ozawa et al., 1977).

Field measurements of natural communities have demonstrated that although the absolute values of AEC were more variable than those of pure cultures and individual organisms (see Table 4-5), they were lower under less favourable conditions (Table 4-7). For both salt marsh sediments and certain zooplankton, values of AEC were lower in winter than summer. The AEC's of thermophilic blue-green algae decreased with a decrease in temperature from ambient. Only a few studies have been carried out to examine the effects of man-made pollutants on AEC. Ivanovici (1977, 1980b) found that in two molluscan species, lower AEC's correlated with man-made perturbations. In the gastropod *Pyrazus ebeninus*, values were significantly less in animals transferred to mudflats that were contaminated with hydrocarbons (Ivanovici, 1977). This effect occurred within 24 h and was reversible, with normal values of AEC being established on return to a clean site. In the bivalve *Trichomya hirsuta*, lower AEC's were found in individuals that were in the hot water outlet of a power station than individuals from the inlet side (Ivanovici, 1980a). Decreases in AEC were seen in *Corbicula fluminea* with exposure to cadmium (5 μg litre^{-1}) (Giesy et al., 1978) and in the isopod *Cirolana borealis* with exposure to toluene (0.14 mM) (Skjoldal and Bakke, 1978).

Ivanovici and Wiebe (1981) concluded that the adenylate energy charge may be used to detect stress in organisms and to indicate the severity of the stress. Deflections exceeding 0.3-0.4 units from values typical of healthy organisms are considered indicative of critical or non-recoverable stress, while deflections less than this are considered indicative of a recoverable stress. Cited advantages of the technique are as follows (Ivanovici, 1980a):

1. Reduction in AEC was consistent with stressful environmental conditions: an increase in AEC under such conditions has never been demonstrated.
2. Variability between individuals was sufficiently low to require sample sizes of no more than 6 animals to detect significant differences between treatments. Variability levels were not greater in the field than under laboratory conditions.
3. Response times of AEC were fast (minutes to 24 h or less) and more rapid than physiological measurements.
4. The response was found in a wide variety of species.

A number of limitations of the method are recognised as existing at present and are as follows (Ivanovici, 1980a):

1. Methodology. The highly labile nature of ATP in biological samples necessitates careful handling and careful evaluation of each stage of the analyses.
2. Exceptions to the general pattern of values for adenylate energy charge are known. Values of less than 0.8 have been measured in actively growing cells (e.g. Eigener, 1975) and in the different tissues of individual animals, e.g. *M. edulis* (Wijsman, 1976): some organisms remain viable despite AEC's below 0.5 (Ball and Atkinson, 1975), while high AEC's have been measured in moribund organisms under lethal conditions (Chapman and Atkinson, 1973; Ivanovici, unpublished data); in a comparison of the effects of reduced salinity

TABLE 4–5. Adenylate Energy Charges Measured in a Variety of Organisms Exposed to Known Environmental Perturbations

	Adenylate energy charge		Environmental perturbation	Reference
	Optimal condition	Non-optimal condition		
A. MICRO-ORGANISMS				
Escherichia coli	0.83	0.58 (rev.) 0.50 (irrev.)	glucose depletion	Chapman et al. (1971)
Escherichia coli	0.91	0.6	anoxia	Anderson & von Meyenburg (1977)
Peptococcus prevotii	0.82	0.55 (rev.) 0.50 (irrev.)	starvation	Montague & Dawes (1974)
Chromatium	0.85	0.65	dark	Miovic & Gibson (1973)
B. ALGAE AND PLANTS				
Diatom	0.80	0.60	nitrogen limitation	Falkowski (1977)
Tortula ruralis	0.76	0.52	dessication	Bewley & Gwozdz (1975)
		0.36	anoxia, dark	
Soybean plants	0.89	0.63	dark	Ching et al. (1975)
Soybean modules	0.83	0.40	anoxia	Ching (1976)
Acer saccharum	0.80	0.52	anoxia	Simmonds & Dumbroff (1974)
C. INVERTEBRATES				
Zooplankton				
Meganyctiphanes norvegica	0.79	0.69	handling	Skjoldal & Bamstedt (1976)

Euchaeta norvegica	0.74			Skjoldal & Bakke (1978)
Cirolana borealis	0.73	0.23	anoxia	
		0.55 (rev.)		
		0.25 (irrev.)		
		0.30	0.14 mM toluene	
Annelid				
Moniezia expansa	0.71	0.66	hypotonicity	Behm & Bryant (1975)
Molluscs				
Mytilus edulis	0.91	0.67	anoxia	Wijsman (1976)
Trichomya hirsuta	0.89	0.63	anoxia	Ivanovici (1977)
Anadara trapezia	0.35	0.69	hypotonicity	Rainer et al. (1979)
Pyrazus ebeninus	0.88	0.64 (rev.)	hypotonicity at 29°	Ivanovici (1977, 1980b)
		0.53 (irrev.)		
Pyrazus ebeninus	0.82	0.63	hydrocarbon	Ivanovici (1977)
D. VERTEBRATES				
Human sperm	0.88	0.68	heat (50° F)	Chulavatnatol & Haesungcharern (1977)
		0.66	caffeine	
Rat brain	0.81	0.60 (rev.)	anoxia	Ridge (1972)
		0.17 (irrev.)		
Rat liver	0.84	0.52 (rev.)	hemorrhagic shock	Ozawa et al. (1977)
		0.33 (irrev.)		
Fetal mouse heart	0.85	0.48	anoxia	Kaufman et al. (1977)
Goldfish	0.92	0.75	anoxia	Thillart et al. (1976)

From Ivanovici (1980a).

Note: Where data is available, the response of AEC to the environmental perturbation is listed as reversible (if organisms recovered) or irreversible (if organisms did not recover) (rev: reversible; irrev: irreversible).

103

TABLE 4-6. Values of Adenylate Energy Charge, Their Association with Specific Environmental Conditions, and the Characteristics of Organisms under such Environmental Conditions

Adenylate energy charge	Environmental condition	Organisms characterised by
0.80–0.90	non-limiting (no stress)	High growth rates Reproduction Viability
0.50–0.75	limiting (partial stress)	Slow or zero growth rate No reproduction Viability maintained
~0.50	severely limiting (severe stress)	No growth No reproduction Viability lost, even after transfer to non-stress conditions

From Ivanovici (1980a).

TABLE 4-7. Adenylate Energy Charges Measured in Microbial and Natural Communities

Community type	Environmental factor	Adenylate energy charge	Reference
Saltmarsh sediments	summer	0.68	Wiebe & Bancroft (1976)
	winter	0.32	
Thermophilic algae	normal high temperature (39°C)	0.46	
	abnormal decrease in temperature (23°C)	0.19	
Zooplankton	summer	0.76	Skjoldal & Bamstedt (1976)
	winter	0.62	

From Ivanovici and Wiebe (1981).

on three estuarine molluscs, the least change in AEC was recorded in the species least capable of withstanding such conditions (Rainer et al., 1979). Some of these differences may have been due to poor methodology (resulting in loss of ATP), but some may represent specialised situations.

3. The predictive power of AEC measurements is limited because of the lack of detailed information in multicellular organisms on the effects of both short-term and long-term decreases of AEC on biological performance, i.e. growth, reproductive capacity and the viability of offspring.

Because of these limitations, Ivanovici and Wiebe (1981) recommended that the adenylate energy charge be used in conjunction with other sublethal indices of stress. They considered it a *general index of stress*, but one that can be used for the early and rapid detection of stress in polluted environments. They also interpreted it as having potential for the elucidation of the mechanisms of response to stress.

The adenylate energy charge appears to fulfill the two main criteria of an index of sublethal stress—it decreases in response to a deterioration in environment and reduced values are associated (at least in microorganisms) with low growth rates and impaired reproduction. In higher organisms, decreased values were associated with environments that on the basis of experience would be likely to result in impaired biological performance, i.e. hydrocarbons and thermal stressors. The lack of information on the relationship between AEC and measures of biological performance, such as scope for growth, limit its application at present. Without such information, it is difficult to assess over what part of the sublethal range of effects it operates. If an organism will "strongly resist any deviations from an AEC value of 0.85," it may require a considerable stress to affect a new steady-state value less than this.

If the concepts of Atkinson are correct and the instant regulation of the metabolic processes of energy production and utilisation can be viewed in terms of AEC, then the AEC must represent the most *primary* of biochemical responses to environmental change. Change in any environmental parameter should effect at least a transient change in AEC and may or may not result in a new steady-state. AEC would therefore appear to be, theoretically as well as empirically, a *general index of stress*. Initial problems may be encountered in the analyis of samples, but once these have been resolved the enzymatic part of the methodology at least offers the possibility of automation. The question of sensitivity of the index is difficult to assess because of the lack of information on its relationship with biological performance. However, if a long-term effect on properties of ecological consequence (e.g. reproduction) can be demonstrated, and if a new steady-state of AEC can be established within 24 h or less, then AEC would represent one of the most sensitive biochemical indices of stress available at present.

Finally, it may be worthwhile to consider the significance of a reduced steady-state value of AEC in an organism. Such considerations may be useful from the point of view of the assessment of AEC data in the absence of any other biological effects information and in understanding the mechanisms of responses to stressful environments, as suggested by Ivanovici and Wiebe (1981). A low steady-state value of AEC can be considered both in terms of the energy status of the cell and in terms of the regulation of the pathways of energy production and utilisation:

1. Energy status of the cell. A cell with a low AEC will have less energy available in the adenylate system for potential use. However, in the absence of an energy input, the amount of energy in the adenylate system of a healthy cell would be completely utilised in a matter of seconds. AEC, therefore, says nothing about the amount of energy that may be stored in other forms (e.g. phosphagens, such as creatine phosphate and arginine phosphate, and macromolecules, such as glycogen and lipid).

2. Regulation of the pathways of ATP production and utilisation. The AEC also does not reflect the actual absolute rates of the ATP-generating reactions and the ATP-requiring processes. For example, the same decrease in AEC ($0.85 \rightarrow 0.73$) is observed in the catch adductor muscle of the giant scallop *Plactopecten magellanicus* during both swimming and valve closure, although the resulting rates of glycolysis (ATP-producing reactions) differ by more than one order of magnitude, i.e. 1.03 and 0.03 μmol min^{-1} gm^{-1} wet weight, respectively (De Zwaan et al., 1980). A temporary imbalance between energy-producing and energy-requiring reactions presumably may occur during transient changes in AEC. However, if a new steady-state of AEC is established, then the two processes must be balanced. This could be achieved either by the activities of the processes lying along different lines than those depicted in Fig. 4-1, with intersection at values of AEC below 0.85 (see also Ridge, 1972) or by the operation of some other metabolic control signal which would counteract the signal given by a

decrease in AEC—e.g. during aerial exposure the AEC in the tissues of *M. edulis* declines but the glycolytic rate (ATP-production) decreases due to the drop in pH ($7.4 \rightarrow 6.7$) which inhibits the key regulatory enzymes of glycolysis (Wijsman, 1976; De Zwaan, 1977). In either case, the significance of a reduced steady-state AEC is that energy-metabolism will be less tightly regulated and integrated, because the rates of the two processes will change less (the response times will be slower) for a given change in AEC away from the steady-state value (see Fig. 4-1— compare the effect on energy-consuming and energy-requiring processes of changes in AEC of say $0.85 \rightarrow 0.75$ and $0.6 \rightarrow 0.5$). This aspect is reflected in the observation that AEC is often highest in tissues that are energetically active and have to respond quickly to altered situations, e.g. the posterior adductor muscle of *M. edulis* (AEC: 0.91) compared with the mantle (0.88) and hepato-pancreas (0.69) (Wijsman, 1976) and the phasic adductor muscle of *P. magellanicus* (AEC: 0.92) compared with the mantle rim muscle (0.81) and the residue (0.78) (De Zwaan et al., 1980).

Enzyme Activities

Many enzymes from a variety of organisms have been studied in relation to the effects of pollutants. However, with the exception of the mixed-function oxidase system (considered separately below), it would appear from the information to date (Table 4-8) (see also Uthe et al., 1980; Lee et al., 1980) that in marine invertebrates, and probably also in fish, none of the enzymes and their responses are sufficiently well understood to be applicable as sublethal indices of stress. The enzymes of fish have been the most thoroughly studied; however, although a number have been suggested for diagnostic uses, in each case there are problems (see references in Table 4-8 for details), namely brain acetylcholinesterase to detect organophosphorous compounds, δ-aminolevulinate dehydrase to detect lead and other heavy metals, serum aspartate aminotransferase as an indicator of cell destruction and ATPase as a sensitive response to DDT and PCBs. In more recent years, marine invertebrates have been examined, but the diversity of the studies has been such that the information is limited for any one enzyme. Variability of some of the findings (Table 4-8)— although likely to be explainable by tissue differences, time-course of the response, etc—reflects the complex nature of the problems.

TABLE 4-8. Studies of the Responses (Specific Activities) of Enzymes to Pollutants*

Enzymes	Fish
1. Alcohol dehydrogenase (E.C.1.1.1.1)	no change (Cd)
2. α-Glycerophosphate dehydrogenase (E.C.1.1.1.8)	—
3. Lactate dehydrogenase (E.C.1.1.1.27)	no change (PH,Cd)
4. Malate dehydrogenase (E.C.1.1.1.37)	variable[a] (PH,Cd)
5. NADP$^+$-malate dehydrogenase (decarboxylating) (E.C.1.1.1.40)	—
6. NADP$^+$-isocitrate dehydrogenase (E.C.1.1.1.42)	no change (Cd)
7. Xanthine oxidase (E.C.1.2.3.2)	variable (M)
8. Succinate:cytochrome c oxidoreductase (E.C.1.3.9.9.1)	no change (Cd)
9. Glutamate dehydrogenase (E.C.1.4.1.3)	—
10. NADPH:cytochrome c oxidoreductase (E.C.1.6.2.3)	no change (PH)
11. Glutathione reductase (E.C.1.6.4.2)	no change (Cd)
12. Cytochrome oxidase (E.C.1.9.3.1)	no change (PH,Cd)
13. Catalase (E.C.1.11.1.6)	decrease (M)
14. γ-Glutamyl transpeptidase (E.C.2.3.2.2)	—
15. Aspartate aminotransferase (E.C.2.6.1.1)	no change (PH), increase (CH) or variable (M)
16. Alanine aminotransferase (E.C.2.6.1.2)	variable (PH)
17. Hexokinase (E.C.2.7.1.1)	—
18. Phosphofructokinase (E.C.2.7.1.11)	—

*In the majority of the studies, animals were exposed to pollutants in the laboratory (see references for details of species, tissues, exposure levels, exposure times etc.). In a few studies, the changes represent comparisons between different field populations. Key: Cd: cadmium; Pb: lead; Hg: mercury; M: variety of metals; PH: polyaromatic hydrocarbons; CH: chlorinated hydrocarbons; OP: organophosphorous compounds; I: industrial organic effluent.

[a]Variable = both increases and decreases observed.

Crustaceans	Bivalves	Polychaetes	References
—	—	—	27
—	—	no change or increase (I)	1,2
no change (PH) or increase (PH,Cd)	no change (PH) or increase (CH)	no change (I)	1,6,7,8,9,12,15 27
variable (PH,Cd)	variable (PH)	no change or increase (I)	1,2,6,7,8,12,15, 27
—	—	no change (I)	1
—	no change or increase (PH)	no change (I)	1,12,27,26
—	—	—	19
—	—	—	27
—	—	no change (I)	1
no change (PH)	no change (PH)	—	6,15
—	—	—	27
no change (PH)	no change (PH)	—	6,15,27
—	—	—	19
no change and decrease (PH)	—	—	6, 13
no change (PH,M) or increase (PH,M)	no change (PH)	decrease (I)	1,4,6,12,13,14, 15,22,23,24, 27,29
variable (PH)	variable (PH)	no change (I)	1,6,7,8,15,27
—	no change (PH,CH)	no change (I)	1,9,35
—	no change (PH) or increase (PH,CH)	decrease (I)	1,2,3,9,35

(continued)

TABLE 4-8. *(Continued)*

Enzyme	Fish
19. Pyruvate kinase (E.C.2.7.1.40)	—
20. Ribonuclease (E.C.2.7.7.16)	variable (M)
21. Acetylcholinesterase (E.C.3.1.1.7)	no change (PH) or decrease (OP)
22. Alkaline phosphatase (E.C.3.1.3.1)	variable (M) or no change (PH)
23. Acid phosphatase (E.C.3.1.3.2)	no change (PH) or decrease (M)
24. Fructose diphosphatase (E.C.3.1.3.11)	—
25. β-Glucuronidase (E.C.3.2.1.31)	variable (PH)
26. Leucine aminopeptidase (E.C.3.4.1.1)	decrease (PH) or increase (Cd)
27. ATPase (E.C.3.6.1.3)[b]	decrease (CH) or variable (Hg)
28. Phosphoenolcarboxykinase (E.C.4.1.1.32)	—
29. Citrate Synthase (E.C.4.1.3.7)	—
30. Carbonic anhydrase (E.C.4.2.1.1)	increase (Cd)
31. δ-Aminovulinate dehydrase (E.C.4.2.1.24)	decrease (Pb,Hg)
32. Phosphoglucose isomerase (E.C.5.3.1.9)	—

[b] A number of these studies are *in vitro* enzyme studies.

References

1. Blackstock (1978)
2. Blackstock (1980a)
3. Blackstock (1980b)
4. Bell (1968)
5. Caldwell (1974)
6. Chambers et al. (1978)
7. Chambers et al. (1979a)
8. Chambers et al. (1979b)
9. Engel et al. (1972)
10. Gibson et al. (1969)
11. Gould (1979)
12. Gould (1980)
13. Gould & Karolus (1974)
14. Gould et al. (1976)
15. Heitz et al. (1974)
16. Holland et al. (1967)
17. Jackim (1973)
18. Jackim (1974)

Crustaceans	Bivalves	Polychaetes	References
no change (Cd)	no change (PH) or decrease (CH)	decrease (I)	1,2,9,12,35
—	—	—	18,19
no change (PH)	no change (PH)	—	7,8,10,15,16,25, 31,32,33,36
variable (PH)	no change (PH)	—	6,7,8,15,19
no change (PH)	no change (PH)	—	6,15,19
—	decrease (CH)	decrease (I)	1,9
no change or decrease (PH)	no change or increase (PH)	—	6,7,8,15
no change (PH)	no change (PH)	—	6,11,15
decrease (CH)	—	—	5,20,21,26,28, 29,30,36
—	no change and increase (PH)	no change (I)	1,35
—	—	decrease (I)	1
—	—	—	11
—	—	—	17,19
no change and increase (Cd)	—	—	12

19. Jackim et al. (1970)
20. Janicki & Kinter (1971)
21. Kinter et al. (1972)
22. Lane & Scura (1970)
23. MacInnes et al. (1977)
24. McKim et al. (1970)
25. Nicholson (1967)
26. Renfro et al. (1974)
27. Roberts et al. (1979)
28. Schmidt-Nielsen et al. (1977)
29. Thurberg et al. (1977)
30. Tucker (1979)
31. Weiss (1958)
32. Weiss (1959)
33. Weiss (1961)
34. Weiss (1965)
35. Widdows et al. (1982)
36. Yap et al. (1971)

An aspect that has emerged is that structural and other properties of enzymes, as well as the specific activities, can be affected by exposure of the animals to pollutants (Gould et al., 1976; Gould, 1977; Thurberg et al., 1977). Gould has suggested that because of the reduced sensitivity of such enzymes to modulation, there will be a loss of metabolic flexibility in these organisms.

Two aspects are important in considering future studies of enzymes as sublethal indices of stress—the choice of enzyme, and the interpretation of the response. Several rationales have been used to select the enzyme for study:

1.   It is used as a clinical diagnostic test in higher vertebrates (e.g. see Heitz et al., 1974).
2.   It is inhibited *in vitro* by the pollutant or is anticipated to be a target *in vivo*, e.g. ATPases are inhibited by PCBs (Yap et al., 1971; Caldwell, 1974) and cadmium is anticipated to affect metalloenzymes and enzymes requiring similar metal ions for maximal activity (Gould, 1977).
3.   It is known to be important in a particular aspect of metabolism, e.g. fructose diphosphatase and gluconeogenesis (Engel et al., 1972) and aspartate aminotransferase and amino acid turnover (Gould et al., 1976).

The interpretation of the responses, particularly in marine invertebrates, has been largely circumstantial, with a heavy dependence on mammalian biochemistry. In only a few instances have attempts been made to correlate a change in enzyme activity with a change in metabolic function, e.g. ATPase and osmoregulation (Kinter et al., 1972; Caldwell, 1974; Schmidt-Nielsen et al., 1977).

In using marine invertebrates for monitoring studies, it is important to appreciate that their biochemistry differs in many aspects from that of vertebrates and differences also exist between and within the invertebrate phyla: such factors will obviously affect the choice of enzyme and interpretation of the response. The same enzyme may perform a different metabolic function in two organisms, and an index developed for one may not necessarily be applicable to another. For example, pyruvate kinase functions at the branch point of aerobic and anaerobic metabolism in sessile bivalves but not in crustacea (De Zwaan, 1977; Ebberink and De Zwaan, 1980); lactate dehydrogenase is the terminal dehydrogenase in crustacea but is generally replaced by octopine dehydrogenase (E.C.1.5.1.a) in swimming bivalves and cephalopods (Gäde,

1980); glutamate dehydrogenase is a key enzyme in the amino acid metabolism of crustacea (Schoffeniels, 1976), but its function is undefined in bivalves (Zurburg and De Zwaan, 1981). A second important consideration is that many aspects of the metabolism of marine invertebrates, particularly sessile organisms, are seasonally variable (see Livingstone, 1980, 1981). This seasonality is often linked to the reproductive cycle and the storage and utilisation of energy reserves. For example, for some tissues of *M. edulis*, seasonal changes are seen in pyruvate kinase (Livingstone, 1975), cytoplasmic L-malate dehydrogenase (Livingstone, 1976), glycogen synthetase (E.C.2.4.1.11) (Gabbott et al., 1979), glucose-6-phosphate dehydrogenase (E.C.1.1.1.49) (Livingstone, 1981) and hexokinase (Livingstone, 1980). A difference in enzyme activities between two populations may therefore indicate that they are simply at different stages of the reproductive cycle rather than that there is a difference in health.

While knowledge of the biochemistry of the organism is important for interpretation of the response, the interpretation can only be unequivocal if it is demonstrated that the change in enzyme activity results in an altered metabolic function. For example, it can be argued that change in activity of an enzyme catalyzing a near-equilibrium reaction will have little or no effect on the rate of flux through the pathway because it is not the rate-limiting enzyme (see below). Also, if the response is to be used as a sublethal index of stress, this altered metabolic function must be deleterious to the organism, as applies to ATPase and osmoregulation. Weber (1963) suggested two criteria to aid in identifying whether a "statistically significant" enzyme change is a "biologically significant" one: (1) the demonstration of changed metabolic flux, e.g. liver tumours with low activities of fructose diphosphatase and glucose-6-phosphatase (E.C.3.1.3.9) have low rates of gluceoneogenesis (Sweeney et al., 1963), and (2) the enzyme activity falls outside the normal physiological range of values. In marine environmental studies, the latter approach would include the establishing of "baseline" data for the enzyme by examining field populations that are well characterised in terms of other indices of condition.

The development of sublethal indices of stress for a particular organism and enzyme will depend upon the degree to which the considerations that have been discussed are fulfilled. An approach that may have some general application, however, is the measurement of the specific activities of enzymes that represent the maximum potential fluxes through particular metabolic pathways.

TABLE 4–9. Enzymes That Are Indicators of the Maximum Potential
Flux through Metabolic Pathways*

Enzyme	Pathway
1. Phosphorylase (E.C. 2.4.1.1)	Glycogen utilisation
2. Hexokinase	Glucose utilisation
3. Phosphofructokinase	Glycolysis
4. Triglyceride and diglyceride lipases (E. C. 3.1.1.3)	Glyceride utilisation

*See Newsholme and Start (1973).

The theory of using specific enzymes as indicators of metabolic
flux has been discussed by Crabtree and Newsholme (1975) and can
be summarised as follows: Reactions can be divided into readily
reversible (i.e. close to equilibrium) and irreversible (i.e. far
displaced from equilibrium) reactions. For a readily reversible
reaction, the rates of both forward and reverse processes are
greater than the net flux. The enzyme catalyzing the reaction is
not saturated with substrate *in vivo*, with the result that the
measured maximum catalytic activity *in vitro* (where saturating
concentrations of substrate are used) is much greater than the
maximum flux through the pathway. In contrast, the rate of the
reverse process for an irreversible reaction is negligible, so that the
rate of catalysis in the forward direction equals the rate of the
pathway. The enzyme catalyzing an irreversible reaction may be
saturated with substrate *in vivo* so that the maximum activity
measured *in vitro* is similar to the maximum rate of the pathway.
Certain enzymes catalyzing irreversible reactions have therefore
been shown to provide a reasonable assessment of the maximum
flux through particular pathways (Table 4-9). Although these
experiments have largely been carried out on the muscle tissues of
vertebrates and insects, it is likely that where the same enzymes
occur in marine invertebrates, they will be rate-limiting (see
Zammit and Newsholme, 1976; De Zwaan, 1977; De Zwaan et al.,
1980). In the case of *M. edulis*, pyruvate kinase can be similarly
considered because it has been shown to be the rate-limiting step
of the anaerobic pathway during the later stages of anaerobiosis
(Ebberink and De Zwaan, 1980). Phosphofructokinase would
appear to offer potential for future study because differences have
been observed in *M. edulis* exposed to polyaromatic hydrocarbons
(Widdows et al., 1982), in field populations of *M. edulis* (Living-

stone, unpublished data) and in field populations of the polychaete *Glycera alba* (Blackstock, 1978, 1980a, 1980b). The advantage of choosing such enzymes for study is that where a change in enzyme activity is considered significant, it can at least be interpreted in terms of an altered potential flux of the pathway.

To summarise, the study of enzymes offers potential for the development of both general and specific sublethal indices of stress, but more research is required before a practicable index is likely. A certain amount is known about a large number of enzymes, but more detailed studies of individual enzymes are now required. It may be that, in environmental monitoring programmes, a few such indices could be used routinely with a larger number being available where a detailed analysis of a population is required.

SPECIFIC INDICATORS OF STRESS

Mixed-Function Oxidase Systems

The ability of organisms to tolerate the stress effects of chemical pollutants may depend on the availability of a variety of protection mechanisms (e.g. see Slater, 1979). Many such foreign chemicals (xenobiotics) are hydrophobic and lipid soluble and are therefore readily removed from potential sites of toxic action by partitioning into lipid pools (Allen et al., 1974, 1976; Whittle et el., 1977). The apolar pollutants such as hydrocarbons may then be transported with blood lipids to the liver or equivalent organ where they are sequestered into lipid vacuoles (Allen et al., 1974, 1975). Metabolic conversion of the organic pollutants will depend upon the presence of a number of enzymes or enzyme systems that generally function to convert the chemicals into more polar metabolites which are easily excreted. A large literature exists on hepatic drug and steroid metabolism in mammals (Conney, 1967; Schenkman and Kupfer, 1982), and the detoxification pathways available to invertebrates have been reviewed by Khan et al. (1974).

The first enzyme of polycylic hydrocarbon metabolism is *aryl hydrocarbon mono-oxygenase* [reaction(1)], which introduces a single oxygen atom into its substrates to produce epoxides (De Pierre and Ernster, 1978) (R = remainder of the ring system):

$$(1)$$

The epoxide (arene oxide) can rearrange non-enzymatically to hydroxy compounds (phenols) [reaction(2)] or can be further metabolised by two main pathways [see below, reactions (3) and (4)]:

$$(2)$$

Before the existence of the epoxide intermediate was realised, the name *aryl hydrocarbon hydroxylase* was used to describe the relevant enzyme system. Mono-oxygenases use molecular oxygen, and a third substrate is therefore required to donate electrons for the reduction of the second oxygen atom to water. Hence the mono-oxygenases are also called *mixed-function oxygenases*. The general equation of such reactions is:

$$RH + XH_2 + O_2 \rightarrow ROH + H_2O + X$$

where RH is the substrate undergoing hydroxylation and XH_2 is the electron donor.

In mammalian tissues the enzyme system reponsible for the aryl hydrocarbon mono-oxygenase activity is the microsomal *mixed-function oxidase system* (MFO) (De Pierre and Ernster, 1978). The MFO system is a membrane-bound non-phosphorylating electron-transport complex that is usually part of the endoplasmic reticulum. It participates in a wide variety of reactions, including desaturation and hydroxylation reactions, and it will metabolise both xenobiotic (drugs, pesticides, hydrocarbons) and endogenous (steroids, fatty acids) substrates. The MFO system contains at least two protein components: an iron-containing haem protein called *cytochrome P-450* (actually a family of different cytochromes—the name derives from its carbon monoxide difference spectrum maximum observed at approximately 450 nm; see Hodgson, 1976 for a review of its role in comparative toxicology) and a flavoprotein called NADPH-cytochrome P-450 reductase (also called NADPH-cytochrome *c* reductase). The reaction mechanisms of the system are not completely clear even in mammalian systems, but some aspects appear to be common among

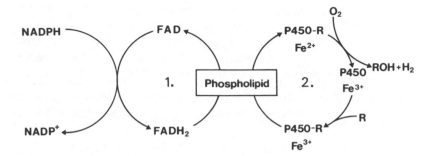

FIG. 4-4. Diagram representing the electron transport nature of the mixed function oxidase system. 1: NADPH-cytochrome P-450 reductase, 2: cytochrome P-450, R: organic substrate, ROH: hydroxylated product.

various species. The electron-donor for the hydroxylation reactions is NADPH (reduced nicotinamide adenine dinucleotide phosphate). Electrons are transferred to the flavoprotein, reducing it completely (see Fig. 4-4). The substrate combines with the oxidised form of cytochrome P-450 [i.e. Fe(iii)] which is then reduced by electrons from the reduced flavoprotein to the Fe(ii) form. Finally, the reduced Fe(ii) form of P-450 reacts with molecular oxygen in such a way that one of the oxygen atoms is reduced to water and the other is introduced into the substrate. The pathway is available to a variety of substrates, facilitating a variety of reaction types (Hodgson, 1976).

The intermediate arene oxides, in addition to spontaneously rearranging to phenols [reaction (2)], can be further metabolised to trans-dihydrodiols by the action of epoxide hydrases [reaction (3)] or converted to glutathione conjugates [reaction (4)], either by the action of particular *glutathione S-transferases* or spontaneously; conjugation with amino acids is also possible (DePierre and Ernster, 1978; Hutson, 1976; Jakoby, 1978):

$$R\text{-arene oxide} + H_2O \longrightarrow R\text{-diol (OH, OH)} \longrightarrow \text{further metabolism} \quad (3)$$

$$R\text{-arene oxide} + GSH \longrightarrow R\text{-(OH, SG)} \longrightarrow \text{further metabolism} \quad (4)$$

where GSH = glutathione (i.e. L-γ-glutamyl-L-cysteinylglycine). Further metabolism of these products is possible. The dihydrodiols may be acted on again by the aryl hydrocarbon mono-oxygenase [reaction (5)] or conjugated with glucuronic acid and sulphate, and the glutathione conjugates may be converted to mercapturic acids (see DePierre and Ernster, 1978):

(5)

By these series of reactions, hydrophobic and lipid-soluble xenobiotics such as hydrocarbons are converted to hydrophilic, non-toxic and readily excretable compounds. A feature of the detoxication system, however, is that in the course of the metabolic transformations, reactive electrophilic intermediates may be formed which are often more toxic, carcinogenic or mutagenic then the original substrates (Jerina and Daly, 1974; Yang et al., 1977; Kinoshita and Gelboin, 1978). Oxidised intermediates of aromatic hydrocarbons, such as the benzo(a)pyrene diolepoxides [formed by reaction (5)], have been demonstrated to bind to DNA and to be strongly mutagenic (see Osborne, 1979). MFO must therefore be viewed as a component of a detoxication/toxication system, the value of which rests on the balance between bioactivation [reactions (1) and (5)] and further conjugation and excretion mechanisms [reactions (3), (4) and further metabolism].

High levels of MFO have been shown to confer resistance to certain drugs and pesticides in both mammals and insects (Conney, 1967; Fukami et al., 1969; Schonbrod et al., 1965). Higher MFO levels can be induced in these animals as a result of exposure to drugs and environmental contaminants. Fish have an inducible MFO system (Payne and Penrose, 1975; Bend et al., 1976; Burnss, 1976a; Pederson et al., 1976; Stegeman and Sabo, 1976; Kurelec et al., 1977; Payne, 1977; Addison et al., 1978; Elcombe and Lech, 1978; Stegeman, 1978; Walton et al., 1978; Payne and May, 1979), but it is uncertain whether induction represents a synthesis of more or different forms of P-450 or represents a faster rate of substrate turnover. In marine species as in mammals, recent evidence has demonstrated the presence of multiple forms of P-450 with different spectral characteristics (Bend et al., 1977a;

Elmamlouk et al., 1977). Insects appear to exhibit elevated levels as a result of genetic selection of populations (Khan, 1970; Khan et al., 1970; Plapp et al., 1976), and the same has recently been suggested for the polychaete *Capitella capitata* (Lee and Singer, 1980). A number of marine invertebrates, particularly crustaceans and polychaetes, possess MFO activity (Burns 1976b; Bend et al., 1977a; Payne, 1977; Singer and Lee, 1977; James et al., 1979; Lee and Singer, 1980; Lee et al., 1977; Payne and May, 1979) but examples of inducible activity are few (Lee and Singer, 1980; Walters et al., 1979; Lee et al., 1981); other studies have failed to demonstrate induction (Burns, 1976b; Payne, 1977; Payne and May, 1979). It has been argued that bivalve molluscs do not have the capability to metabolise organic xenobiotics (Carlson, 1972; Lee et al., 1972a; Payne, 1977; Vandermeulen and Penrose, 1978; Payne and May, 1979). However, recent studies have shown that the complete MFO detoxication system is present in bivalves in activities comparable to other marine invertebrates (Ade et al., 1982; Livingstone and Farrar, 1984). Benzo(a)pyrene hydroxylase has been reported in *M. edulis* (Stegeman, 1980, 1981a, 1981b; Mix et al., 1981) and *Crassostrea virginica* (Anderson, 1978a. 1978b), and the epoxidation of aldrin to dieldrin by MFO has been reported in *Anodonta* sp. (Khan et al., 1972b), *M. californianus* (Gee et al., 1979; Krieger et al., 1979) and *M. edulis* (Bayne et al.,1979; Moore et al., 1980). Other enzyme activities have also been demonstrated, namely epoxide hydrase (*M. edulis*: Bend et al., 1977a); O-demethylation of *p*-nitroanisole (*M. californianus*: Trautman et al., 1979) and hydroxylation of antipyrine (*M. californianus*: Krieger et al., 1979).*

The ability to oxidise xenobiotics appears to be widespread among marine animals, but the rates of conversion clearly are very different. Some fish show levels of P-450 and MFO activity approaching that of mammals, while crustaceans and some other marine invertebrates have shown high P-450 levels but MFO activity orders of magnitude lower than fish (e.g. James et al., 1979). Levels of conjugating enzymes such as the glutathione S-transferase appear high in most species examined (e.g. Bend et al., 1977a) but inducibility appears to be less marked (or absent) than for MFO (DePierre and Ernster, 1978). Environmental contaminants that are inducers (or depressors) of MFO activity will

---

*For a review of the distribution and properties of mixed-genases in marine invertebrates, see Lee (1981).

therefore alter the balance between the production of toxic inter-mediates and their conjugated products, and in vastly different manners in different species. Individual species also show different metabolic capacities for various toxicants, suggesting that several different substrates should be used when assaying MFO activity.

Comparative studies of the MFO systems aid in the understanding of animals that can effectively clear their body tissues of contaminants as against others which store high concen-trations of chemicals that can be activated to possible carcinogens (bioconcentration phenomenon). Such studies should be useful in understanding the distribution of tumours and other histopatho-logical conditions in relation to polluted environments. Because the MFO system also metabolises endogenous compounds such as steroid hormones, elevated levels of MFO can have other conse-quences. Induction of MFO by environmental contaminants has been shown to alter plasma levels of steroids in fish (Sivarajah et al., 1978). Hormonal imbalance may account for observations, such as that by Krebs (1973), that fiddler crabs exposed to fuel oil after an accidental spill displayed mating behaviour and colours in-appropriate for the time of the year. Singer and Lee (1977) showed that high MFO activity in blue crabs was tied to moulting and reproductive cycles. Steroids such as cholecalciferol (Vitamin D_3) are also MFO substrates, and changes in these would be expected to affect calcium metabolism in an animal (Villereale et al., 1974).

MFO as a Specific Index of Sublethal Stress

The MFO enzymes are part of a metabolic system that, for some animals at least, can be used as an adaptive mechanism for tolerating chemical pollution. *In vivo* studies show that rates of detoxication in certain fish are high enough to be functional as a mechanism for clearing body tissues of some xenobiotics. By contrast, rates in invertebrates generally seem too low to make a significant impact on pollutant body burdens, e.g. fiddler crab, *Uca pugnax* (Burns, 1976b). However, in the case of both groups of animals, the use of elevated MFO activity as an index of the presence and possible effects of organic pollution has been suggested.

Most research has been carried out on fish, and a number of workers have recognised the potential of MFO activity measurements for the detection of hydrocarbon pollution and the assessment of the area and duration of biological impact (Payne and Penrose, 1975; Payne, 1976; Kurelec et al., 1977; Penrose, 1978). A role in the detection of biological change has also been emphasised (Stegeman, 1980). In some instances, species of fish suitable as monitor organisms (i.e. territorial, ubiquitous and easy to catch) have been proposed such as the cunner, *Tautogolabrus adspersus* (Penrose, 1978), and species of the family Blenniideae (Kurelec et al., 1977); factors pertinent to such a use (sex, nutritional state, response time, etc.) have been investigated (Walton et al., 1978; Stegeman, 1980). In contrast, the studies on marine invertebrates are limited, and although a sessile, ubiquitous invertebrate would be an ideal indicator animal (see Stegeman, 1980), no particular species has yet seemed suitable. Possible exceptions to this are the bivalve molluscs. The capacity of these organisms to accumulate hydrocarbons and polychlorinated biphenyls from solution in seawater and in the particulate phase is now well documented (Lee et al., 1972a; Stegeman and Teal, 1973; Farrington and Quinn, 1973; Stegeman, 1974; DiSalvo et al., 1975; Fong, 1976; Neff et al., 1976; Boehm and Quinn, 1976; Langston, 1978; Fossato et al., 1979). Although there is no definitive evidence of induction of MFO activity in bivalves, there is, however, evidence of the induction of components of the system—namely NADPH-neotetrazolium reductase and the NADPH-producing enzymes—and the possible use of such observations as specific indices of stress has been suggested (Moore et al., 1980). Induction of the cytochromes b_5 and P-450 has also been observed in *M. galloprovincialis* (Guillaume et al., 1984).

In a recent assessment of the potential and the problems of using MFO measurements, the following points were made (see Lee et al., 1980): (1) Induction of MFO seems to be a response that is limited to particular types of compounds including aromatic hydrocarbons and some halogenated biphenyl isomers. (2) Interactive effects of other pollutant types could possibly severely limit the MFO response. For example, certain pollutants can result in the destruction of P-450 (Glende, 1972), and it has been suggested (Stegeman, 1980) that such a process could have been responsible for the lowered MFO activity observed by Ahokas et al. (1976a) in fish from a polluted environment. Similarly, a number of studies have shown that Cd and Hg inactivate the P-450 system (Johnston et al., 1974; Pani et al., 1976; Yoshida et al., 1976). A lack of an evident MFO response should therefore be assessed carefully. (3) The response to inducers can be rapid in fish, occurring within 24 hours, but slower for lower doses of pollutants and possibly slower still for invertebrates. There is reason to believe that the response following a single exposure might persist for days to weeks, and that chronic low-level exposure might yield a sustained response. (4) Seasonal and sex-linked differences could contribute to a high variance in a field sample and mask low-level induction. Similarly, low temperature can diminish the induction response. (5) Technical training to perform MFO assays is not great and costs are quite low. However, interpretation will require a thorough familiarity with cytochrome P-450 systems generally and with the details of the particular species in question.

The induction of MFO activity fulfills the first criterion of an index of sublethal stress in that it is a response to change in an environmental factor, in this case hydrocarbon or other organic pollution. This has been demonstrated both in the laboratory and in the field (e.g. Kurelec et al., 1977). It is a *primary biochemical response* that is specific to this environmental stressor. Although at present the specificity is limited to a large group of compounds, the possibility exists that with a more complete characterisation of the many components of the MFO system, the specificity can be made more selective. For example, it may be that different cytochromes are induced by different molecular types; similarly, the use of different substrates in the *in vitro* assay may aid selectivity.*

MFO is a sensitive index both in terms of response time and pollutant levels. For example, Payne and Penrose (1975) recorded a 4-fold increase in MFO activity towards benzopyrene with the exposure of capelin and brown trout to about 1 ppm of petroleum. Moore et al. (1980) recorded increases in NADPH-neotetrazolium reductase with the exposure of *M. edulis* to 8–68 μg litre^{-1} concentrations of the water-accommodated fraction of North Sea crude oil. These levels of hydrocarbons are similar to those encountered in the field (Table 4-10; also see footnote to Table 4-10). Problems may arise in the application of the index in the form of assay difficulties and the previously mentioned background interference from seasonal variation and sex differences. Dose-response information is also limited. However, many of these problems should be resolved for a particular species by preliminary and

---

*It has been stated that in capelin and rainbow trout, benzopyrene MFO activity is induced by oil but not by polychlorinated biphenyls (Penrose, 1978); however, Elcombe and Lech (1978) observed a 10-fold increase in this activity in the rainbow trout *Salmo gairdneri* following injection of commercial polychlorinated biphenyl mixtures.

TABLE 4-10. Hydrocarbon Concentrations Determined in Subsurface (1 m to 5 m) Water Samples During Field Studies

Concentration μg litre^{-1}	Location, study, duration	Analytical procedure[a]	Reference
1. 1.6–9.3	Bedford Basin, Nova Scotia, Canada	fluorescence	Keizer et al. (1977)
2. 2–13.5	North Sea, Ekofisk oil spill, 2–6 days after spill	fluorescence	Mackie et al. (1978)
0.55–7.80	"	GLC[b]	"
3. 2.8–44.5	Brittany, France, Amoco Cadiz oil spill, 7–8 days after spill	fluorescence	Mackie et al. (1978)
0.69–6.34	"	GLC	"
4. 0.8–200	Amoco Cadiz spill, 22–93 days after spill	fluorescence	Law (1978)
5. 19–560	Eastern England (North Sea), Eleni V. oil spill, 12–351 days after spill	fluorescence	Blackman & Law (1980)

[a] Differences in the type of compound detected and in the standardisation procedures may result in differences of two-fold in the concentrations determined by fluorescence and GLC techniques.
[b] GLC: gas liquid chromatography (aromatics and alkanes).

baseline studies. In some instances, immediate application of the index has been recommended (see Penrose, 1978, and Walton et al., 1978; also Kurelec et al., 1977, and Kurelec et al., 1979).

The second criterion for a biochemical response to be acceptable as an index of biological effect is that it must lead to or be associated with decreased animal performance. Two possibilities exist for MFO, namely the presence of the xenobiotic may (1) result in decreased animal performance (e.g. a reduction in scope for growth) but by mechanisms not associated with MFO activities or (2) cause a decline in cellular condition through the biotransformation of the xenobiotic by the induced MFO system to compounds that are mutagenic and carcinogenic. Neoplasms have been observed in M. edulis from a polluted environment (Lowe and Moore, 1978) and in other marine organisms (Farley and Sparks,

1970). The formation and sources of mutagenic compounds are now topics of some interest, and although petroleum hydrocarbons do contain small amounts of such compounds, a number of workers believe that they are unimportant as a source of mutagenic activity in the marine environment (King, 1977; Payne et al., 1979). More likely sources are suggested to be sewage, industrial waste and the products of petrol combustion (Payne et al., 1978; Payne et al., 1982). A correlation between induced MFO activities and increased mutagenicity has recently been observed in *Mugil cephalus* taken offshore from an industrial environment (Kurelec et al., 1979). The decision as to which of possibilities (1) or (2) may have occurred would be made on the basis of a consideration of the particular physiological, cytological and biochemical studies.

NADPH-producing Enzymes

The electron-donor for the hydroxylation reactions catalyzed by the MFO system is NADPH. The major enzymes thought to be responsible for the formation of NADPH for the MFO system are glucose-6-phosphate dehydrogenase (G6PDH) (E.C.1.1.149), phosphogluconate dehydrogenase (decarboxylating) (E.C.1.1.1.44), malic enzyme (E.C.1.1.1.38) and NADP-dependent isocitrate dehydrogenase (E.C.1.1.1.42). It is well established for mammalian tissues that treatment with compounds such as phenobarbital, which will result in an increase in MFO activity, will also lead to an increase in G6PDH activity and in the activities of other NADPH-producing enzymes (Altman, 1972). The results are less definitive for the effects of polycyclic hydrocarbons, with both increases (Koudstaal and Hardonk, 1972) and no change (Bresnick and Yang, 1964) in G6PDH activity being recorded. However, such differences may have arisen because the different techniques used by different workers either measure cytosolic or microsomal G6PDH activities or both; it is now thought that in vertebrates the two enzymes are genetically distinct with different properties and different functions, the cytosolic isoenzyme having a major role in the pentose phosphate pathway and the microsomal isoenzyme being important in MFO reactions (Kimura et al., 1979; Stegeman and Klotz, 1979). The latter enzyme is identical with the enzyme formerly known as glucose dehydrogenase (E.C.1.1.1. 47) and has now been retermed hexose-6-phosphate dehydrogenase (Hori and Takahashi, 1974). The possibility therefore exists that, if the same systems operate in the tissues of marine organisms, G6PDH and other NADPH-producing enzymes may be responsive to the presence of organic xenobiotics and therefore offer potential as a specific index of sublethal stress.

Studies of *M. edulis* indicate that changes in G6PDH occur in response to aromatic hydrocarbons. However, the responses were variable and different from the mammalian system (Moore et al., 1980; Livingstone, unpublished data). The main observations were: (1) Specific activity (S.A.: activity per mg protein) in the blood cells increased with exposure of mussels to water-accommodated fraction of North Sea crude oil (WAF) and following injection of 2,3-dimethylnaphthalene but not with exposure of mussels to increased temperature. (2) The number of blood cells increased greatly (activity of G6PDH per ml increased up to ×6) but in response to both WAF and temperature. (3) The digestive gland contains cytosolic and microsomal G6PDH which increased in S.A. (activity per fresh weight) following injection of 2,3-dimethyl-naphthalene; the combined fractions ("post-40,000 g supernatant") did not increase with the exposure of mussels to WAF. (4) The digestive gland cytosolic and microsomal enzymes have similar properties (substrate specificity, electrophoretic mobility) which are intermediate between those of the mammalian isoenzymes. The blood cells of *M. edulis* in particular appear to offer potential for future study. In addition to being important in MFO reactions they may be involved in other detoxication reactions which are critically dependent on NADPH, e.g. reactions involving reduced glutathione (Meister, 1975). Future studies of these and other tissues will need to examine the seasonal variability of G6PDH (Livingstone, 1981) and its functional relationship with the detox-ication system. The latter will have a bearing on the second criterion of an index of sublethal stress, i.e. that the change in the biochemical process causes or is associated with decreased animal performance.

Metallothioneins

Many marine organisms have a large capacity for trace metal ac-cumulation, the consequences of which may be deleterious to the organism (for a review of the uptake, fate and effects of trace metals in marine organisms, see Moore, 1981). However, as in other organisms, potentially toxic trace metals can be detoxified intracellularly by partitioning into lysosomes (Moore, 1980) or by binding to the protein metallothionein.

Upon entering the cell many metal ions are bound by metallothioneins. The metallothioneins are a group of specific non-enzyme proteins that are increasingly being demonstrated to play a central role in metal metabolism. They were first discovered by Margoshes and Vallee (1957) and are now recognised as low molecular weight proteins [approximately 10,000 daltons (gel filtration studies: Kägi and Vallee, 1960, 1961); 6,000 to 7,000 daltons (amino acid composition: see Kojima and Kägi, 1978)] of unusual structure. Cysteine constitutes one-third of the amino acids, and there are approximately 24 cysteine residues per metallothionein molecule (Bremner and Davies, 1975; Winge et al., 1975). Each three cysteine residues bind 1 metal ion with a resultant 8 metal ions bound to each metallothionein molecule; metallothionein appears always to occur in the saturated state (Kägi and Vallee, 1960, 1961; Pulido et al., 1966; Bremner and Davies, 1975). Aromatic amino acids are absent or low, and sequencing studies indicate the preservation of the metal-binding residues in different species (Kojima and Kägi, 1978).

Metallothionein is apparently ubiquitous, having been described in mammals (Margoshes and Vallee, 1957), fish (Olafson and Thompson, 1974), bivalves (Noël-Lambert, 1976; Talbot and Magee, 1978; George et al., 1979), zooplankton (Brown and Parsons, 1978) and phytoplankton (Maclean et al., 1972). Metallothionein may exist to some level in most or all animal tissues since it has been found to occur in liver, kidney, gills, testes, intestine, muscle, plasma, erythrocytes, tissue cultured skin epithelial cells and urine (Jakubowski et al., 1970; Nordberg, 1972; Nordberg and Piscator, 1972; Bouquegneau et al., 1975; Rugstad and Norseth, 1975; Sugawara and Sugawara, 1975). In mammals and fish, metallothionein appears to be concentrated in liver and kidney tissue (Jakubowski et al., 1970; Nordberg, 1972), while in fish (Bouquegneau et al., 1975) and bivalves (Roesijadi, 1979) high levels of metallothionein are also found in gill tissue. Metallothionein is described as a cytoplasmic protein (e.g. Winge et al., 1975), although there is some evidence that an insoluble protein polymer of metallothionein-amino acid composition is found within lysosomes (Porter, 1974); this is consistent with the known partitioning of metals into lysosomes (Moore, 1977) and the apparent marked resistance of metallothionein to degradation by proteolytic enzymes (Webb, 1972).

Natural tissue levels of metallothionein can be greatly increased (up to 40 times: Piscator, 1964; Piotrowski et al., 1973) by exposure of the organisms to various trace metals, namely mercury, cadmium, copper, zinc, silver, and tin (Winge et al., 1975; Sabbioni and Marafante, 1975). The induction of metallothionein may occur at the translational level (increased synthesis of protein from a given mRNA) for low metal exposures, or at the transcriptional level (increased synthesis of mRNA) for higher metal exposures (Webb, 1972; Squibb and Cousins, 1974). The metallothionein binds the metal ions, so preventing them from exerting toxic effects through binding to enzymes or other sensitive sites (Goldman, 1970; Brown et al., 1977; Brown and Parsons, 1978; see also Moore, 1981). If, however, the rate of influx of metals into the cell exceeds the rate at which metallothionein can be synthesised, there may be a "spillover" of metals from metallothionein into the enzyme pool (Brown et al., 1977; Brown and Parsons, 1978; Engel and Fowler, 1979; Pruell and Engelhart, 1980; Roesijadi, 1979). Toxic effects can then be due to the displacement of essential metals from metalloenzymes* by non-essential metals (Friedberg, 1974). This displacement can change the conformational shape of the enzyme so that the substrate molecules no longer fit the binding sites in the enzymes, resulting in the loss of enzyme activity (Friedberg, 1974).

The metal composition in the naturally occurring metallothionein is variable and depends on the tissue of origin; e.g. Zn is the principal constituent in metallothionein from liver. This composition can change and will reflect the metals to which an organism has been exposed. It appears that increased tolerance to trace metals may be mediated by the production of metallothionein with a portion of binding sites occupied by a relatively nontoxic and readily displaceable metal. Leber (1974) found that rats, pre-injected with Cd, synthesised metallothionein with Zn in approximately half of its binding sites. If a further dose of Cd was administered, then the Cd displaced Zn from the metallothionein. Similarly, pretreatment with Zn increased tolerance to subsequent

---

*Metalloenzymes are enzymes that require specific metal ions to be catalytically active. In such enzymes the metal ion may serve as (1) the primary catalytic centre; (2) a bridging group, to bind substrate and enzyme together; or (3) an agent stabilising the conformation of the enzyme in its catalytically active form.

exposure to cadmium since Cd could then displace Zn from Zn-containing metallothionein. This suggests that the increased tolerance in both cases results from the presence of high levels of Zn in metallothionein binding sites with subsequent displacement of Zn from metallothionein by Cd. Free cytoplasmic Zn is much less toxic than Cd as it is a natural component of over 70 metalloenzymes (Riordan, 1977). Similarly, exposure to Ag, Cu or Hg results in the synthesis of metallothionein containing approximately equimolar levels of Zn and the exposure metal (Winge et al., 1975). Therefore, it would appear that exposure to any one of Cd, Hg, Ag, Cu or Zn should result in increased tolerance to any of the other metals upon subsequent exposure. However, it is also important to realise that sometimes large concentration differences are required before one metal will displace another, due to the greater affinity of metallothionein for the original metal. Such concentration differences may not be environmentally realistic.

As discussed previously, the toxic effects of trace metals usually occur only when the binding capacity of the metallothionein has been exceeded and there is a resultant interaction of the toxic trace metals with the enzyme pool. However, in addition to this, high levels of toxic trace metals may occur in the enzyme pool before metallothionein becomes saturated if there is a deficiency of an essential trace metal in the enzyme pool. For example, it has been demonstrated by Brown and Chatel (1978), for duck liver and kidney tissues, that when the enzyme pool was replete with Zn, over 75% of cytoplasmic Cd was bound to metallothionein. However, when the enzyme pool was apparently Zn deficient, only 25% of the Cd was bound to metallothionein with 75% occurring in the enzyme pool. This increase of the portion of cytoplasmic Cd in the enzyme pool of Zn-deficient ducks was attributed to an increased ability of Cd to compete for binding sites in the enzyme pool. Conversely, if the enzyme pool was Zn-replete, then Cd would be out-competed for the enzyme binding sites. In the latter situation, the Cd would be more likely to bind to mRNA coded for metallothionein, resulting in translational induction of metallothionein (Webb, 1972).

In the light of the types of metal interactions described above, it is becoming apparent that a proper understanding of metal metabolism will be possible only when several metals have been examined simultaneously in any given study. Furthermore, understanding of the interactions of metals with metallothionein will be clear only if the relative levels of competing metals in the

metalloenzyme pool are examined. Zn appears to play a particularly important role in toxic metal metabolism and should always
be considered.

Metallothionein as a Specific Index of Sublethal Stress

The role of metallothionein in detoxifying metals has been identified as a promising area for the development of a stress index
specific for metals as a pollutant (Bayne et al., 1980b; Lee et al.,
1980). The types of information that such a study might provide
are discussed later. There are a few examples of the application of
metallothionein studies in the field, but a relationship between
metallothionein and pollution has been demonstrated for mussels.
For example, in M. edulis, Brown et al. (1977) found that the ratio
of total metal (Cd, Cu and Zn) in the metallothionein pool to total
metal in the enzyme-containing pool increased with increased
levels of pollution; similarly, Brown (1978; also see Bayne et al.,
1980b) demonstrated that the levels of metallothionein bound Cd,
Cu and Zn increased with exposure to increasing levels of metals
in the vicinity of a sewer outfall, and that at the site of highest
exposure (the mussel population here was sparse) there was a
dramatic increase in the amount of Cd, Cu and Zn in the enzyme-
containing pool. Viarengo et al. (1982) found that the level of
metallothionein-like Cu-binding protein was three times higher in
the digestive gland of M. galloprovincialis from a polluted environment than in the tissue of those from a clean environment; also, the
rates of protein and RNA synthesis and amino acid uptake were
reduced in the animals from the polluted environment. Induction
of metallothionein in the tissues of mussels has also been indicated
in laboratory studies, namely for M. edulis in response to Cd (whole
tissues: Nöel-Lambert, 1976; digestive diverticula: George et al.,
1979) and to a mixture of Cd, Cu and Zn (whole tissues: Brown,
1978), and for M. galloprovincialis in response to Cu (gills:
Viarengo et al., 1980; mantle and hepatopancreas: Viarengo et al.,
1979). These studies indicate that several Cd-binding proteins
exist in M. edulis and can be isolated as monomers [molecular
weight of between 10,000 (Nöel-Lambert, 1976) and 13,000 (Talbot
and Magee, 1978)] or dimers [molecular weight of 25,000 ± 5,000
(George et al., 1979)]. The most complete analysis to date of these
proteins indicates that they have many properties in common with
mammalian metallothionein (George et al., 1979).

From the studies described above it is clear that metallo-thionein fulfills the first criterion of an index of sublethal stress, namely that the changes in the profile of metal binding are a response to change in an environmental factor, i.e. metals. It is a *primary biochemical response* that is likely to be specific to this environmental stressor. The specificity with respect to the metal (in the sense of identifying the particular metal that is being bound and eliciting a response) is theoretically absolute as the metallothionein is identified by its molecular weight range and by the identified bound metal. Changes in the metal composition of the metallothionein pool presumably will identify the environmental metal that is eliciting the response (Leber, 1974). The limited information on the time-course and sensitivity of the metallothionein response in marine organisms includes the following points: (1) The response time appears to be short; although most studies have only examined the changes after several weeks of exposure, Viarengo et al. (1980) recorded a change in the metal binding of the metallothionein pool of the gills of *M. galloprovincialis* between 24 and 48 hours after exposure of the mussels to Cu. (2) Although knowledge of the effective concentrations of metals in the marine environment is limited because of the problems of bio-availability (see Moore, 1981), the indications are that the levels of metals used in laboratory experiments to elicit a response are environmentally realistic; e.g. Cu: 0.015 ppm (Viarengo et al., 1979); a mixture of Cd, Cu and Zn: 0.001, 0.09 and 0.07 ppm, respectively (total 0.161 ppm) (Brown, 1978). (3) The amount of induction of metallothionein may be difficult to estimate because it is unlikely that an increase of the relevant protein will be detected and because an increase in binding of a specific metal could represent displacement of another metal.* However, a measure of induction can be obtained from the increase in the amount of total metal bound to metallothionein. In this case, the induction observed for mussels (increase in bound Cd, Cu and Zn) varies from ×1.3 (Brown, 1978) to ×10 or greater (Nöel-Lambert, 1976). Another more exacting and precise method for the determination of the level of induction is the measurement of the incorporation of radio-labelled amino acids into the metallothionein pool

---

*The displacement of one metal by another requires time, and it may be that, given sufficient background knowledge, changes in the binding of a single metal may be employable as a measure of induction.

(Premakumar et al., 1975; Olafson et al., 1979; Viarengo et al., 1980). With this method, Viarengo et al. (1980) recorded a 7- to 10-fold increase in the incorporation of ^{35}S-cysteine into the 12,000 molecular weight fraction from the gills of copper-exposed mussels. No information appears to be available on the time-course of the induced changes, i.e. on the formation of a new steady state.

The second criterion for a biochemical response to be acceptable as an index of sublethal stress is that it must lead to or be associated with decreased animal performance.* Metallothionein is a detoxication system that functions initially by binding the toxic metal. Continuing or pre-exposure to the metal can lead to increased synthesis of metallothionein and therefore to an acquired tolerance to increasing metal levels (e.g. Bouquegneau, 1979). However, at a particular high concentration of a metal, according to the "spillover" theory, there will be toxic effects when the binding capacity of metallothionein is exceeded and the metal then interacts with the enzyme-containing pool or other sensitive sites. This movement of metal into the high molecular weight pool has been observed for a number of species including bivalves (Brown, 1978) and appears to coincide with the appearance of pathological effects (Winge et al., 1973; Brown, 1977; Brown et al., 1977; Irons and Smith, 1976). Therefore, the metallothionein-associated changes can eventually result in decreased animal performance. Although the decreased performance will have to be assessed by other criteria (e.g. cytological, physiological), observing changes in the metal-binding characteristics of the protein profile would appear to offer a very strong tool for the detection of events (metal-mediated) leading up to and resulting in decreased animal performance. Three stages are potentially discernable in the pattern of events: (1) displacement of "endogenous" bound metal from metallothionein by the foreign metal, (2) induction of metallothionein (increase in total bound metal) and (3) spillover of foreign metal into the high molecular weight pool (and resultant decreased animal performance). Application of metallothionein studies to the field will presumably require information on possible sex differences and seasonal changes. Similarly, the choice of tissue may

---

*There have been a few studies which suggest that induced levels of metallothionein may themselves have deleterious consequences for an animal; e.g. injection of isolated Cd-metallothionein into rats resulted in necrosis of kidney proximal renal tubular cells (Cherian et al., 1976).

require preliminary studies. Interactions of the metals with other pollutants are also possible and may lead to different patterns of binding. For example, it has been suggested that Cd in tumor-bearing flounders (*Parophrys vetulus*) may be alkylated by "bioactivated" organic carcinogens to form an alkyl Cd which is then no longer bound by metallothionein but interacts with the high molecular weight proteins (Brown, 1977).

5

Bioassay

RATIONALE FOR THE BIOASSAY APPROACH

Water quality is often assessed chemically in terms of the concentrations of known toxic contaminants. This method may be satisfactory when there are a limited number of contaminants whose biological effects are well known and predictable, but effluents are often extremely complex and may contain numerous synthetic organic compounds, for example, besides the better known contaminants like metals and ammonia. Effluents from a modern industrial complex entering a bay or an estuary may include thousands of individual elements and compounds, making it impractical to define and monitor water quality by chemical analysis alone. Furthermore, it is well known that many factors influence the toxicity of contaminants on entering seawater (Bryan, 1976). Some may degrade quickly into harmless products; indeed, increasing numbers of consumer products are designed to break down quickly in seawater. Some toxicants may become bound by organic matter or particulates, with consequent changes in their biological availability, and some may interact chemically to become more, or less, toxic in combination than separately.

The kinds of problem that arise in the estimation of biological water quality from a knowledge of chemical constituents alone are best illustrated by considering metals and the toxicity of different forms or "species" of metals that are found in seawater. Metals are the best known of marine contaminants because in recent years much work has been devoted to identifying the different species, their proportions and the factors that determine their equilibria. Metals may become incorporated in the lattice structure of clay particles, such as kaolinite or montmorillonite, or merely attached to particulates by the force of their charges. Metal ions may be complexed in specific chemical associations by fulvic or humic acids (Mantoura et al., 1978), large organic molecules which constitute the bulk of dissolved organic matter in seawater. Metals may be chemically transformed to form more toxic organic compounds, as in the case of mercury or lead (Bryan, 1976).

What is important in the present context is that the form in which a metal occurs profoundly affects its biological availability, and it follows that the toxicity of a metal cannot be predicted from a knowledge of concentration of total metal alone. A further complication is that it is almost impossible to duplicate natural environmental conditions in laboratory experiments with metals and other contaminants. This observation is justification for the view that toxicants have a "laboratory toxicity" and an "environmental toxicity" and that it is difficult to predict the latter from the former.

Since the ultimate concern is the capacity of the sea to support life, it is clearly desirable to measure water quality in terms of biological response, and that is the aim of this manual. Among other things the responses of suitable organisms in the laboratory to water samples taken from polluted areas can be used as an index of water quality. In this way all the biologically relevant variables that affect water quality are integrated in terms of the responses of individual organisms. Among the advantages of this approach is the integration it provides, not only of the effects of toxicants and modifying variables that are known and understood, but also of those that are not yet known. At present the environmental chemist may detect new toxicants or transformations in seawater, but since there is no continuous and systematic search for them, it is largely fortuitous how widely distributed they become before they are discovered. Routine bioassays of water quality provide a realistic means of detecting the effects of new toxicants in seawater, and of monitoring the integrated biological effects of contaminants and the variables that influence their toxicity in seawater.

BIOASSAY TECHNIQUES—ACTUAL AND POTENTIAL

The origins of the bioassay approach lie in the accidental discovery that the developmental success of invertebrate larvae (polychaetes and echinoderms) used for experimental work on settlement behaviour and metamorphosis changed when the seawater used came from different water masses, identified by characteristic planktonic indicator organisms (Wilson, 1951). The larvae were then used to provide an index of water quality, and the technique was applied to the problem of identifying the factors responsible for the differences in water quality (Wilson and Armstrong, 1961).

Similar techniques using other larvae have been applied to the problem of assessing water quality in the context of marine pollution. In Japan, Kobayashi (1971) developed a bioassay using echinoderm larvae. Gametes are obtained from adults collected from local populations, and their development over 12–24 h is then followed in the water sample for the bioassay. Three species of echinoderm are used which breed at different times, so that experiments can be conducted at most times of the year. One index of response to poor water quality is the increased frequency of abnormal larvae, such as exo-gastrulae. The formation of a fertilisation membrane, the two-cell stage and the gastrula are normal developmental stages at which success is assessed. Kobayashi et al. (1972) found marked geographical variations in water quality in a large-scale experiment involving 200 samples from the waters of the Inland Sea of Japan. Sometimes the effects on larvae of water collected near the bottom appeared to be related to elevated metal levels in the sediments, but the researchers were not able to establish the causes of the responses observed.

Woelke (1967, 1968, 1972) developed an oyster larval bioassay in which the index of depressed water quality is the percentage of larvae that develop abnormally at 48 h after fertilisation. Apart from its use in assessing the toxicity of specific contaminants, the oyster larval bioassay has been used extensively to assess the quality of polluted water samples (Woelke, 1967, 1972) and specifically waters polluted by pulp mill effluents and from the area of oyster beds (Woelke, 1968) (Fig. 5-1).

Larval bioassays are extremely sensitive to variations in water quality, and so they can be used in short-term experiments. Connor (1972), in a series of comparative experiments with a range of invertebrate larvae, showed that they were generally sensitive

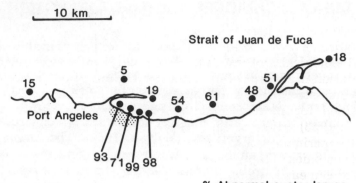

FIG. 5-1. The response of oyster larvae to water samples from a polluted area. High frequencies of larval abnormality occur in water samples from near Port Angeles, but decrease along the coast to the east and west. (From Woelke, 1968.)

to toxicants at concentrations about two orders of magnitude lower than their adults. Many larval stages have the advantage that they are lecithotrophic, thus avoiding the problem of providing food and thereby avoiding experimental stress due to lack of food. However, sensitivity to low levels of toxins is related in part to the duration of exposure, so in longer experiments with planktotrophic larvae it is necessary to feed the larvae.

One problem in the use of larvae is the availability of adult organisms. In some ways it is best if these can be drawn from laboratory cultures, or from natural populations that are unstressed, because it is known that the poor condition of adults can be passed on to their larvae (Bayne, 1972). In some cases it is possible only to initiate larval release twice in a lunar month at the time of spring tides (Knight-Jones, 1951; Kobayashi, 1971), which may limit their use for some purposes.

Convenient larval responses in short-term experiments are those used by Woelke and Kobayashi, but larval growth rate (Davis and Hidu, 1969) and the rate of development have often been used (Crisp, 1974). A complication in the interpretation of these data is that growth and development rates are frequently increased by toxins that are inhibitory at higher concentrations (Crisp, 1974; Benifts-Claus and Benifts, 1975).

In order to avoid some of these difficulties of working with larvae, a new bioassay technique has been developed using hydroids. The culture of hydroids, the experimental methods and the handling of data are described fully in Chapter 11; the advantages and disadvantages of using hydroids for this kind of work will be considered here.

Hydroids have long been used for experimental work on general biological problems since Trembley's early experiments on regeneration in *Hydra* (1740), although the culture of hydroids did not become straightforward until it was found that they could be maintained for indefinite periods with *Artemia salina* nauplii (Loomis, 1953). Hydroids are sessile, which simplifies their handling in experiments. Furthermore, as they reproduce asexually forming colonies of replicated members, material for a complete experiment can easily and quickly be grown from a single hydranth. We have used a single clone of *Campanularia flexuosa* (Stebbing, 1976) for over 10 years, and clones of *Hydra* isolated by Loomis (1954) are cultured in laboratories in a number of countries (Stebbing and Pomroy, 1978). The advantage of using a single clone for improving the precision of experimental data is, of course, well known in microbial and botanical work, but the opportunities of doing so are limited among the metazoa.

Hydroids are sensitive to stress partly because they are small and therefore have a large surface area, relative to their volume, across which exchange with the environment occurs. Apart from invertebrate larvae, hydroids are the only other kind of organism which has been used to bioassay water samples from the field (Stebbing, 1979). However, those who manage environmental levels of contaminants are not as concerned with the survival of hydroids, as with ecologically or economically more important species. This raises the question of how readily one might translate the responses of one organism into the responses of another. A systematic study of the effects of different toxicants on a range of organisms showed that the relative toxicities of metals remained constant for each organism (Shaw, 1961), while also having chemical meaning as the Irving-Williams order (Irving and Williams, 1953). This suggests that translation of sensitivities to toxicants might be possible.

CHEMICAL MANIPULATIONS TO IDENTIFY TOXIC CONTAMINANTS

It is clearly not enough to correlate the distribution of a contaminant in space and time with a bioassay reponse in order to establish a causal relationship between contaminant and response, because any other contaminant sharing the same distribution could have the same effect. One way of establishing causal relationships is to demonstrate that water quality improves when the discharge of a specific effluent ceases. Woelke (1972) examined the effect of pulp mill effluent on the biological quality of the receiving waters by observing changes in developmental success of oyster larvae in samples before, during and after a period when the pulp mill was closed (Fig. 5-2). Within two weeks of the mill closing, 99% of the larvae developed normally in the receiving water, but when the mill re-opened developmental success fell to zero.

Opportunities for determining the effects of specific effluents in this way are uncommon. However, various methods of changing seawater chemically have been used in conjunction with bioassay techniques to identify the determinants of biological water quality. In their work on natural variations in water quality, Wilson and Armstrong (1961) attempted to identify the causes of poor larval development in water samples by supplementing them with trace

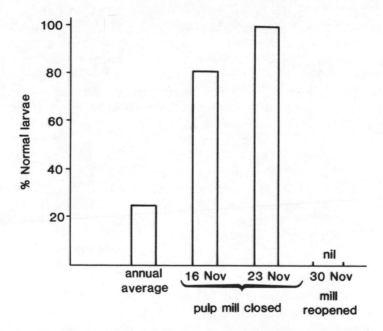

FIG. 5-2. The response of oyster larvae to samples from waters receiving pulp mill effluent. When the pulp mill closed, increase in the frequency of normal larvae indicates improved water quality, but there is rapid deterioration on reopening the mill. (From Woelke, 1972.)

TABLE 5-1. Echinoid Larval Bioassay Results

	Control water	Boiled control water	Osaka Harbour water	Boiled Osaka Harbour water
Fertilisation membrane	100	98	16.3	96.2
Two-cell stage	100	97.8	12.8	96.05
Gastrula	100	98.7	23.6	94.8

From Kobayashi (1971).

metals, chelating agents or extracts of seawater in which larval development was often more successful. However, in the context of marine pollution, poor water quality is not usually due to deficiencies, but to the presence of contaminants that have deleterious effects, and these effects can be demonstrated by selectively removing the agent(s) responsible.

Kobayashi (1971) showed that the quality of polluted water from Osaka Harbour could be restored almost to that of clean seawater by boiling the water (Table 5-1), suggesting that volatile pollutants might be important. However, so many changes to the seawater are likely to be caused by this treatment that it is difficult to interpret the relevance of these results, although it is important to note that boiling the control water apparently did not change its biological quality.

Other manipulative techniques are being developed in conjunction with the hydroid bioassay, although they can obviously be used in conjunction with any bioassay that is responsive to variations in the quality of polluted water. The techniques for the removal or breakdown of organic compounds and the removal of volatile constituents or divalent metals will be described in detail in Chapter 11, and it will be most useful to consider next the development and application of this approach in the context of marine pollution.

It is not possible to manage pollution levels in relation to biological effects, unless pollutants can be associated unambiguously with their effects in the environment. The linear form and constant direction of flow of fluvial systems makes it possible to establish without difficulty the source and therefore the nature of any effluent having deleterious effects on the biota. In the sea the problem is not so simple, because many effluents discharge into tidal water masses. It may therefore be necessary to use techniques to remove contaminants selectively. One may therefore imagine a series of chemical manipulations of a water sample of increasing specificity with which one would determine with a bioassay whether a biologically significant contaminant was inorganic or organic, volatile or non-volatile, metal or non-metal (Stebbing, 1980a). Techniques for removing single contaminants from seawater do not yet exist, but this is because there has not been good reason for developing them, rather than the inherent technical difficulties of doing so.

6

Ecological Consequences
of Stress

The techniques discussed in this manual are all concerned with
biochemical, cytological or physiological measures of the response
to stress, or with the use of bioassay procedures to assess water
quality; the measurement of possible ecological effects of pollution
on populations or on communities is not considered. However, it is
an often-stated (and sound) maxim of research on the effects of
pollution that unless such effects are likely (or are shown) to result
in damaging consequences for the population, it is arguable
whether pollution can be truly said to have occurred. This
necessary link between effects on the individual and consequences
for the population was incorporated by Bayne (1975) into a definition of the stress response, and it was subsequently stated by
McIntyre et al. (1978) as follows: "from a strictly biological point
of view it is the population and not the individual that is important
and it is argued that unless an effect has consequences at the
population level it is insignificant." The possibilities for measuring
population and community effects directly have been considered
by McIntyre et al. (1978), Gray (1979, 1980), Heip (1980) and Gray
et al. (1980), amongst others. We argue later for the combined use
of as wide a suite as possible of measurement indices in monitoring
programmes; here we are concerned with responses by the individual that can be shown to have direct consequences for population
and/or community attributes.

Sub-lethal effects on the individual that might be expected to
have damaging consequences for the population include depressed

rates of growth, reduced fecundity, reduction in egg viability and negative effects on competitive ability; all are inter-related. Reduced rates of growth will depress population production, limit fecundity (where this is size-related) and also reduce competitive ability, particularly where space may be limiting. Reduced fecundity will ultimately damage population survival, as would greatly reduced reproductive effort. When the environmental stress is severe enough to reduce egg viability as well as egg numbers, there may be even more serious implications for population survival.

Effects on populations may in turn have repercussions on the community, particularly in circumstances where the population in question is considered a "key" species. The concept of key species in community organisation is controversial. Nevertheless, in many communities a limited number of species may be numerically and competitively dominant. This is the situation in some temperate, inter-tidal, hard-substrate, epifaunal communities where *Mytilus edulis* is dominant in terms of abundance and space utilisation and where the individual mussels provide much of the secondary space available for colonisation by other species (Dayton, 1971; Paine, 1974). In these circumstances, changes to the population structure and production of *Mytilus* can be expected to affect community attributes such as species richness, niche breadth and overlap, the impact of predators and the partitioning of energy flow.

In this section, therefore, we will briefly consider some of the evidence, from studies on *M. edulis*, that demonstrates relationships between environmental stress and the properties of growth, fecundity, larval survival and reproductive effort (see also Bayne, 1984). These studies support the general premise that effects on the individual may indeed be reflected at the population level, and they illustrate the extent to which natural populations of the species in different environments may differ in the extent of ecological impact from environmental stressors.

GROWTH

The measurement of the scope for growth and its application as an index of the stress response is discussed in Chapter 1. Studies by Bayne et al. (1978, 1981) and by Bayne and Worrall (1980) compared estimates of growth from physiological measurements (the scope for growth) with estimates (1) from length-to-weight regressions before and after various experimental treatments in the laboratory (Fig. 6-1) and (2) from measured rates of growth in two naturally occurring populations of mussels (Fig. 6-2). In all three cases there was very good agreement between measured and calculated rates of growth. Evidence of this agreement enables confidence to be placed upon scope for growth measurements as an index of true physiological condition. The advantages of using physiological estimates of growth potential, rather than more direct measurements of growth, include the ability to analyse the components of the energy budget (absorption, respiration, excretion) for possible causes of disturbance to growth. Nevertheless, direct growth measurements have an important place in pollution effects studies.

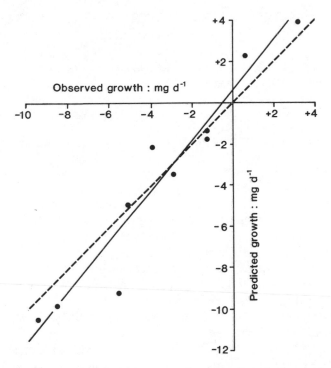

FIG. 6-1. The relationship between growth as predicted (from physiological measurements) and as observed (from length to weight regressions) in *M. edulis* in laboratory experiments. The solid line is fitted to the data by least-squares regression; the dashed line assumes an exact equivalence between observation and production.

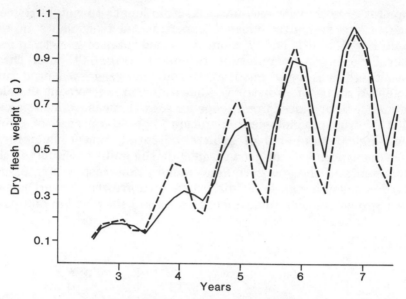

FIG. 6-2. Comparison of growth in weight for *M. edulis* as calculated from age-class analysis (broken line) and from physiological estimates of the scope for growth (solid line). (From Bayne and Worrall, 1980.)

Studies of growth in bivalve molluscs usually take the form of measurements of length which are subsequently converted to equivalents in flesh weight with the use of length/weight regression equations. Growth in length may be estimated by analysing annual growth rings, by measurements of marked individuals, by the analysis of size-classes in the population, or by a combination of these procedures (Haskin, 1954). More recently, examination of microscopic growth features, within the shells of molluscs, by the use of acetate peels of polished and etched sections of the shell, has made it possible to measure growth on time scales from days to years (comprehensively reviewed by Lutz and Rhoads, 1980; see also Richardson et al., 1980). Kennish (1980), working with *Mercenaria mercenaria*, has shown how these techniques may be employed in the analysis of the population dynamics of the species and in the detection of environmental impacts on growth.

Figure 6-3 shows the growth in weight of individuals from two populations of mussels. Growth was markedly seasonal, with weight gains in the summer and weight losses in the winter; in one population (the Cattewater) the period of weight loss was pro-

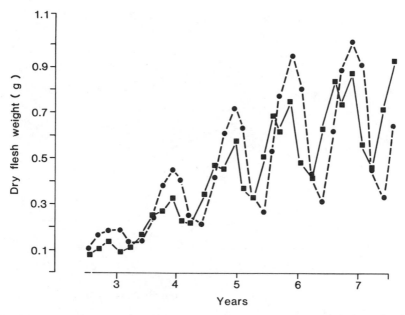

FIG. 6-3. Growth in weight of *M. edulis* over 5 years in two populations: Lynher, solid line; Cattewater, broken line. (From Bayne and Worrall, 1980.)

longed, lasting from October to March, but in the Lynher population the winter period of negative growth was of shorter duration. The net annual rates of growth in both populations can be converted into production in energy units (1 mg dry flesh weight ≡ 21.8 ± 1.7 J) incorporating both somatic and gamete production (see later). Figure 6-4 illustrates the greater production by a single cohort in the Lynher than in the Cattewater population.

Cohort production estimates arrived at in this way can be informative in comparing different sites, but they are incomplete for assessing net production differences. For a more complete assessment of production, differences in mortality between populations must be considered. Freeman and Dickie (1979) used *M. edulis* in such a study to compare the production potential of two bays in Nova Scotia, Canada. Marked individuals were held in cages at the two sites and regularly monitored for growth and mortality. Average growth rates differed only slightly between the two bays (although rates differed markedly between individuals), but mortality differences were more evident and resulted in significant net production differences between the bays. Freeman and

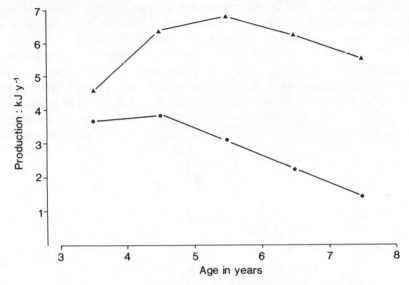

FIG. 6-4. Production as kJ per year in two populations of *M. edulis.* triangles, Lynher; circles, Cattewater.

Dickie (1979) point out the difficulties that might arise in applying procedures of this kind; e.g. the existence of genetic differences between individuals (possibly explaining individual growth differences) and the size-dependence of both growth and mortality. The extent to which mortality differences such as those observed by Freeman and Dickie might be linked to physiological differences, as measured in scope for growth determinations, is also a problem for future research. Nevertheless, "an environmental index using growth and mortality rates of *Mytilus edulis* may well provide a sensitive measure of relative productivity between areas" (Freeman and Dickie, 1979, p. 1249).

In comparing growth rates between different populations, use is often made of parameters in the Bertalanffy or Gompertz growth models. Caution is necessary when basing such comparisons on individual parameters only (Haukioja and Hakala, 1979), although the parameters may be estimated to include a measure of variance (Bayley, 1977). Richardson et al. (1980) discussed the use of the rate constant k (from the Bertalanffy equation), incorporating a correction constant ($L_\infty - l$, where L_∞ is also a fitted parameter estimating maximum body size and l is length), for such comparisons. These authors pointed out the potential use of short-term estimates of k in species such as the cockle *Cerastoderma edule* to identify possible environmental effects on growth over periods less than the normally used annual cycle.

The seasonal changes in the growth in weight of *Mytilus* (e.g. Fig. 6-5) have already beeen emphasised. In most populations growth in length ceases, or proceeds extremely slowly, during the winter, when food may become limiting and the mussel loses weight. An example of the amplitude of this seasonal weight change in a hypothetical mussel of constant shell length is given in Fig. 6-5. This is a natural phenomenon, brought about by natural variability in environmental resources, and not the result of anthropogenic stress. The occurrence of these periods of negative growth (and negative scope for growth) in the natural growth cycle of the mussel (and other bivalves) must be appreciated when assessing the results of physiological or other measurements of the stress response. If the making of such

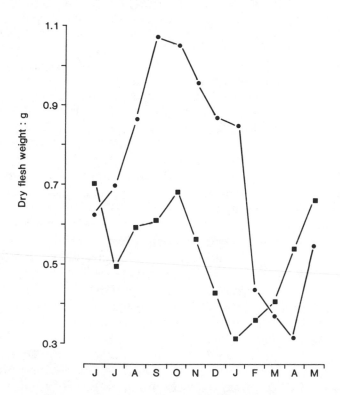

FIG. 6-5. Dry flesh weight of *M. edulis* of 6 cm shell length individuals in two populations; squares, Lynher; circles, Cattewater.

measurements has to be limited to one period of the year, this should be mid-summer, when growth would normally be positive. Different species may show different seasonal patterns, however (e.g. *Macoma balthica* in the Dutch Wadden Sea has periods of negative growth in the summer, due to high temperatures; Lammens, 1967; De Wilde, 1975), and there is no substitute for a general understanding of seasonal variability before any programme of physiological monitoring is initiated.

FECUNDITY

Fecundity—the number, weight or energy content of reproductive products of either males or females—may be measured by direct or indirect means. Direct methods involve the collection of sperm or eggs released by adults in the laboratory; indirect methods involve estimates of the weight of the gonad before and after spawning, with subsequent conversion from weight units to numbers and/or to energy content. In both cases it is necessary to conduct parallel histological studies and autopsies to confirm that spawning has been complete and to assess the number of spawnings per annum; the quantitative stereological techniques described in Chapter 8 can be used to provide this information. Two examples of a direct and an indirect assessment of fecundity of *Mytilus edulis* will illustrate the types of procedure available.

For direct measurements of fecundity, adults are brought into the laboratory and artificially induced to release their gametes (i.e. to spawn), which are collected and counted, weighed or analysed for energy content. Although mussels may sometimes be induced to shed gametes at a time of year when spawning would not normally occur, the animals are usually refractory to spawning stimuli unless they possess ripe gametes ready to be shed normally. A knowledge of the normal seasonal cycle (see Chapter 2) is important in judging the optimal time for spawning inducement. Various means for the stimulation of spawning have been used with bivalve molluscs.

Mussels from a population at Swansea were collected in March and held in the laboratory at 5°C, with adequate food, for between 4 and 14 days. On five occasions, batches of 15 individuals were removed to flowing seawater at 15°C for 1.5 h and the water temperature was then gradually raised to 20°C. Of 75 individuals treated in this way 32 (43%) spawned; 21 of these were females. The eggs were washed in isotonic ammonium formate, dried and weighed, and fecundity was then calculated as the weight of eggs released by each female (also of known weight). Autopsies on the post-spawned females confirmed that spawning was complete in all cases.

The results of this experiment (Fig. 6-6) suggest an allometric relationship between adult body weight and the weight of eggs released, with a fecundity of 40 mg eggs spawned by an adult of 1 g dry flesh weight. For this population, the weight of 10^6 eggs was determined as 29.1 ± 5.5 (S.D.) mg.

Worrall (pers. comm) used an indirect method to establish the fecundity of a different population of mussels. In *Mytilus* much of the ripe gonad is found in the mantle tissue, and weight losses at spawning, due to decline in mantle weight, may be used as an indirect fecundity measurement (Fuji and Hashizume, 1974; Thompson, 1979; Griffiths and King, 1979; Bayne and Worrall, 1980). Worrall determined, by stereology, that spawning occurred between April and June; the dry weight of the mantle for mussels

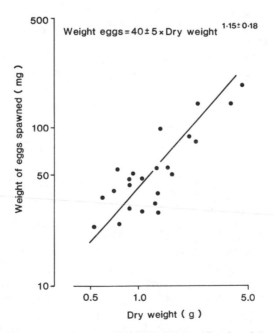

FIG. 6-6. Fecundity (as total weight of eggs spawned) related to adult size (dry flesh weight) in *M. edulis* from one population.

TABLE 6-1. Equations Describing Annual Dry Weight Loss on Spawning (W^*, mg) Related to Total Dry Body Weight before Spawning (W, g) for *M. edulis* from Different Populations

Population	Allometric equation	Authority
Bellevue	max: $W^* = 398 \times W^{1.124}$	Thompson (1979)
	min: $W^* = 294 \times W^{1.124}$	Thompson (1979)
Long Island	$W^* = 308 \times W^{1.269}$	Thompson (1979)
Petpeswick	max: $W^* = 471 \times W^{1.481}$	Thompson (1979)
	min: $W^* = 277 \times W^{1.481}$	Thompson (1979)
Lynher	$W^* = 208 \times W^{1.40}$	Bayne & Worrall (1980)
Cattewater	$W^* = 21 \times W^{1.29}$	Bayne & Worrall (1980)
Mothecombe	$W^* = 193 \times W^{1.51}$	Worrall (unpublished)

of 1.003 g dry weight was 314 mg in April and 155 mg in June. The calculated weight loss on spawning was therefore 159 mg. Earlier studies on this population had established a mean weight of 10^6 eggs as 52.5 mg (Bayne et al., 1975) so that the fecundity as numbers of eggs spawned by a female of 1 g dry weight was $155/52.5 = 2.95 \times 10^6$ eggs.

Worrall (pers. comm.) was also able to establish, by stereological techniques, a total change in volume of follicles with ripe gametes (see Chapter 8) from 0.54 cm^3 in April to 0.05 cm^3 in June. The calculated volume loss on spawning was therefore 0.49 cm^3. The mean diameter of the eggs of *M. edulis* is 70 μm, with a volume of 1.79×10^5 μm^3. These values can be used to estimate the number of eggs spawned:

$$\frac{0.49 \times 10^{12} \mu m^3}{1.79 \times 10^5 \mu m^3} = 2.74 \times 10^6 \text{ eggs}$$

The two estimates, by weight (2.95×10^6 eggs) and by volume (2.74×10^6 eggs) are in good agreement. In routine surveys, careful monitoring of weight changes in the gonad tissue can serve as an indirect assessment of fecundity.

Thompson (1979) used both direct and indirect techniques to measure the fecundity of *M. edulis* from various populations in Nova Scotia. He recorded considerable annual variation within populations; our own studies have demonstrated similar variation between populations. Some of these results are summarised in Table 6-1 as regression equations fitted to the data. In all cases there is an accelerated fecundity with increase in body size (i.e. the slopes of the allometric equations are all greater than 1.0).

The question follows, to what extent are these variations in fecundity due to environmental stress? Laboratory studies with *Mytilus* have indicated that environmental stress may indeed reduce fecundity in mussels. Mussels were held at different temperatures and different ration conditions for up to 9 weeks, in order to induce different values for the scope for growth from + 125 to − 220 J d^{-1}. The mussels were then stimulated to spawn, all eggs collected and the total energy content of the spawned eggs determined by biochemical analysis. The results (Fig. 6-7) indicate a linear relationship between the scope for growth and fecundity. This relationship cannot be applied directly to animals in natural

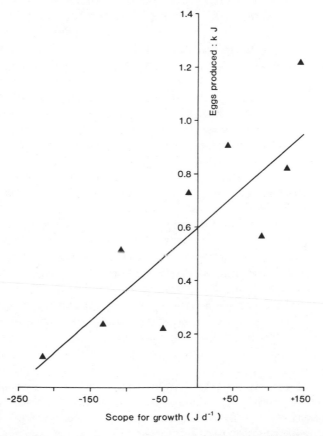

FIG. 6-7. Fecundity (as total energy content of eggs spawned) in *M. edulis* related to the scope for growth, as determined in laboratory experiments.

populations, since an undetermined proportion of the eggs spawned in these experiments would have been produced before the mussels were brought into the laboratory. Nevertheless, the implications are clear; under conditions of stress during which the growth potential of the individual is reduced, fewer eggs are produced for spawning.

Bayne et al. (1978) studied some of the cytological processes in the connective and germinal tissues of the mantle accompanying gametogenesis in mussels under conditions of high temperatures and reduced ration levels. When mussels with developing gametes were placed under stress, enhanced autolysis of the connective tissue cells followed, detected as a reduced latency of lysosomal enzymes (see Chapter 2) and a general increase in free lysosomal enzyme activity. There was evidence also of a lysosomally based autolysis of ripe gametes, followed by infiltration of granulolytic haemocytes (blood cells) which eventually phagocytosed the degrading gametes. At the same time as these processes were occurring, young germinal cells continued to develop into oocytes and spermatocytes. This "generation" of gametes, however, produced under conditions of a negative scope for growth, was fewer in number, and the oocytes smaller in size, than that produced in animals not subjected to stress. Concomitant with these changes there was a decline in glycogen from the storage cells of the mantle tissue, some of which was utilised in the production of gametes (Bayne et al., 1975). Under very severe stress, glycogen utilisation and gametogenesis became uncoupled (Bayne et al., 1982), gametes were not produced and the glycogen was all directed towards maintenance energy metabolism.

These studies have provided a cytological description of the course of events that leads, during stressful environmental conditions, to reduced fecundity. They illustrate some of the processes that result in a decline in gamete production and provide a link between observations of lysosomal latency, reduced scope for growth, the utilisation of glycogen and a reduction in spawned products. The suggestion emerges that musssels subjected in nature to temperature or nutritive stress during gametogenesis would similarly be expected to produce fewer gametes than mussels in more optimal environments.

In a companion study, Bayne and Widdows (1978) and Bayne and Worrall (1980) examined two mussel populations, one (from the Lynher estuary) a normal estuarine population, the other (from the Cattewater region of the Plym estuary) subjected in the winter, during the normal period for gametogenesis, to low food levels and unseasonally high temperatures caused by the cooling-water effluent from a local electricity generating station. Mussels from the Cattewater showed reduced fecundity compared with those from Lynher, with an average weight loss on spawning some five times less than the normal population (Table 6-1). In addition, mussels from the Lynher population spawned twice during the year, those from the Cattewater only once; the latter mussels were apparently unable to produce gametes during the winter due to the environmental stresses experienced.

To a large extent, the available evidence suggests that reductions in fecundity of the type discussed here are due to a competition between maintenance metabolism, somatic production and gamete production for the finite amount of energy made available from the diet. Under normal circumstances not only is surplus energy available after the maintenance requirement has been met (i.e. the scope for growth is positive) but there is also sufficient energy in this surplus (1) to replace body mass lost at other times of the year, (2) to produce a net increase in mass over the year and (3) to produce gametes. Under sub-optimal environmental conditions the mean annual maintenance energy demand must, of course, be met, with some surplus for net growth; there may be little energy remaining for gamete production. This appears to be the situation in the Cattewater population, and possibly at other sites subjected to pollution. The partitioning of energy between these various demands may be indexed by measures of the reproductive effort.

REPRODUCTIVE EFFORT

Two measures of reproductive effort are discussed here. In the first, the energy allocated to gamete production (P_r) is stated as a proportion of total production (P), which is itself the sum of somatic growth (P_g) and P_r. This is the simplest meaningful measure of reproductive effort. Results from the Lynher and Cattewater populations are plotted in Fig. 6-8A and show the increase in reproductive effort with age in both populations and the much lower effort made by the mussels under stress in the Cattewater. Thompson (1979) and Griffiths and King (1979) reported similar trends for M. edulis and Aulacomya ater, respectively.

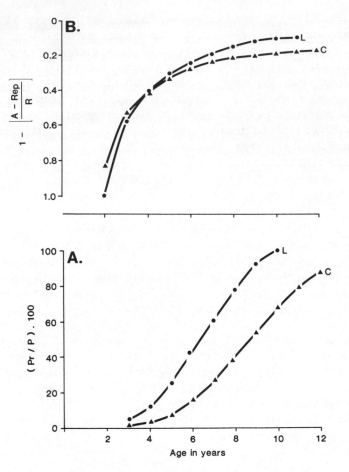

FIG. 6-8. *A.* Reproductive effort as P_r (gamete production) as a proportion of total production (P) in *M. edulis* from two populations. L, Lynher; C, Cattewater. *B.* Reproductive effort, calculated following Calow (1979) in *M. edulis* from two populations. L, Lynher; C, Cattewater.

The second measurement of reproductive effort, due to Calow (1979), incorporates the maintenance energy requirement in the proportioning of energy to gamete production; the greater the difference between the absorbed ration (*A*; see Chapter 1) and the energy allocated to reproduction (*Rep*), scaled as a proportion of the routine metabolic expenditure (*Rest*), the lower is the reproductive effort:

$$\text{Effort } (E) = 1 - \frac{A - Rep}{Rest}$$

If $E = 0$, reproduction makes no demands on other aspects of metabolism. If $E > 1$, reproduction does make such demands and the animal is said to be reproductively "reckless." If $E < 1$, the amount of energy left to the animal after reproduction is more than enough for the rest of metabolism, and reproduction is said to be "restrained." There are problems associated with the correct values for $Rest$ as discussed by Calow (1979). In the following calculations for $Mytilus$, $Rest$ is taken as the energy equivalent of respiration, calculated as an annual mean value measured under field ambient conditions; A is the absorbed ration and Rep is the fecundity, both calculated as energy units and annual means.

Values for Calow's (1979) index are plotted in Fig. 6-8B. There is now very little difference between the two populations (cf. Fig. 6-8B) in reproductive effort. A comparison between the two indices of effort emphasises the overwhelming respiratory demands in these animals. When the respiratory requirement is excluded from the index and the reproductive effort is assessed simply in terms of somatic versus gamete production, population differences emerge that indicate how different degrees of environmental stress may bring about significant differences in fecundity and the proportion of surplus energy available for reproduction (Bayne et al., 1983).

EGG QUALITY AND LARVAL SURVIVAL

The results of laboratory studies suggest that not only fecundity but also the viability of the gametes may be reduced when produced under stress. A decline in egg viability may in turn affect the chances of larval survival and so represent a further negative ecological consequence to the population. Bayne et al. (1978) recorded a reduction in the organic matter per egg of $M. edulis$ under stress in the laboratory. The biochemical composition of the eggs (i.e. the *proportions* of lipid, carbohydrate and protein per unit egg weight) remained relatively constant, but eggs produced by adults showing negative scope for growth were smaller, with less organic matter per egg than those produced by mussels with a positive scope for growth. The result was a positive correlation between the scope for growth and the energy *content* per egg, varying from 2×10^{-3} J egg^{-1} at positive scope for growth to 0.5×10^{-3} J egg^{-1} when the adults showed a scope for growth of -200 J d^{-1}.

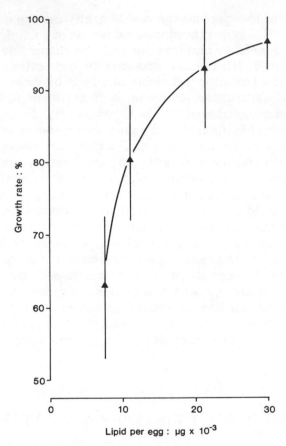

FIG. 6-9. The rate of growth of *M. edulis* larvae developing from eggs of different lipid content. Results from laboratory experiments, mean ± S.E.

Of the biochemical components of the eggs, the one that showed greatest variation was the lipid content, which changed by a factor of 6 between the extreme values for scope for growth. Helm et al. (1973) studied the relationship between the rate of growth of newly released oyster (*Ostrea edulis*) larvae, their lipid composition (as % by weight) and the conditions under which the parents were kept prior to larval release. Larvae liberated (*O. edulis* broods its larvae within the mantle cavity until the straight-hinge stage) by adults maintained at low ration (unsupplemented natural seawater) had a slower rate of growth and lower lipid content than larvae released from adults held at high ration (seawater with algae added). A similar relationship between the lipid content of the egg and the rate of growth of the larvae holds in *M. edulis* (Fig. 6-9). Planktotrophic larvae such as these suffer considerable mortality and loss due to "over dispersion" whilst in the plankton (Bayne, 1976). Presumably any extension of the duration of the larval period, brought about by reduced rates of growth, represents an added drain on recruitment potential and hence on ecological fitness.

In the bivalve molluscs, the glycogen reserves of the adult are used, in part, to provide lipid in the eggs (Gabbott, 1976; Holland, 1978); during stress, when the glycogen available for gametogenesis becomes limiting, eggs are produced with a reduced lipid content, which in turn reduces the viability of the eggs and the vigor of the larvae that develop. If part of the fundamental reproductive behavior of *Mytilus* is to produce the greatest possible number of eggs, each provisioned with a minimal viable energy reserve, as argued on theoretical grounds by Vance (1973) and Crisp (1975), then reduced fecundity and egg lipid, caused by environmental stresses, represent very significant ecological consequences to the population (see Bayne et al., 1981).

PART **II**

PROCEDURES

7

Physiological Procedures

EXPERIMENTAL DESIGN

Previous studies have applied three different experimental approaches to the measurement of physiological stress indices (See Chapter 1) of mussels acclimatized to different environmental conditions, namely:

1. Measurement of native mussel populations in the field under ambient conditions (Bayne and Widdows, 1978).
2. Measurement of transplanted mussels in the field under ambient conditions (Salkeld and Widdows, unpublished data).
3. Measurement of transplanted mussels after transfer to standard laboratory conditions (Widdows et al., 1981b).

If the objective is concerned less with understanding the bioenergetics or providing a good prediction of growth for a native population, but more with the comparison of growth potential or degree of stress experienced at different sites where animals are exposed to different environmental conditions, then the transplantation of organisms from a "clean base-line" population to selected sites is to be recommended. The advantages of transplanting organisms are (1) that animals can be placed at selected sites along a pollution gradient or at specific "hot-spots" and clean sites in a bay or estuarine system, and there is no reliance on the sporadic distribution of naturally occurring populations of the indicator species and (2) that the animals all originate from the same population and therefore are of similar genetic constitution, similar reproductive condition, and have experienced a similar environmental history at an "unpolluted" site, which ultimately reduces variability and so improves the chances of detecting an effect of pollution.

If the facilities provided by a mobile laboratory (e.g. vessel or converted minibus) are available, then the field measurement of physiological stress indices under ambient conditions is to be recommended. Seawater is pumped from within a few metres of the mussel population to a reservoir and thence through experimental apparatus in the mobile laboratory. Physiological measurements can then be made under conditions that very closely resemble those experienced in the environment (similar or identical temperature, salinity, oxygen, suspended particulate load and contaminant levels).

In a recent study by Salkeld and Widdows (unpublished data), the validity of returning animals to the laboratory for physiological measurement (respiration, feeding, excretion and absorption efficiency) was evaluated. Three mussel populations were visited and physiological determinations made using a mobile laboratory within a few metres of the natural population on the shore. Individuals were then transported to a laboratory seawater system where physiological rates were measured under standard conditions of temperature and salinity, approximating the field situation, and algal diet (*Isochrysis galbana* and *Phaeodactylum tricornutum*) at a particle concentration of 3×10^3 cells ml^{-1}. The results showed that there were no significant differences between field and laboratory measurements if the latter were made within 24 hours of animals entering the laboratory. Absorption efficiency proved to be the exception, because this parameter is immediately altered by the change in diet. However, this alteration in absorption efficiency is followed by a new steady state within ca. 2 days.

Body size is an important variable affecting most physiological responses (see Fig. 1-1) but one that can be excluded by selecting and transplanting animals of similar body size. It is inevitable, however, that there will be some differences in the dry body mass of animals before and after transplanting. This effect can be removed by correcting rates of metabolism, feeding, excretion and growth to a "standard body size" by means of the allometric equation:

$$Y = aX^b \tag{1}$$

or $$\log_{10} Y = \log_{10} a + b \log_{10} X \qquad (2)$$

where Y = physiological rate, X = dry body mass in grams, and a and b are the intercept and slope, respectively. Physiological rates are converted to an appropriate weight-specific rate using the exponent b.

The equations describing the relationship between each physiological rate and dry body mass are first established for the "base-line population" used in the transplant programme. Approximately 30 individuals covering a wide size range are measured and the data are then analysed by linear regression of the logarithmically (base 10) transformed values (X, Y).

Example: Relationship between oxygen consumption and body size

Population: Sullom Voe.

Animal	X = Dry mass (g)	Y = Oxygen consumption rates (ml O_2 h^{-1})
1	1.601	0.698
2	1.184	0.631
3	0.985	0.482
⋮	⋮	⋮
34	0.209	0.209
35	0.154	0.138

These data are then transformed by $\log_{10}$ and analysed by least-square linear regression with the following result (where Y is transformed oxygen consumption and X is transformed dry body mass):

Source	D.F.	Sums of sq.	Mean sq.	F
Regression	1	1.101	1.101	91.5
Residual	34	0.409	0.012	
Total	35	1.510		

Correlation coefficient = 0.85
Standard deviation of Y on X = 0.110
Regression equation:

$$\log Y = -0.294 + 0.65 \,(\log X)$$
$$\text{S.D.} \pm 0.044 \quad \text{S.D.} \pm 0.068$$

or
$$Y = 0.508 X^{0.65}$$
$$\text{S.D.} \pm 0.051$$

The weight exponent or slope of each equation is then used to correct for the differences in dry body mass found within the sample of transplanted animals. If animals of approximately 1 g dry mass are selected and measured, then the rates can be corrected to a "standard 1-g animal." The following example shows the calculations involved.

Example: The slope ($b = 0.65$) describing the relationship between oxygen consumption and dry body mass is substituted in Eq. (2). Therefore, if animal 1 has an oxygen consumption of 0.698 ml O_2 h^{-1} and a dry mass of 1.601 g then:

$$\log a = \log Y - b \log X$$
$$\log a = \log 0.698 - 0.65 (\log 1.601)$$
$$a = 0.154$$

However, if the average body mass of transplanted animals measured is markedly different from 1 g dry mass, then a standard body size equivalent to the mean body mass is chosen and the corrections for any weight differences are made in a similar manner but using the following equation:

$$\log Y_c = \log Y_o - (b \log X_o - b \log X_c) \tag{3}$$

where Y_c is the corrected value for a standard body mass (X_c) and Y_o and X_o are the individual's measured rate and body mass, respectively.

Further data analysis using weight-corrected physiological rates will be discussed after the procedures for determining each physiological rate have been outlined.

SCOPE FOR GROWTH

The physiological measurements necessary for the calculation of scope for growth include: (1) clearance rate, (2) food absorption efficiency, (3) respiration rate and (4) ammonia excretion rate.

The sampling and handling procedure is as follows: Collect at least 20 animals of a standard body size (preferably with a body mass of approximately 1 g) and immediately place them in tanks of flowing seawater. Before any physiological measurements are made, all individuals should be cleaned of epibiotic growth. After the completion of all physiological measurements the animals' body tissues are removed from their shells and dried to constant weight at 90°C (for 24 h) so that each measured rate can be corrected for any differences in dry tissue mass. It is preferable to measure the clearance rate, food absorption efficiency, respiration and excretion rate on the same individuals (minimum of 15) so that the scope for growth can be calculated on an individual basis with an estimate of the variance about the mean.

Clearance Rate

Clearance rate, defined as the volume of water cleared of particles per hour, is estimated by measuring the removal of suspended particles larger than 4 μm in diameter as water at a known flow rate passes through an experimental chamber containing a mussel. The suspended particles can be either natural particulates if field measurements are being undertaken or algal cells (e.g. *Phaeodactylum tricornutum*, *Tetraselmeis suecica* or *Isochrysis galbana*) added to pre-filtered seawater if measurements are being carried out in the laboratory.

Individuals are placed in five (or more) experimental chambers with the inflow at the bottom and the outflow from an overflow tube at the top (Fig. 7-1). An additional chamber without an animal acts as a "control."

Seawater is pumped from a reservoir to a mixing chamber and then through each chamber at a flow rate of at least 150 ml min^{-1}. The mixing chamber is necessary to ensure that the particle concentrations entering each of the experimental chambers are not significantly different. This should be tested before placing animals in the chambers.

The animals are left undisturbed for at least 60 min to allow the valves to open, ventilation to be resumed and the system to establish an equilibrium. The flow rate through each chamber is recorded.

Water samples are collected simultaneously from the outflow of all chambers, and the particle concentrations are measured by means of a Coulter counter (Model ZB or TAII) using a 140-μm orifice tube (mean of several counts per sample). The sensitivity settings of the Coulter counter should be adjusted so that only particles larger than 4 μm are counted and there is no coincidence counting.

The water sample from the control chamber represents the inflowing particle concentration (C_I), and the water sample from

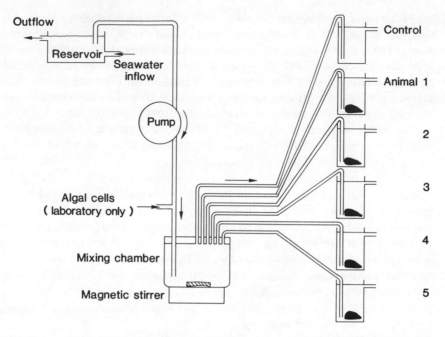

FIG. 7-1. Apparatus for the measurement of clearance rate. If flow rate is insufficient to maintain required temperature then the apparatus should be held in a temperature-controlled water bath.

each experimental chamber containing a mussel represents the outflow particle concentration (C_o). Clearance rate is then calculated as follows:

$$\text{Clearance rate (litre } h^{-1}) = \frac{C_I - C_o}{C_I} \times \text{flow rate (litre } h^{-1}) \quad (1)$$

Example: Clearance rate $= \dfrac{4,500 - 3,000}{4,500} \times 9.6$ litre $h^{-1} = 3.2$ litre h^{-1}

Correct clearance rate to a standard body size.

Experimental Flow Rates

Accurate estimates of clearance rate (and ventilation rate) are only achieved if the flow rate through each experimental chamber is sufficient to prevent any significant recirculation of water by the animal. Any such recirculation will result in an underestimate of the clearance rate (Bayne et al., 1976a; Hildreth and Crisp, 1976; Riisgard, 1977). The minimum flow rate required will depend on the size and geometry of the experimental chamber and the clearance rate of the animal, which will vary with body size, population, species and environmental conditions. Clarification of this potential artefact should therefore precede any study of clearance rates using flow-through techniques. The adequacy of a given flow rate can be demonstrated either by measuring no change in clearance rate with increasing flow rates (Riisgard, 1977; Møhlenberg and Riisgard, 1979), or by comparing the clearance rate measured in a flow-through system with that determined in a static system (see Chapter 1).

If the high flow rates necessary to prevent recirculation of water by the animal are unobtainable with the equipment available, then an alternative method is to accept a lower flow rate (e.g. 50 ml min^{-1}) through a larger experimental chamber (>1 litre) and to use aeration to circulate the water in order to provide a homogeneous particle concentration in the chamber. Under these circumstances the outflow concentration is equivalent to the concentration surrounding the animal and the following equation is used to calculate clearance rates (Hildreth and Crisp, 1976):

$$\text{Clearance rate (litre h}^{-1}) = \frac{C_1 - C_o}{C_o} \times \text{flow rate (litre h}^{-1}) \qquad (2)$$

When using this approach it is necessary to ensure that the water surrounding the animal is thoroughly mixed, otherwise the clearance rate may be over-estimated (unpublished observations). One disadvantage of this method is that the food concentration surrounding the animal will be reduced as the animal's clearance rate is increased, which may lead to some difficulty in maintaining constant ration levels in all experimental chambers. Consequently, there may be some slight errors associated with the estimate of food absorption efficiency and the calculation of scope for growth.

In many suspension feeding bivalves, where exhalent and inhalent siphons are mobile or close to one another, e.g. *Cardium*, it is difficult to prevent recirculation of water and under these circumstances this alternative procedure, using Eq. (2), is preferable.

Comparison of Three Methods
for Determining Clearance Rate

In a comparative study, the clearance rates of *Mytilus edulis* (Whitsand population, $n = 10$, mean dry mass $= 0.6$ g) were determined by three different methods:

1. The exponential decline in cell concentration in a static system (5-litre volume).
2. The removal of particles in a flow-through system (volume of chamber = 0.4 litre; flow rate = 160 ml min^{-1}) using Eq. (1) to compute clearance rate.
3. The removal of particles in a flow-through system (volume of chamber = 1.6 litre; flow rate = 60 ml min^{-1}; aeration) using Eq. (2) to calculate clearance rate.

The results showed no significant differences between the three procedures (t-test, paired comparisons):

Method	1	2	3
Clearance rate (litre h^{-1})	4.22	4.25	4.17
S.E.	± 0.33	± 0.17	± 0.24

Food Absorption Efficiency

Seston Concentration

The amount of suspended particulate material or seston concentration (mg litre^{-1}) in the inflowing water is sampled in duplicate at approximately 2-hourly intervals. A known volume of water is filtered through a washed, ashed and pre-weighed 4.5-cm GFC glass fibre filter (see Strickland and Parsons, 1972) and the salts washed out of the filter with distilled water (3×10 ml). Care is also taken to wash salts out of the edge of the filter. When sampling natural particulates the water should pass through a ca. 150-μm sieve before membrane filtering to prevent copepods and any large debris being sampled on the filter. The filters are oven dried at 90°C and weighed in order to calculate the total dry weight of particulate matter per litre of seawater. The filters are then ashed for several hours at 450°C in a muffle furnace and weighed again in order to calculate the weight of material combusted. This value is referred to as the weight of particulate organic matter (POM) or ash-free material. It is important that the GFC filters are thoroughly washed in distilled water before ashing and determining the initial dry weight, otherwise there may be a considerable weight loss during sampling. Blank GFC filters should also be weighed at each stage. All filters should be handled with forceps and stored in desiccators during cooling and transfer from ovens to balance for weighing.

Faeces

Mussels of standard body size are maintained in separate flow-through chambers (see clearance rate measurements) where they receive seawater and suspended particulates from a reservoir. Faeces and, where present, pseudofaeces are collected at intervals by pipetting onto washed, ashed and pre-weighed glass fibre filters. The salts are then washed out of the filters with distilled water (3 × 10 ml), and the filters are dried at 90°C and weighed before and after ashing at 450°C.

The absorption efficiency (e) is measured by the ratio method of Conover (1966) and represents the efficiency with which mussels absorb material cleared from suspension. This method depends upon the assumption that only the organic component of food is significantly affected by the digestive processes. Therefore, the percentage organic matter or the ash-free dry weight:dry weight ratio is lower in the faeces than in the food.

The Conover ratio for absorption efficiency is calculated as follows:

$$e = \frac{F - E}{(1 - E)F}$$

where F = ash-free dry weight:dry weight ratio of food (seston), and E = ash-free dry weight:dry weight ratio of faeces. It is recommended that the mean absorption efficiency of 10 animals is used in the calculation of scope for growth.

Respiration Rate

An individual mussel is introduced into the respirometer chamber (modified Quickfit flask; volume ca. 500 ml) and allowed to attach by byssus threads to a perforated glass plate over a stirrer bar (Fig. 7-2). Water in the chamber is stirred by means of a magnetic stirrer at a speed sufficient to provide a steady reading on an oxygen meter. Animals are left undisturbed for at least 45–60 min before isolating the chamber from the flowing water (by turning the taps marked F in Fig. 7-2).

The decline in oxygen tension in the chamber is then monitored with a Radiometer oxygen electrode (E5046) and amplifier (Model PHM 72) which is coupled to a 100-mV chart recorder. The rate of oxygen consumption is measured over a period of 45–60 min. Oxygen tension should not fall below ca. 100

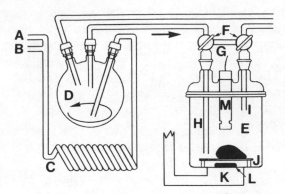

FIG. 7-2. Apparatus for the measurement of rates of oxygen consumption. A, seawater inflow; B, algal cell inflow (laboratory use only); C, temperature equilibration coil; D, mixing chamber; E, experimental chamber; F, two-way taps; G, bypass; H, inflow; I, outflow; J, perforated base plate; K, magnetic stirrer; L, stirring bar; M, oxygen electrode. Apparatus is held in a temperature-controlled water bath.

mmHg because *Mytilus* becomes an oxygen-conformer (i.e. rate of oxygen consumption is dependent on oxygen tension) at lower oxygen concentrations.

It is advisable to use two experimental chambers in conjunction with each oxygen probe, so that a second animal can be opening its valves and resuming normal activity during the 45–60 min period of measurement of the first animal. After completing the oxygen consumption measurements of animal 1, the probe is carefully transferred to the chamber containing animal 2, the chamber is isolated from the flowing water and the decline in pO_2 is recorded. Meanwhile, a new animal is introduced into the first chamber and allowed to open and resume normal pumping activity. Approximately 15 individuals of standard body size should be measured. Before obtaining the animal's dry tissue mass, the displacement volume of each individual should be determined with a measuring cylinder.

Use of Radiometer Oxygen Meter

The Radiometer probe is calibrated in solutions of known oxygen tension. After renewing the membrane on the oxygen probe, the probe should be placed in pO_2 zero solution and the meter adjusted to zero. Before using the new probe it should be left to stabilize overnight with the polarizing current on. Each day the probe should be calibrated in oxygen-saturated water at the required experimental temperature (water sampled from the surface of a tank with flowing seawater is usually within a few percent of full saturation). The oxygen meter is then set at 155 mmHg.

A silicone tubing sleeve (or several layers of parafilm wrapped round the probe 1–2 cm from the end) provides an airtight seal between the probe and the orifice in the respirometer chamber.

Calculation of Rate of Oxygen Consumption

The rate of oxygen consumption ($\dot{V}_{O_2}$) should be calculated for a period of linear decline in pO_2 from the start of the test (t_o) to the completion of the test (t_1), as follows.

On the basis of the O_2 saturation value (C) at specific temperature and salinity (see Table 7-1), convert mmHg into ml O_2 litre^{-1}:

$$\frac{\text{mmHg at } t_o}{160 \text{ mmHg}} \times C \text{ (ml } O_2 \text{ litre}^{-1}) = \text{ml } O_2 \text{ litre}^{-1} \text{ at } t_o = A$$

$$\frac{\text{mmHg at } t_1}{160 \text{ mmHg}} \times C \text{ (ml } O_2 \text{ litre}^{-1}) = \text{ml } O_2 \text{ litre}^{-1} \text{ at } t_1 = B$$

(note that 160 mmHg is equivalent to 21.33×10^3 Pa). The rate of oxygen consumption is then given by:

$$\dot{V}_{O_2} = \text{ml } O_2 \, h^{-1} = (A - B) \times (\text{Vol. of respirometer}$$

$$- \text{Vol. of animal)} \times \frac{60}{t_1 - t_o (\text{min})}$$

where the volumes of the respirometer and animal are in litres. Correct oxygen consumption rate to a standard body size.

Ammonia Excretion Rate

Five litres of seawater are filtered through Millipore membrane filters (0.45 μm). The batch of filtered seawater is then returned to full oxygen saturation by aeration.

Animals are placed in individual beakers containing 200 ml of membrane-filtered seawater (300 ml may be necessary for large mussels of 8–9 cm length). An additional beaker containing 200

TABLE 7-1. Solubility of Oxygen (C) in Seawater (ml litre^{-1}) with Respect to an Atmosphere of 20.95% Oxygen and 100% Relative Humidity at a Total Atmospheric Pressure of 760 mmHg

T (°C)						Salinity (‰)								
	0	5	10	15	20	25	30	31	32	33	34	35	36	37
0	10.22	9.87	9.54	9.22	8.91	8.61	8.32	8.27	8.21	8.16	8.10	8.05	7.99	7.94
1	9.94	9.60	9.28	8.97	8.68	8.39	8.11	8.05	8.00	7.94	7.89	7.84	7.78	7.73
2	9.67	9.35	9.04	8.74	8.45	8.17	7.90	7.85	7.79	7.74	7.69	7.64	7.59	7.53
3	9.41	9.10	8.80	8.51	8.23	7.96	7.70	7.65	7.60	7.55	7.50	7.45	7.40	7.35
4	9.16	8.86	8.57	8.29	8.02	7.76	7.51	7.46	7.41	7.36	7.31	7.26	7.22	7.17
5	8.93	8.64	8.36	8.09	7.83	7.57	7.33	7.28	7.23	7.18	7.14	7.09	7.04	7.00
6	8.70	8.42	8.15	7.89	7.64	7.39	7.15	7.11	7.06	7.01	6.97	6.92	6.88	6.83
7	8.49	8.22	7.95	7.70	7.45	7.22	6.98	6.94	6.89	6.85	6.81	6.76	6.72	6.67
8	8.28	8.02	7.76	7.52	7.28	7.05	6.82	6.78	6.74	6.69	6.65	6.61	6.57	6.52
9	8.08	7.83	7.58	7.34	7.11	6.89	6.67	6.63	6.59	6.54	6.50	6.46	6.42	6.38
10	7.89	7.64	7.41	7.17	6.95	6.73	6.52	6.48	6.44	6.40	6.36	6.32	6.28	6.24
11	7.71	7.47	7.24	7.01	6.80	6.58	6.38	6.34	6.30	6.26	6.22	6.18	6.14	6.10
12	7.53	7.30	7.08	6.86	6.65	6.44	6.24	6.21	6.17	6.13	6.09	6.05	6.01	5.98
13	7.37	7.14	6.92	6.71	6.50	6.31	6.11	6.07	6.04	6.00	5.96	5.93	5.89	5.85
14	7.20	6.98	6.77	6.57	6.37	6.17	5.99	5.95	5.91	5.88	5.84	5.80	5.77	5.73
15	7.05	6.84	6.63	6.43	6.24	6.05	5.87	5.83	5.79	5.76	5.72	5.69	5.65	5.62
16	6.90	6.69	6.49	6.30	6.11	5.93	5.75	5.71	5.68	5.64	5.61	5.58	5.54	5.51
17	6.75	6.55	6.36	6.17	5.99	5.81	5.64	5.60	5.57	5.53	5.50	5.47	5.43	5.40
18	6.61	6.42	6.23	6.05	5.87	5.69	5.53	5.49	5.46	5.43	5.40	5.36	5.33	5.30
19	6.48	6.29	6.11	5.93	5.75	5.59	5.42	5.39	5.36	5.33	5.29	5.26	5.23	5.20
20	6.35	6.17	5.99	5.81	5.64	5.48	5.32	5.29	5.26	5.23	5.20	5.17	5.14	5.10
21	6.23	6.05	5.87	5.70	5.54	5.38	5.22	5.10	5.16	5.13	5.10	5.07	5.04	5.01
22	6.11	5.93	5.76	5.60	5.44	5.28	5.13	5.10	5.07	5.04	5.01	4.98	4.95	4.92
23	5.99	5.82	5.65	5.49	5.34	5.18	5.04	5.01	4.98	4.95	4.92	4.89	4.87	4.84

ml of filtered seawater, but with no animal, acts as a control. Following a 2-h incubation period in a water bath at the field ambient temperature, samples are taken from each beaker and analysed for ammonia using the phenol-hypochlorite method of Solorzano (1969).

Elevated ammonia concentrations (above approx. 10 μM NH_4-N litre^{-1}) can inhibit the rate of NH_4 excretion. The incubation time and volume of water should therefore be adjusted when necessary.

Ammonia Test

Into each tube place:

    10 ml seawater sample
    0.4 ml phenol solution
Mix well; add
    0.4 ml nitroprusside solution
Mix; add
    1 ml oxidising solution (made fresh)
Mix well
Cap tubes and place in dark.

Read on spectrophotometer at 640 nm after 2–24 h. Carry out analysis in duplicate with clean test tubes (acid-wash tubes or heat tubes at 450°C in muffle furnace).

For standards, with deionized–distilled H_2O (DW) as blank, use:

    1 μM (10 μl stock in 10 ml DW)
    5 μM (50 μl stock in 10 ml DW)
  10 μM (100 μl stock in 10 ml DW)
  20 μM (200 μl stock in 10 ml DW)
  40 μM (400 μl stock in 10 ml DW)

Use 10 ml of standards and treat same as samples.

Reagents

1.   Phenol solution:
    Dissolve 10 g phenol in 100 ml of 95% v/v ethyl alcohol. Store at 5°C.

2. Sodium nitroprusside:
   Dissolve 1 g of sodium nitroprusside in 200 ml DW. Store in amber bottle at 5°C for not more than 1 month.
3. Oxidizing solution:
   Mix 25 ml fresh domestic bleach (commercial hypochlorite) with 100 ml alkaline solution. This solution is only stable for ca. 12 h and has to be made up fresh each day.
4. Alkaline solution:
   Dissolve 100 g trisodium citrate and 5 g NaOH in 500 ml DW. Store at 5°C.
5. Standard stock solution:
   1 mM NH$_4$Cl = 0.05349 g NH$_4$Cl per litre. Add a few drops of chloroform to preserve.

Calculation of Ammonia Excretion Rate

Construct a standard curve and convert optical density (O.D.) readings for samples and control to μM NH$_4$Cl. Subtract the control from the samples and express rate of excretion as μg NH$_4$-N h^{-1}.

Example:
When

$$1 \ \mu M \ \text{NH}_4\text{Cl} = 0.05349 \ \text{mg litre}^{-1} \text{ or } 14 \ \mu\text{g NH}_4\text{-N litre}^{-1}$$

Then:

$$\mu\text{g NH}_4\text{-N excreted h}^{-1} = (\text{test } \mu M - \text{control } \mu M) \times \frac{14}{1,000/V} \times \frac{1}{t}$$

where V = volume of seawater in which animal is incubated (200 ml) and t = incubation time (2 h).

Correct excretion rates to a standard body size.

Calculation of Scope for Growth

To calculate the scope for growth, the physiological components of the energy equation are first converted to energy equivalents (J h^{-1}) as follows:

1. Energy consumed (C):
   C = clearance rate (litre h^{-1}) $\times$ POM (mg litre^{-1}) $\times$ energy content of POM (J mg^{-1})
   The energy content of particulate organic matter (POM) is approximately 23.5 J mg^{-1} (Widdows et al., 1979b), a typical energy value for most organisms and food materials (Slobodkin and Richman, 1961).
   Under conditions where pseudofaeces are produced, the "energy consumed" (C) is not equivalent to the energy ingested by the animal but is the energy filtered from suspension by the gills.
   When physiological measurements are performed in the laboratory using cultured algal cells as food, it is necessary to establish conversion factors for:

   (a) algal cell numbers to algal dry mass (i.e. 10^6 cells = ? mg), and

   (b) algal dry mass to energy content (i.e. 1 mg = ? J).

   This enables the algal concentration (cells litre^{-1}) in the inflow water to be converted to mg litre^{-1} and thence to J litre^{-1}. Energy consumed (C) is therefore the clearance rate (litre h^{-1}) multiplied by the energy content of the algal cells per litre (J litre^{-1}).
2. Energy absorbed from the seston (A):
   $A = C$ (J h^{-1}) $\times e$
   where e = absorption efficiency.
3. Energy respired (R):
   $R = \dot{V}_{O_2}$ (ml O$_2$ h^{-1}) $\times$ 20.33
   Note that the oxygen consumption is converted to Joules by multiplying ml O$_2$ h^{-1} by 20.33.
4. Energy excreted (U):
   $U = $ NH$_4$ excretion (μg NH$_4$-N h^{-1}) $\times$ 0.0249.
   Note that the ammonia excretion is converted to Joules by multiplying μg NH$_4$-N h^{-1} by 0.0249.

On the basis of the above energy equivalents, the scope for growth (P) can now be calculated from the equation

$$P \text{ (J h}^{-1}) = A - (R + U)$$

Examples of the method are shown in Table 7-2.

TABLE 7-2. The Calculation of Scope for Growth of *M. edulis* of 1 g Dry Flesh Weight

					C	e	$A = (C \times e)$	R	E	$A - (R + E)$
Animal	Clearance rate (litre h^{-1})	×	P.O.M. × 23.5 (mg $litre^{-1}$) (J mg^{-1})	=	Energy consumed (J h^{-1})	Absorption efficiency	Energy absorbed (J h^{-1})	Energy respired (J h^{-1})	Energy excreted (J h^{-1})	Scope for growth (J h^{-1})
1	4.603	×	5.08	=	23.38	.58	13.56	7.22	0.39	+5.95
2	4.349	×	5.08	=	22.09	.58	12.81	8.27	0.40	+4.14
3	4.673	×	5.08	=	23.74	.58	13.77	5.57	0.52	+7.68
4	4.358	×	5.08	=	22.14	.58	12.84	5.77	0.34	+6.73
.	.		.		.	.	.	.	.	.
.	.		.		.	.	.	.	.	.
.	.		.		.	.	.	.	.	.

From Widdows et al. (1981a).
Note: Data obtained from study at Ronas Voe, October 1978.

NET GROWTH EFFICIENCY

The net growth efficiency, K_2, is a measure of the efficiency with which food is converted into body tissues. It is calculated from components of the balanced energy equation as follows:

$$K_2 = \frac{A - (R + U)}{A}$$

where A is the energy absorbed from the food (J h^{-1}), R is the energy respired (J h^{-1}) and U is the energy excreted (J h^{-1}).

Example:
Site: Ronas Voe; date: October 1978 (from data in Table 7-2).

Animal	A	R	U	$K_2 = \dfrac{A - (R + U)}{A}$
1	13.56	7.22	0.39	0.44
2	12.81	8.27	0.40	0.32
3	13.77	5.57	0.52	0.56
4	12.84	5.77	0.34	0.52
⋮	⋮	⋮	⋮	⋮

THE OXYGEN TO NITROGEN RATIO

The rate of oxygen consumed to nitrogen excreted is calculated in atomic equivalents:

1. Multiply the rate of oxygen consumption in ml O_2 h^{-1} by 1.428 to convert to mg O_2 h^{-1} and then divide by the atomic weight (16).
2. Divide the rate of nitrogen excretion in mg NH_4-N h^{-1} by the atomic weight (14).

$$\text{Then } O:N = \frac{\text{ml } O_2 \times 1.428}{16} : \frac{\text{mg } NH_4\text{-N h}^{-1}}{14}$$

Example:
Site: Ronas Voe; date: October 1978.

Animal	Oxygen consumption (ml O_2 h^{-1})	Ammonia excretion (mg NH_4-N h^{-1})	Atomic equivalents		Ratio O:N
			O	N	
1	0.355	0.016	0.0317	0.0011	28.8
2	0.407	0.016	0.0363	0.0011	33.0
3	0.274	0.021	0.0245	0.0015	16.3
4	0.284	0.014	0.0253	0.001	25.3
⋮	⋮	⋮	⋮	⋮	⋮

Calculate the mean and the variance about the mean.

BODY CONDITION INDEX

The body condition index based on dry tissue mass is calculated as follows:

$$\text{B.C.I.} = \frac{\text{Dry tissue mass (g)}}{\text{Shell cavity volume (ml)}} \times 1{,}000$$

The shell cavity volume is the total displacement volume of a completely closed bivalve, minus the displacement volume of the shell, after opening and removing the body tissues.

The dry tissue mass is determined by drying the soft tissues in pre-weighed containers to constant weight (ca. 24 h) at $90°C$.

Example:
Dry mass of tissues = 1.048 g
Total displacement volume of animal = 21 ml
Displacement volume of shell = 3 ml

$$\text{B.C.I.} = \frac{1.048}{21 - 3} \times 1{,}000$$

$$= 58.2$$

Calculate mean and variance about the mean ($n > 10$).

8

Cytological and Cytochemical Procedures

PREPARATION
OF TISSUE SECTIONS
FOR CYTOLOGY

The preparation of tissues for the examination of cell structures demands the use of specialized methodology. Relevant techniques are described in the following section, where particular emphasis is placed on the preparation of tissues for subsequent quantitative analysis of the cell composition of the tissues, cellular structure and enzyme cytochemistry. The ability to make the types of observations discussed in Chapter 2 demands the preparation of high-quality stained sections. Such sections can be prepared in a variety of ways depending ultimately on the type of observations to be made, but for the most part the sequence of events leading to the finished product is very similar.

In this chapter all observations are related to either wax-embedded or frozen material, and it is these preparative techniques that will be described. The preparation of wax-embedded sections has several distinct phases—fixation, dehydration, embedding, sectioning and finally staining—and each stage is critical for the preparation of good sections.

Fixation

Fixation is perhaps the most important stage: incorrect fixation will result in tissue breakdown—making reliable observations almost impossible—or, if the wrong fixative has been used, certain techniques may not be applicable. Several factors must be taken into consideration in the choice of fixatives for any particular application. The number of fixatives available is extensive, and each has its own merits and disadvantages. Some fixatives fix nuclei in preference to cytoplasm, and vice versa. Certain solutions are good lipid and carbohydrate fixatives, others are superior for protein-rich connective tissues. The final choice, therefore, is governed by the nature of the material to be examined and the components to be demonstrated.

For our observations reported to date, the main fixative used has been Baker's formol calcium (2.0% sodium acetate, 10% formalin) with 2.5% sodium chloride added to render it isosmotic with the body fluids of the animals examined. The use of this fixative makes it possible to cut both wax and frozen tissues, and fixation is usually carried out at 4°C for 24 h. The maximum size of a piece of tissue to be fixed should not exceed 5 × 5 × 5 mm and the ratio of tissue to fixative should not be greater than 1:10. Following fixation, the tissue block is cut into two pieces, rinsed in distilled water and stored in gum sucrose at 4°C prior to either wax embedding and/or preparation of frozen sections.

The demonstration of lipids in frozen sections and carbohydrates (mainly glycogen) in wax sections is frequently necessary, and Baker's formol calcium has proved to be suitable for both purposes, causing minimal streaming artifacts in the glycogen-rich cells. It may also be necessary to demonstrate metal ions in tissues, which makes it imperative to employ a fixative (such as Baker's) that does not iteself contain any metal ions; Helly's and Zenker's solutions do not meet this criterion. However, a single fixative will not suffice for all animal types and tissues. For example, when Baker's formol calcium was used on *Chlamys* a great deal of shrinkage of the reproductive tissues resulted; it was therefore necessary to employ Davidson's fixative (Shaw and Battle, 1957). This fixative contains—in addition to formalin, glycogen and 95% alcohol—acetic acid which causes tissues to swell, thereby counteracting any effects due to shrinkage. The solution is made up in filtered seawater to achieve the necessary osmotic balance.

Dehydration and Embedding

The preparation of frozen tissues is discussed later; this section will concentrate exclusively on the preparation of wax-embedded material. The sequence of events required for a processing schedule leading to wax embedding is very simple. Basically, water is removed from the tissues by an ascending alcohol series, the alcohol is then removed by a solvent which is miscible with both alcohol and wax (e.g. xylene or Histosol, Shandon Southern products) and then the tissue is placed in wax. Many schedules exist and most of them differ from one another in several ways, usually in terms of the time spent in the solutions, the concentrations of the alcohol series and the nature of the de-alcoholizing ("clearing") agent.

Prior to dehydration, the tissues are washed in distilled water to remove the gum sucrose; the processing schedule is then as follows:

70% alcohol	2 h
90% alcohol	1 h
absolute alcohol (4 changes)	1 h each
50:50 absolute alcohol/xylene	1 h
xylene (2 changes)	1 h each
wax (2 changes)	1 h each

This schedule is run overnight on an automatic tissue processor. If no processor is available then alternative schedules may be used; e.g. a wax vacuum oven can shorten the time in wax to about 30 min. Time can also be saved by reducing the number of absolute alcohol changes; however, as a general rule the shorter the dehydration time used the smaller the piece of tissue which can be processed. Several leading authorities advocate that the ascending alcohol series should commence at 30% alcohol, then to 50%, 70%, 90% and so to absolute alcohol; this is particularly recommended for fragile tissues.

Having impregnated the tissues with wax, they must be made up into wax blocks for presentation to the microtome knife. There are numerous methods for preparing wax blocks, and the choice is very much one of preference and convenience depending on several factors including the type of microtome to be used. Whatever the choice of mould used, one point is common to all systems: the specimens must be picked up and placed in the mould with hot forceps, otherwise (1) the specimens will stick to the forceps and (2) air bubbles will gather around the specimen and make sectioning more difficult. In our laboratory two blocking systems are used, one of which utilises rubber moulds (Cambridge Instruments); the other is a complete dehydration and blocking system in one comprehensive cassette (Ames) which also contains the identity number of the sample. Having prepared the wax block, it must be allowed to set solid before any cutting can be undertaken. The method often employed with open type moulds such as those produced by Cambridge Instruments is to wait until a skin has formed on the surface of the wax mould (ca. 3 min) and then slowly and gently lower the mould into still, cold water. This will instantly set the surface solid, and the mould can then be released and allowed to sink into the water where the wax will solidify. Alternatively, the mould can be left on a cool part of the bench for 1 h or more where it will solidify slowly; we have found this to be a better method. With the Ames moulds a chilled plate can be employed; this has the effect of solidifying the wax quickly and also effects an easy release of the wax block from the mould.

Sectioning

The cutting of tissue sections is performed on a microtome. These devices fall into two broad categories—those in which the block moves across a stationary knife and, conversely, those in which the knife moves across a stationary block. There are numerous refinements within these two groups, making some models more desirable than others. Many of the modern microtomes are of the rocking, rotary retracting type which employ the best of the many individual refinements developed over the years (e.g. Bright model 5030/WDM). The cutting angle is all important and there must be some clearance between the block and the cutting facet of the knife (clearance angle) to prevent the cutting facet scraping across the block surface. The whole cutting geometry for any microtome, knife and block complex must be established before reliable and repeatable sections can be obtained. Although the recommended clearance angle lies between 3 and 5°, and there are many theoretical considerations which might be taken into account in assessing the best cutting geometry, the most appropriate angle will probably be arrived at by trial and error.

Once cut, the sections are flattened on a water bath at 40°C and then collected on acid-cleaned, albuminised microscope slides, "frosted" at one end and dried in an oven (50°C) for at least 4 h before routine staining. Whilst frosted-end microscope slides are more expensive than plain slides, they make slide identification easier, as the reference number can be written on the frosted area in pencil. The slides are coated with egg albumen (in dilute glycerol) to improve adhesion of the sections, thereby reducing the likelihood of their floating off during staining.

Staining

A vast number of stains are available to the histologist to demonstrate tissues and their component cells. Listed below are the three stains and their schedules that we have employed to demonstrate the various tissue components required in our work with marine bivalves.

Papanicolaou Method (Non-specific, General-purpose Stain)

Dewax sections in xylene	5 min
Rinse in absolute alcohol	2 min
Rinse in 70% alcohol	2 min
Rinse in tap water	5 min
Stain in Harris's haematoxylin	3 min
Wash in tap water until sections are blue	5 min
Differentiate in 0.1% hydrochloric acid solution	
Blue in ammonia water	
Wash in tap water	2 min
Rinse in 70% alcohol	1 min
Rinse in 95% alcohol	1 min
Stain in Papanicolaou O.G.6. solution	3 min
Rinse in 95% alcohol	1 min
Stain in Papanicolaou E.A.50 solution	3 min
Rinse in 95% alcohol	1 min
Rinse in absolute alcohol	2 min
Clean in xylene	2 min
Mount in colophonium resin or DPX	

Results in *Mytilus* section: Nuclei, blue; muscle, red; connective tissues, green; adipogranular cells, orange; sperms, blue; oocytes, blue to mauve.

Feulgen Reaction (DNA-specific Stain)

Dewax sections in xylene	5 min
Rinse in absolute alcohol	2 min
Rinse in 70% alcohol	2 min
Rinse in tap water	5 min
Treat with 1 N HCl at 60°C	10 min
Wash in tap water	5 min
Rinse in distilled water	1 min
Treat with Schiff reagent at room temperature	45 min
Wash in tap water	15 min
Rinse with 3 N HCl	1 min
Wash in tap water	2 min
Counterstain with 0.1% light green	30 sec
Rinse with tap water	1 min
Rinse in 70% alcohol	1 min
Rinse in absolute alcohol	2 min
Clean in xylene	2 min
Mount in colophonium resin or DPX	

Results: Nuclear material, magenta; all other tissues, green.

Periodic Acid–Schiff Reaction (Glycogen-specific Stain, with Amylose Controls)

To verify that a stain can be attributed to the presence of glycogen it is necessary to stain slides in pairs. In conjunction with the complete schedule below, one of each pair is treated, just prior to the periodic acid stage, with 0.1% malt diastase at 37°C for 40 min and rinsed in distilled water for 1 min.

Dewax both sections in xylene	5 min
Rinse in absolute alcohol	2 min
Rinse in 70% alcohol	2 min
Rinse in tap water	5 min
Rinse in distilled water	1 min
Treat with 1% periodic acid solution	10 min

Wash in tap water	2 min
Rinse in distilled water	1 min
Treat with Schiff reagent at room temperature	20 min
Wash in tap water	15 min
Rinse with 3 N HCl	1 min
Wash in tap water	2 min
Counterstain nuclei in Coles haematoxylin	5 min
Wash in tap water until nuclei blue	5 min
Differentiate in 1% hydrochloric acid	
Blue nuclei in ammonia water	
Wash in tap water	2 min
Rinse in 70% alcohol	1 min
Rinse in absolute alcohol	2 min
Clear in xylene	2 min
Mount in colophonium resin or DPX	

Results: Magenta staining in the non–diastase-treated slide which is not present in the other slide can be attributed to glycogen.

QUANTITATIVE ANALYSIS OF TISSUES AND CELLS BY MORPHOMETRIC TECHNIQUES

Stereology has been defined as the extrapolation from two dimensional to three-dimensional space (Freere, 1967; Briarty, 1975). Information regarding cell volumes can be derived, assuming certain sampling criteria are met, from point counts on a two-dimensional surface. The resulting statistic is termed the volume fraction and is usually expressed as a percentage of the total volume analysed. That is, the volume fraction relates to that proportion or percentage of a tissue mass composed of cell x or cell y. For example, in the reproductive tissues in mussels, volume fractions of ripe and developing gametes as well as the adipogranular cells and vesicular connective tissue cells (and blood spaces) can be obtained from simple point counts using a Weibel graticule as a sampling matrix (Bayne et al., 1978; Lowe et al., 1982). The theory behind this technique has been discussed by Elias et al. (1971), Weibel and Elias (1967) and Weibel (1969); only the methodology used for mussels (*M. edulis*) is described here.

Mantle tissue

The mantle tissue of mussels is essentially composed of connective tissue storage cells, blood spaces and at certain times of the year germinal cells (Lowe et al., 1982). All of these cells ramify throughout the mantle lobes with no predisposition towards any particular part of the mantle. This is an important requirement, since in applying stereological principles it is necessary to have tissue sections that are truly representative of the tissue mass. The spatial homogeneity of the cell types within the mantle signifies that a section from any part of the mantle lobe is equally representative of the overall cellular composition. Figure 8-1 is a schematic representation of a typical section of mantle tissue with a Weibel graticule superimposed. Point counts are scored where the end of the test line (⊢) falls on a cell or group of cells under examination. Therefore, in Fig. 8-1, 9 counts (or "hits") are scored on ripe sperm, 15 counts on developing sperm, 6 counts on adipogranular cells and 12 counts on vesicular connective tissue cells. This procedure is repeated for a number of fields, and the sum of counts per cell type is determined and expressed as a percentage of the total possible. Table 8-1 is an example of such an analysis on eight mussels, scanning 5 fields per animal, using a Weibel sampling matrix as shown in Fig. 8-1, which has 42 end points (⊢) from which observations can be taken. The maximum number of possible counts on 5 fields is therefore 210 (i.e. 5 × 42). The volume fraction for any cell type is given by

$$\frac{\text{Number of counts per cell type}}{210} \times 100$$

In order to relate changes in cell volume fraction to the whole tissue, it is necessary to measure the total tissue weight or volume prior the fixation of samples. In the mantle, for example, the ripe gamete fraction may decline with time, but the total volume of ripe gametes may increase due to an overall increase in mantle size.

Digestive Tubules

The main morphological difference between the four different stages of digestive tubules of *M. edulis* (Langton, 1975) is the height of the epithelial cells (Lowe et al., 1981). This variable can be used as an index for the condition of the tubules which can be measured on photomicrographs or projected images of digestive gland sections within a mussel. Figure 8-2 shows a schematic draw-

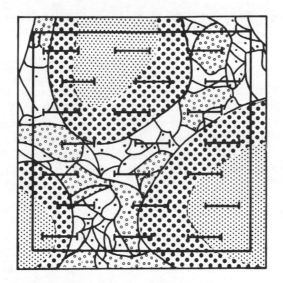

FIG. 8-1. Weibel point-counting graticule for determination of volume fractions of reproductive cells.

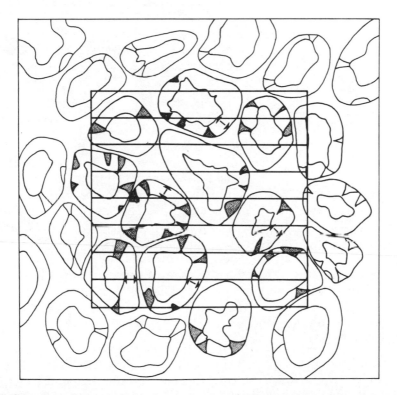

FIG. 8-2. Sampling matrix for determination of intercept points for measurement of digestive epithelium height.

TABLE 8–1. Stereological Assessment of Gametogenesis in the Mantle Tissue of *M. edulis*

Animal	Ripe	V.F.	Developing	V.F.
1	15 7 15 23 5	31.0	18 14 13 13 14	34.3
2	12 6 29 3 6	26.6	14 15 9 21 9	32.4
3	9 14 9 5 5	20.0	16 9 13 6 11	26.2
4	12 24 0 3 22	29.0	8 4 13 6 14	21.4
5	14 4 9 15 15	26.2	17 9 22 14 9	33.8
6	6 6 7 19 11	23.3	7 10 7 9 14	22.4
7	6 20 7 9 18	28.6	6 7 15 7 9	21.0
8	25 0 9 5 9	22.9	12 5 3 8 8	17.1
	$\bar{x}$	25.95	$\bar{x}$	26.08
	S.D.	3.67	S.D.	6.64
	S.E.	1.30	S.E.	2.35
	All morphologically ripe eggs and sperms		All developmental stages of eggs and sperms	

ing of digestive tubules in various stages as they might appear during a digestive cycle (Langton, 1975), and over this a parallel-line sampling grid has been superimposed from which measurements of intercept lengths of epithelial cells are made. The measurements taken represent the shortest distance between the point of intersection of the apical cell surface with a test line to the nearest point on the basement membrane. If a tubule has been sectioned obliquely, giving the appearance of being more oval than circular, then the epithelium may be several cell layers deep, in which case it is not measured. Intercept lengths made on 50 individual tubules from each of five animals in the various treatment groups are then used to calculate the mean epithelial cell height and the standard deviation. A two-way analysis of variance, with one stage of subsampling, can then be used to examine the variance both within and between animals for the detection of treatment, time and treatment × time interaction effects on the mean epithelial cell height (Lowe et al., 1981).

In addition, tissue sections prepared as described in this section can be screened for the presence of the following histopathological conditions:

1. Granulocytomas.
2. Haemapoetic neoplasms.
3. Haemacytic infiltrations.
4. Parasitic infestations.

Evacuated	V.F.	Adipogran	V.F.	V.C.T.	V.F.
0 0 0 0 3	1.4	6 11 9 1 5	15.2	3 5 4 3 6	10.0
0 0 0 0 0	0	10 11 2 9 24	26.7	3 8 0 6 2	9.0
0 0 0 0 0	0	11 12 15 20 8	31.4	3 3 5 9 14	16.2
0 0 0 0 0	0	15 4 12 17 3	24.3	4 4 7 2 3	9.5
1 0 0 0 0	0.5	3 7 2 4 8	11.4	3 5 4 3 4	9.0
3 0 0 4 1	3.8	9 9 8 3 6	16.7	4 4 6 4 4	10.5
2 1 0 0 2	2.4	7 2 5 8 6	13.3	7 5 5 9 3	13.8
0 0 0 0 0	0	2 6 13 6 5	15.2	2 6 4 6 11	5.2
$\bar{x}$	1.01	$\bar{x}$	19.28	$\bar{x}$	10.40
	S.D. 1.42		S.D. 7.22		S.D. 3.32
	S.E. 0.50		S.E. 2.55		S.E. 1.17
Spaces in follicles resulting from spawning activity		Adipogranular cells		Vesicular cells	

PREPARATION OF TISSUE SECTIONS FOR ENZYME CYTOCHEMISTRY

For cytochemical examination, small pieces (3–4 mm^3) of freshly excised tissues are placed on an aluminium cryostat chuck (e.g. up to 5 pieces of tissue in a straight row across the centre). The chuck is then placed for 1 min in a small bath of hexane (aromatic hydrocarbon-free; boiling range 67–70°C) which has been pre-cooled to −70°C (using a surrounding bath of liquid nitrogen or a mixture of crushed solid CO_2 and acetone). The chuck plus the supercooled solidified tissues are then sealed by double-wrapping in parafilm and stored at −30°C or, preferably, at −70°C until required for sectioning. Tissues may be stored for 4–6 months at −70°C. By following this procedure there is no formation of ice and hence no structural damage to the subcellular components (Bitensky et al., 1973). Cryostat sections (10 μm) are cut in a Bright's Cryostat (preferably with motorised cutting) with the cabinet temperature below −25°C and with the knife cooled with crushed solid CO_2. The sections are transferred to "warm" slides (i.e. 20°C, or room temperature), which effectively flash-dries them (Bitensky et al., 1973), and the slides can be stored in the cryostat for at least 4 h. Cryostat sections that are required for concurrent structural or non-enzymic cytochemistry can be post-fixed in calcium formol.

LYSOSOMAL STABILITY

Demonstration of Latent Activity of Lysosomal Hydrolases for Assessment of Lysosomal Stability

Latent lysosomal activity of the lysosomal enzymes N-acetyl- β-hexosaminidase, β-glucuronidase and arylsulphatase can be demonstrated in the digestive cells of bivalve molluscs using naphthol AS-BI substrates and post-coupling with diazonium salts to prevent inhibition by the coupler.

Method for N-Acetyl-β-hexosaminidase

Serial cryostat sections prepared as described above are pretreated in a staining jar containing 0.1 M citrate buffer (pH 4.5) containing 2.5% NaCl (w:v) at 37°C in order to labilise the lysosomes (Bitensky et al., 1973; Moore, 1976). The pretreatment sequence commences at 26 min down to 2 min, at 3-min intervals. A sequence of 5-min intervals can also be used if less precision is required (i.e. 25, 20, 15, 10, 5 and 2 min). Two minutes is used as the minimal pretreatment time as sections that have undergone zero pretreatment may sometimes show stronger staining than short-term pretreated sections (Moore, 1976). This staining activity is believed to be largely due to non-membrane bound hydrolase which can be lost by diffusion from the section when no polypeptide stabiliser is present. Such activity is frequently localised in large secondary lysosomes or digestive vacuoles which may be damaged in sectioning. Due to this complicating factor, the zero preincubation is usually omitted and the 2-min pretreatment is taken as representing the free lysosomal activity.

The pretreatment procedure can be further refined by first incubating the sections as indicated above to determine the approximate pretreatment time required to labilise the lysosomes, and then carrying out a second series of pretreatments at 1-min intervals in the appropriate time period to obtain greater precision. The alternative is to carry out the full pretreatment sequence at 1-min intervals, although from our experience this degree of precision is not usually necessary (see section below, Determination of Lysosomal Labilisation Period).

Following this pretreatment sequence, the slides are transferred to the substrate incubation medium; this contains 20 mg napthol AS-BI-N-acetyl-β-D-glucosaminide (Sigma, Koch-Light) dissolved in 2.5 ml 2-methoxyethanol which is made up to 50 ml with 0.1 M citrate buffer (pH 4.5) containing 2.5% NaCl (w : v) and 3.5 g of low viscosity polypeptide (Sigma POLYPEP P5115) to act as a section stabiliser (Bitensky et al., 1973; Moore, 1976). Incubation time is 20 min at 37°C in a staining jar, preferably in a shaking water-bath. The slides are subsequently rinsed in 3.0% NaCl at 37°C for 2 min before being transferred to 0.1 M phosphate buffer (pH 7.4) containing a diazonium coupler (1 mg ml^{-1}) at room temperature for 10 min. Suitable diazonium salts are fast violet B (Sigma), fast red violet LB (Difco), fast garnet GBC (Sigma), fast blue BB (Sigma) and fast blue RR (Sigma). The slides are then rinsed rapidly in running tap water, fixed for 10 min in calcium formol containing 2.5% NaCl (w : v) at 4°C, rinsed in distilled water and mounted in aqueous mounting medium (e.g. Difco UV-free aqueous mounting medium).

Methods for β-Glucuronidase and Arylsulphatase

The method for the demonstration of latent activity of lysosomal β-glucuronidase (Moore, 1976) is essentially similar to the method described above, but with the following exceptions: the pretreatment to labilise the lysosomal membranes is carried out using 0.1 M *acetate* buffer (pH 4.5) containing 2.5% NaCl (w : v), and the substrate incubation uses 14 mg naphthol AS-Bl-β-D glucuronide (Sigma, Koch-Light) as substrate dissolved in 0.6 ml 50 mM NaHCO$_3$, which is made up to 50 ml with 0.1 M acetate buffer (pH 4.5) containing 2.5% NaCl (w : v) and 3.5 g of polypeptide (Sigma POLYPEP P5115) at 37°C for 20 min.

For the demonstration of latency of arylsulphatase (Moore, 1980b; Moore et al., 1982), the sections are pretreated as for β-glucuronidase (see above) to labilise the membranes. The substrate incubation medium contains 30 mg naphthol AS-BI sulphate (Sigma) dissolved in 2 ml 2-methozyethanol and made up to 50 ml with 0.1 M acetate buffer (pH 5.5) containing 2.5% NaCl (w : v) and 3.5 g polypeptide (Sigma POLYPEP P5115) at 37°C for 20 min. The substrate forms an opaque microcrystalline suspension when the acetate buffer is added.

Rinsing and coupling solutions for both β-glucuronidase and arylsulphatase are the same as those used for hexosaminidase.

Determination of Lysosomal Labilisation Period

The labilisation period is the time of pretreatment required to labilise the lysosomal membranes fully, resulting in maximal staining intensity for the enzyme being assayed (Fig. 8-3). The staining intensity can be measured using a scanning integrating microdensitometer to obtain an activity plot as shown in Fig. 8-4 (Bitensky et al., 1973). As the organism is stressed (in this instance with phenanthrene) the peak of activity would be moved towards the y axis and the decreased labilisation period determined from the x axis (Fig. 8-4).

Alternatively, if a microdensitometer is not available, then the labilisation period can be accurately determined by microscopical assessment of the maximum staining intensity in the preincubation series (Fig. 8-3).

As mentioned above, this technique does not usually require the degree of precision obtained from a pretreatment sequence at 1-min intervals. Intervals of 3 or 5 min are generally satisfactory for most test situations. When 3- or 5-min intervals are used the data can be statistically tested (i.e. test data compared with reference or base-line data) using the Mann-Whitney U-test (Siegel, 1956). When applying this test to our data we have found that there is sometimes a problem with ties, i.e. many of the labilisation periods for one sample (5 animals) are the same and overlap may occur between the data sets being compared. In the situation where there are ties and overlap, a special table of tie vectors has been produced (Table 8-2) which permits the determination of the level of significance for critical values of the U-statistic. Two examples of the use of the table of tie vectors are given below. It should be especially noted that Table 8-2 is designed for *sample sizes of 5*.

Example 1:

Labilisation period (min)	2	5	8	11	14
Sample A	* * *	* *			
Rank	2, 2, 2	5.5, 5.5			
Sample B		* *	* * *		
Rank		5.5, 5.5	9, 9, 9		
Tie vector	3	4	3		

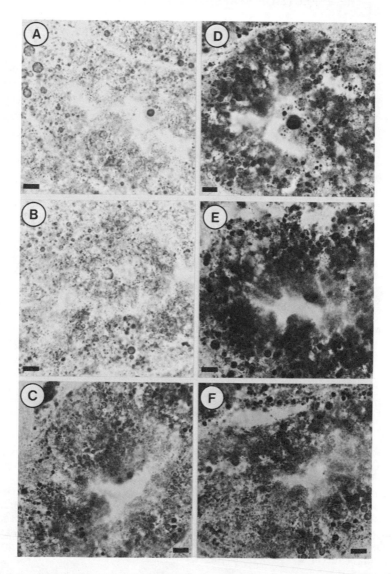

FIG. 8-3. Serial cryostat sections of the digestive gland stained to show N-acetyl-β-hexosaminidase reactivity in the lysosomal vacuolar system of digestive cells in a digestive tubule of *M. edulis*. *A*. Section pretreated at pH 4.5 and 37°C for 2 min. *B*. Section pretreated for 5 min showing a slight increase in the staining intensity of some lysosomes. *C*. Section pretreated for 11 min showing a continuing increase in lysosomal staining intensity. *D*. Section pretreated for 14 min showing a continuing increase in lysosomal staining. *E*. Section pretreated for 17 min showing maximal lysosomal staining intensity; this time of pretreatment represents the labilisation period. *F*. Section pretreated for 23 min showing a decrease in staining intensity indicating a probable loss of enzyme by diffusion from fully labilised lysosomes. (Scale Bar $\equiv$ 10 μm.)

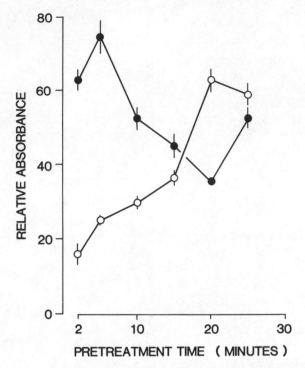

FIG. 8-4. The effect of pretreatment of sections at pH 4.5 and 37°C on the activity of lysosomal N-acetyl-β-hexosaminidase in the digestive cells of *M. edulis*. Open circles: mussels injected with 100 μl of medicinal liquid paraffin (used as a carrier medium for phenanthrene). Closed circles: mussels injected with 100 μl 10^{-2} M phenanthrene in liquid paraffin. Mussels were sampled after 24 h. It is evident that the phenanthrene induces a shift to the left in the maximal activity peak indicating a decreased pretreatment time required to activate latent lysosomal hexosaminidase. A secondary increase in activity is apparent in the phenanthrene treated tissue. Points represent means, bars are ± S.E., $n = 10$ readings. Microdensitometric measurements were made using a Vickers M85 microdensitometer with a measuring spot size of 0.5 μm (×40 objective, spot size 1) and a circular mask diameter of 13 μm. As fast violet B was used as the post-coupling diazonium salt, the wavelength setting was 560 nm.

The tie vector is determined by:

(a) ignoring the difference between A and B;
(b) totalling the numbers of data points (*) in each cell;
(c) omitting any empty cells.

Calculate the Mann-Whitney U-statistic in the normal manner (Siegel, 1956):

$$R_A = 2 + 2 + 2 + 5.5 + 5.5 = 17$$
$$U = n_A \, n_B + \tfrac{1}{2}[n_A(n_A + 1)] - R_A$$
$$= 25 + 15 - 17 = 23.$$

Then calculate $U' = n_A n_B - U \ (= 25 - 23 = 2)$; the U-statistic is defined to be the smaller of U and U'.

The critical value of U for the 3 4 3 tie vector is ≤ 2.0 for significance at the 5% level (Table 8-2). Therefore, A is significantly lower than B at the 5% level.

Example 2:

Labilisation period (min)	2	5	8	11	14
Sample A	*		* *	*	*
Rank	3		7, 7	9	10
Sample B		* * * *	*		
Rank		3, 3, 3, 3	7		
Tie vector	5	0	3	1	1

The empty cell is omitted, giving a tie vector 5 3 1 1.

The Mann-Whitney U statistic is calculated in the normal manner:

$$R_A = 3 + 7 + 7 + 9 + 10 = 36$$
$$U = n_A n_B + \tfrac{1}{2}[n_A(n_A + 1)] - R_A$$
$$= 25 + 15 - 36 = 4$$

Hence, $U' = 25 - 4 = 21$. The critical value of U for the 5 3 1 1 tie vector is 0.0 for significance at both the 5% and 1% levels (Table 8-2). Therefore, there is no significant difference between A and B.

Problems in Assessment of Labilisation Period

Determination of labilisation period is usually quite straightforward, but a complicating situation occasionally arises in which the preincubation series shows two peaks of staining intensity (Moore et al., 1978a), possibly due to differential latent properties of the lysosomal hydrolase concerned (Fig. 8-4). In this situation the first peak of activity is used to determine labilisation period as in our experience it has been the most responsive (Fig. 8-4).

TABLE 8-2. Critical Values* of U for Possible Tie Vectors with $n_1 = 5$ and $n_2 = 5$

Tie vector	Critical values of U at % significance		Tie vector	Critical values of U at % significance	
	5.0	1.0		5.0	1.0
91	—	—	334	4.0	—
82	—	—	325	0.0	0.0
73	—	—	316	2.5	—
64	2.5	—	271	—	—
55	0.0	0.0	262	—	—
46	2.5	—	253	—	—
37	—	—	244	4.5	—
28	—	—	235	0.0	0.0
19	—	—	226	2.5	—
811	—	—	217	—	—
721	—	—	181	—	—
712	—	—	172	—	—
631	2.5	—	163	—	—
622	2.5	—	154	5.0	—
613	2.5	—	145	0.0	0.0
541	0.0	0.0	136	2.5	—
532	0.0	0.0	127	—	—
523	0.0	0.0	118	—	—
514	3.0	0.0	7111	—	—
451	5.0	—	6211	2.5	—
442	4.5	—	6121	2.5	—
433	4.0	—	6112	2.5	—
424	0.5	—	5311	0.0	0.0
415	3.0	0.0	5221	0.0	0.0
361	—	—	5212	0.0	0.0
352	—	—	5131	3.0	0.0
343	2.0	—	5122	3.0	0.0

*The critical values are based on the exact permutation distribution of the two-sample U statistic, under the hypothesis of no difference between the two populations being sampled, allowing fully for tied ranks. A great many tied readings are to be expected using this technique; note that standard tables for the U statistic are therefore not appropriate and can be quite misleading. Computer programs have been written which use combinatoric theory to evaluate the full permutation, distribution and specified critical values for U, for any number of readings in each sample. Copies of these programs, written in BASIC PLUS for a DEC PDP 11/40 machine running under RSTS/E, are available from Dr. K. R. Clarke, IMER, Plymouth.

TABLE 8-2. *(Continued)*

Tie vector	Critical values of U at % significance 5.0	1.0	Tie vector	Critical values of U at % significance 5.0	1.0
5113	3.0	0.0	2233	1.0	—
4411	5.0	—	2224	2.5	—
4321	3.5	—	2215	3.0	0.0
4312	3.0	—	2161	—	—
4231	3.0	—	2152	—	—
4222	2.5	—	2143	2.0	—
4213	2.0	—	2134	3.0	—
4141	2.5	0.0	2125	0.0	0.0
4132	2.0	0.0	2116	2.5	—
4123	1.5	0.0	1711	—	—
4114	1.0	0.0	1621	—	—
3511	—	—	1612	—	—
3421	2.0	—	1531	5.0	—
3412	2.0	—	1522	5.0	—
3331	1.0	—	1513	2.0	—
3322	1.0	—	1441	0.0	0.0
3313	3.0	—	1432	0.0	0.0
3241	0.0	0.0	1423	0.0	0.0
3232	0.0	0.0	1414	2.5	0.0
3223	4.0	0.0	1351	5.0	—
3214	1.5	0.0	1342	4.5	—
3151	2.0	—	1333	1.0	—
3142	1.5	—	1324	3.0	—
3133	3.0	—	1315	3.0	0.0
3124	2.0	—	1261	—	—
3115	3.0	0.0	1252	—	—
2611	—	—	1243	2.0	—
2521	—	—	1234	3.5	—
2512	—	—	1225	0.0	0.0
2431	4.5	—	1216	2.5	—
2422	1.5	—	1171	—	—
2413	1.5	—	1162	—	—
2341	0.0	0.0	1153	—	—
2332	0.0	0.0	1144	5.0	—
2323	0.0	0.0	1135	0.0	0.0
2314	2.0	0.0	1126	2.5	—
2251	5.0	—	1117	—	—
2242	1.5	—	61111	2.5	—

(continued)

TABLE 8-2. *(Continued)*

Tie vector	Critical values of U at % significance		Tie vector	Critical values of U at % significance	
	5.0	1.0		5.0	1.0
52111	0.0	0.0	23311	0.0	0.0
51211	3.0	0.0	23221	0.0	0.0
51121	3.0	0.0	23212	0.0	0.0
51112	3.0	0.0	23131	2.0	0.0
43111	4.0	—	23122	2.0	0.0
42211	2.5	—	23113	2.0	0.0
42121	2.0	—	22411	4.0	—
42112	3.0	—	22321	1.0	—
41311	4.0	0.0	22312	3.0	—
41221	3.5	0.0	22231	2.5	—
41212	3.0	0.0	22222	2.5	—
41131	3.0	0.0	22213	2.5	—
41122	2.5	0.0	22141	2.5	0.0
41113	2.0	0.0	22132	2.0	0.0
34111	2.0	—	22123	1.5	0.0
33211	1.0	—	22114	2.5	0.0
33121	3.0	—	21511	—	—
33112	3.0	—	21421	2.0	—
32311	0.0	0.0	21412	2.0	—
32221	2.0	0.0	21331	3.0	—
32212	2.0	0.0	21322	3.0	—
32131	1.5	0.0	21313	1.0	—
32122	1.5	0.0	21241	0.0	0.0
32113	2.5	0.0	21232	0.0	0.0
31411	1.5	—	21223	2.0	0.0
31321	3.0	—	21214	3.0	0.0
31312	1.0	—	21151	2.0	—
31231	3.0	—	21142	1.5	—
31222	2.5	—	21133	3.0	—
31213	3.5	—	21124	3.0	—
31141	2.5	0.0	21115	3.0	0.0
31132	2.0	0.0	16111	—	—
31123	2.5	0.0	15211	5.0	—
31114	2.0	0.0	15121	2.0	—
25111	—	—	15112	2.0	—
24211	1.5	—	14311	0.0	0.0
24121	1.5	—	14221	0.0	0.0
24112	1.5	—	14212	0.0	0.0

TABLE 8-2. *(Continued)*

Tie vector	Critical values of U at % significance 5.0	1.0	Tie vector	Critical values of U at % significance 5.0	1.0
14131	2.5	0.0	11251	5.0	—
14122	2.5	0.0	11242	1.5	—
14113	2.5	0.0	11233	1.0	—
13411	4.0	—	11224	2.5	—
13321	3.5	—	11215	3.0	0.0
13312	3.0	—	11161	—	—
13231	0.5	—	11152	—	—
13222	2.5	—	11143	2.0	—
13213	3.0	—	11134	4.0	—
13141	2.5	0.0	11125	0.0	0.0
13132	2.0	0.0	11116	2.5	—
13123	1.5	0.0	511111	3.0	0.0
13114	3.0	0.0	121111	3.0	—
12511	—	—	412111	3.0	0.0
12421	2.0	—	411211	2.5	0.0
12412	2.0	—	411121	2.0	0.0
12331	3.5	—	411112	3.0	0.0
12322	1.0	—	331111	3.0	—
12313	3.0	—	322111	2.0	0.0
12241	0.0	0.0	321211	1.5	0.0
12232	0.0	0.0	321121	2.5	0.0
12223	2.0	0.0	321112	2.5	0.0
12214	3.5	0.0	313111	1.0	—
12151	2.0	—	312211	2.5	—
12142	1.5	—	312121	2.0	—
12133	3.0	—	312112	3.0	—
12124	2.0	—	311311	2.0	0.0
12115	3.0	0.0	311221	2.5	0.0
11611	—	—	311212	3.0	0.0
11521	—	—	311131	3.0	0.0
11512	—	—	311122	2.5	0.0
11431	4.0	—	311113	3.0	0.0
11422	4.0	—	241111	1.5	—
11413	1.5	—	232111	0.0	0.0
11341	0.0	0.0	231211	2.0	0.0
11332	0.0	0.0	231121	2.0	0.0
11323	0.0	0.0	231112	2.0	0.0
11314	4.0	0.0	223111	3.0	—

(continued)

TABLE 8-2. *(Continued)*

Tie vector	Critical values of U at % significance		Tie vector	Critical values of U at % significance	
	5.0	1.0		5.0	1.0
222211	2.5	—	131311	2.0	0.0
222121	2.5	—	131221	1.5	0.0
222112	3.0	—	131212	3.0	0.0
221311	2.0	0.0	131131	1.0	0.0
221221	1.5	0.0	131122	2.5	0.0
221212	1.5	0.0	131113	3.0	0.0
221131	2.5	0.0	124111	2.0	—
221122	2.5	0.0	123211	1.0	—
221113	2.5	0.0	123121	3.0	—
214111	2.0	—	123112	3.0	—
213211	3.0	—	122311	0.0	0.0
213121	1.0	—	122221	2.0	0.0
213112	1.0	—	122212	2.0	0.0
212311	0.0	0.0	122131	1.5	0.0
212221	2.0	0.0	122122	1.5	0.0
212212	2.0	0.0	122113	2.5	0.0
212131	3.0	0.0	121411	1.5	—
212122	1.5	0.0	121321	3.0	—
212113	3.0	0.0	121312	1.0	—
211411	1.5	—	121231	3.0	—
211321	3.0	—	121222	2.5	—
211312	1.0	—	121213	2.0	—
211231	2.0	—	121141	2.5	0.0
211222	3.0	—	121132	2.0	0.0
211213	3.0	—	121123	2.5	0.0
211141	2.5	0.0	121114	2.0	0.0
211132	2.0	0.0	115111	—	—
211123	2.5	0.0	114211	4.0	—
211114	3.0	0.0	114121	1.5	—
151111	2.0	—	114112	1.5	—
142111	0.0	0.0	113311	0.0	0.0
141211	2.5	0.0	113221	0.0	0.0
141121	2.5	0.0	113212	0.0	0.0
141112	2.5	0.0	113131	2.0	0.0
133111	3.0	—	113122	2.0	0.0
132211	2.5	—	113113	2.0	0.0
132121	3.0	—	112411	4.0	—
132112	2.0	—	112321	1.0	—

TABLE 8-2. *(Continued)*

Tie vector	Critical values of U at % significance		Tie vector	Critical values of U at % significance	
	5.0	1.0		5.0	1.0
112312	3.0	—	2121121	3.0	0.0
112231	2.5	—	2121112	3.0	0.0
112222	2.5	—	2112111	1.0	—
112213	2.5	—	2112211	3.0	—
112141	2.5	0.0	2112121	3.0	—
112132	2.0	0.0	2112112	3.0	—
112123	1.5	0.0	2111311	2.0	0.0
112114	2.5	0.0	2111221	2.5	0.0
111511	—	—	2111212	3.0	0.0
111421	2.0	—	2111131	2.0	0.0
111412	2.0	—	2111122	3.0	0.0
111331	3.0	—	2111113	3.0	0.0
111322	3.0	—	1411111	2.5	0.0
111313	1.0	—	1321111	2.0	—
111241	0.0	0.0	1312111	3.0	0.0
111232	0.0	0.0	1311211	2.5	0.0
111223	2.0	0.0	1311121	3.0	0.0
111214	3.0	0.0	1311112	2.0	0.0
111151	2.0	—	1231111	3.0	—
111142	1.5	—	1222111	2.0	0.0
111133	3.0	—	1221211	1.5	0.0
111124	3.0	—	1221121	2.5	0.0
111115	3.0	0.0	1221112	2.5	0.0
4111111	3.0	0.0	1213111	1.0	—
3211111	2.5	0.0	1212211	2.5	—
3121111	3.0	—	1212121	2.0	—
3112111	3.0	0.0	1212112	3.0	—
3111211	2.5	0.0	1211311	2.0	0.0
3111112	3.0	0.0	1211221	2.5	0.0
2311111	2.0	0.0	1211212	3.0	0.0
2221111	3.0	—	1211131	3.0	0.0
2212111	1.5	0.0	1211122	2.5	0.0
2211211	2.5	0.0	1211113	3.0	0.0
2211121	2.5	0.0	1141111	1.5	—
2211112	3.0	0.0	1132111	0.0	0.0
2131111	1.0	—	1131211	2.0	0.0
2122111	2.0	0.0	1131121	2.0	0.0
2121211	1.5	0.0	1131112	2.0	0.0

(continued)

TABLE 8–2. *(Continued)*

Tie vector	Critical values of U at % significance		Tie vector	Critical values of U at % significance	
	5.0	1.0		5.0	1.0
1123111	3.0	—	13111111	2.0	0.0
1122211	2.5	—	12211111	2.5	0.0
1122121	2.5	—	12121111	3.0	—
1122112	3.0	—	12112111	3.0	0.0
1121311	2.0	0.0	12111211	2.5	0.0
1121221	1.5	0.0	12111121	3.0	0.0
1121212	1.5	0.0	12111112	3.0	0.0
1121131	2.5	0.0	11311111	2.0	0.0
1121122	2.5	0.0	11221111	3.0	—
1121113	2.5	0.0	11212111	1.5	0.0
1114111	2.0	—	11211211	2.5	0.0
1113211	3.0	—	11211121	2.5	0.0
1113121	1.0	—	11211112	3.0	0.0
1113112	1.0	—	11131111	1.0	—
1112311	0.0	0.0	11122111	2.0	0.0
1112221	2.0	0.0	11121211	1.5	0.0
1112212	2.0	0.0	11121121	3.0	0.0
1112131	3.0	0.0	11121112	3.0	0.0
1112122	1.5	0.0	11113111	1.0	—
1112113	3.0	0.0	11112211	3.0	—
1111411	1.5	—	11112121	3.0	—
1111321	3.0	—	11112112	3.0	—
1111312	1.0	—	11111311	2.0	0.0
1111231	2.0	—	11111221	2.5	0.0
1111222	3.0	—	11111212	3.0	0.0
1111213	3.0	—	11111131	2.0	0.0
1111141	2.5	0.0	11111122	3.0	0.0
1111132	2.0	0.0	11111113	3.0	0.0
1111123	2.5	0.0	211111111	2.0	0.0
1111114	3.0	0.0	121111111	3.0	0.0
31111111	3.0	0.0	112111111	3.0	0.0
22111111	3.0	0.0	111211111	3.0	0.0
21211111	3.0	0.0	111121111	3.0	—
21121111	3.0	—	111112111	3.0	0.0
21112111	3.0	0.0	111111211	3.0	0.0
21111211	3.0	0.0	111111121	3.0	0.0
21111121	3.0	0.0	111111112	2.0	0.0
21111112	2.0	0.0	1111111111	0.0	0.0

STIMULATION OF NADPH-NEOTETRAZOLIUM REDUCTASE

Determination of NADPH-Neotetrazolium Reductase Activity

NADPH-neotetrazolium reductase is demonstrated in 10-μm unfixed cryostat sections prepared as described above. The method is a modification of that of Altman (1972) and employs 100 mM HEPES buffer (pH 8.0) containing 20 mM MgCl$_2$, 20% w:v polyvinyl alcohol (Sigma No. P-8136 Type II, mol wt. ca, 12,000), 6 mM NADPH and 5 mM neotetrazolium chloride (Moore, 1979). This medium is purged with nitrogen for several minutes and incubation of sections is carried out in the dark for 30 min at 37°C in a nitrogen atmosphere in an enclosed container which is kept moist by a bottom lining of damp tissue paper or sponge. The incubation medium is placed within a rectangular rubber or plastic enclosure which surrounds the sections on the slides, thus maintaining a depth of 2–3 mm of medium over the sections during the incubation. Control sections omit NADPH from the incubation medium or else the sections are pretreated with steam for 1 min. Neotetrazolium chloride must be used for this reaction; other salts, such as nitro-blue tetrazolium, are not suitable.

Microdensitometric Measurements

These are made on the cells of interest using a scanning integrating microdensitometer; our investigations have involved the use of a Vickers M85 microdensitometer. Measurement of the reaction products (red and blue formazans) requires a wavelength of 585 nm (Butcher and Altman, 1973) which is the isobestic wavelength for the two formazans produced in the reaction for NADPH-neotetrazolium reductase. Use of the Vickers M85 on mussel blood cells, in cryostat sections of the digestive gland region, requires a measuring spot of 0.5 μm diameter ($\times$ 40 objective, spot size 1) and a circular mask diameter of 8 μm (Mask A2). Ten readings are made per section of one digestive gland and five digestive glands are used per sample, as with the lysosomal techniques. It is preferable to make microdensitometric readings on duplicate sections as a check for errors in section thickness.

TABLE 8–3. Responses of NADPH-Neotetrazolium Reductase Activity in the Blood Cells of *M. edulis* Exposed to Water-accommodated Fraction of North Sea Crude Oil

Experiment	Time (days)	Relative absorbance of NADPH-neotetrazolium reductase activity (machine units of absorbance; mean ± S.E., $n = 5$)	
		Control	Experimental
I (12 μg litre^{-1})[a]	7	18.23 ± 2.00[b]	33.84 ± 3.05
		16.21 ± 2.13[b]	33.09 ± 2.37
	14		32.06 ± 3.23
			30.32 ± 3.07
	35	21.30 ± 1.94	35.63 ± 2.29
		23.94 ± 2.19	42.18 ± 3.91
II (7.7 μg litre^{-1})	3	12.79 ± 1.56	20.80 ± 2.50
II (68 μg litre^{-1})	3		28.41 ± 2.82

Adapted from Moore et al. (1980).
[a]Concentration of total aromatic hydrocarbons.
[b]Duplicate samples in Experiment 1.

An example of the type of results obtained is shown in Table 8-3, which is an experiment on the effect of the water-accommodated fraction of North Sea crude oil on NADPH-neotetrazolium reductase activity in the blood cells of *M. edulis*. The results are expressed as units of relative absorbance or absorption (Chayen, 1978), which if required can be converted to extinction values by reference to a calibration plot of relative absorbance (microdensitometer readings) against extinction as described by Chayen (1978). However, as most results are used for comparison with a reference sample, the units of relative absorbance are all that is required.

9

Cytogenetic Procedures

POMATOCEROS TRIQUETER: A TEST SYSTEM FOR ENVIRONMENTAL MUTAGENESIS

The embryos of the marine tubeworm *Pomatoceros triqueter* (L.) (Serpulidae: Polychaeta) are excellent material for genetic toxicity testing. The cells of the early stage embryos are large, and the chromosomes are correspondingly less condensed than at any other stage in development. *Pomatoceros* has a karyotype consisting of 24 large and mostly metacentric and submetacentric chromosomes (Fig. 9-1). It is a broadcast spawner, producing large numbers of gametes without the marked seasonality which is generally associated with gametogenesis in other groups. These features, together with the worm's tolerance of aquarium conditions, ensure that a continuous supply of embryos can be available for laboratory study. Furthermore, aspects of the ecology and physiology of *Pomatoceros*—namely its sedentary, filter-feeding habit, wide local (eurybathic) and geographical distributions, from cold temperate latitudes to the Equator in the Northern Hemisphere (a close relative, *P. caeruleus*, occupies a similar range in the Southern Hemisphere), and its ability to withstand significant reductions in salinity—enhance the utility of the species for environmental mutagenicity monitoring (Dixon, unpublished).

Table 9-1 is a summary of different tests that have been developed using the gametes and embryos of *Pomatoceros*, indicating the maximum exposure time associated with each life-history stage, the recommended stages for scoring, and the chromosomal or related effects than can be observed. Techniques for inducing spawning and for the examination of material for chromosomal damage and other related cellular effects are described below.

Spawning

Pomatoceros is a protandrous hermaphrodite, but this is of little consequence in the investigation of spawning since the two sexual phases are separated in time. Adult worms will release ripe gametes in response to being removed from their calcereous tubes. To avoid damaging the adult tissues, it is advisable to break open the tube at the narrow end and push the worm out in a posterior direction with a blunt needle applied to the tough operculum at the front end. Mature males have pale green or yellow abdomens, while females are reddish pink.

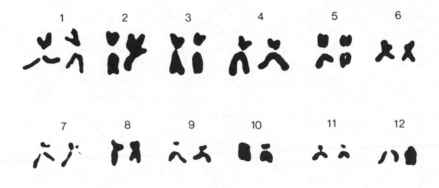

10 μm

FIG. 9-1. Chromosomes of a tubeworm, *Pomatoceros triqueter*. The normal karyotype comprises four groups based on chromosome size and position of the centromere (arm ratio): pairs 1-4 (Group A, submetacentric), pairs 5 and 6 (Group B, metacentric), pairs 7-11 (Group C, submetacentric), and pair 12 (Group D, subtelocentric).

TABLE 9-1. The Different Life-history Stages of *P. triqueter* Which Can Be Used in Testing for Genetically Harmful Agents in Seawater

Material exposed to toxicant	Maximum exposure time	Stage at which scored	Observed effects
Gonad (adult organism)	months	sperm	malformations of head
		oocytes	chromosome damage, e.g. translocation heterozygotes, aneuploids
Gametes	1.5 h (sperm) 6.0 h (oocytes)	fertilisation	reduced rate of fertilisation
Fertilised oocytes	1 h	same or early cleavage	chromosomal and cellular abnormalities, e.g. abnormal polar bodies and vesicle, septate ooplasm
Early stage embryos (< 8 cells)	7 h	same	chromosomal aberrations, i.e. numerical and structural abnormalities; developmental effects, e.g. premature loss of synchrony, malformations

After detubing, the sexes should be placed separately in small dishes containing filtered seawater. Gametes will continue to be released from the genital pores for about 5 min, after which time the adults can be removed from the dish. Oocytes remain viable for up to 6 h after release, whereas sperms remain active for only about a third of this time and ideally should be used within the first hour. After release, the oocytes will settle on the bottom of the dish, from where they can be collected with a pipette; sperms, however, become distributed throughout the water mass.

Gametes in Mutation Testing

Sperm Head Abnormalities

Sperm head malformations, while being of unknown aetiology, show a strong correlation with mutagenicity. While it is not clear whether the effects on sperm morphology reflect gene mutation, chromosome damage, or a mixture of both, the increase in morphological abnormalities of the sperm is dose-related. The proportion of sperm head abnormalities therefore provides a good empirical test of relative mutagenicity (Bruce et al., 1974).

The following is a summary of a convenient test system.

1. Add 1 ml of eosin (1% in seawater) to 9 ml of dilute sperm suspension (from 2 adults).
2. Leave to stain for 30 min before centrifuging down the sperm and resuspending in 3% ammonium formate (10 ml) to remove salt contamination.
3. Make smear peparations by placing a drop(s) of the stained suspension on a clean slide and disperse over the working surface with several passes of a second slide.
4. Leave to air dry, and spray with an aerosol fixative/mountant (e.g. Acrylek, Fisons). Examine under oil using a green filter to increase contrast.

The final concentration may have to be adjusted by centrifugation or further diluted with ammonium formate depending on the quality of the first slide preparations.

Oocytes: Translocation Heterozygotes

Oocytes, in contrast to sperms, are spawned prior to the completion of meiosis at the prophase stage of the first meiotic division (Fig. 9-2A, B). At this stage, a central germinal vesicle and an outer, darker-staining, cortical region can be discerned. The former contains a prominent nucleolus with groups of condensing chromatin arranged as bivalents undergoing synapsis or crossing-over; the latter consists mainly of yolk granules bounded externally by a flexible membrane. Prophase soon continues through to metaphase I, at which stage the bivalents reach their greatest degree of condensation (Fig. 9-2C). By metaphase I the nucleolus and germinal vesicle have dispersed, and development now ceases unless the oocyte is fertilised. Unfertilised oocytes can be scored for chromosome damage (translocation heterozygotes) incurred during their development (Fig. 9-2D), and, as with sperm head malformations, this represents a convenient method for application in field monitoring studies. For general information regarding translocation heterozygosity and its uses in genetic toxicology, see Léonard (1977). The method for slide preparation is the same as that described below for embryos.

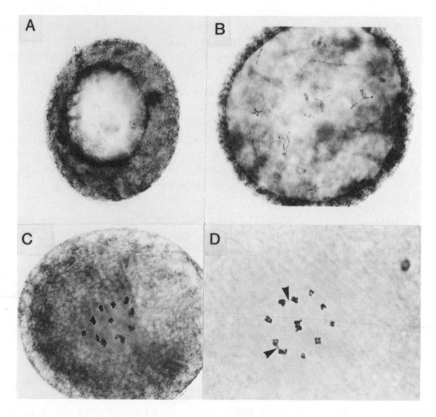

FIG. 9.2. Newly released oocytes. A: Germinal vesicle stage with prominent nucleolus. B: Diplotene, the fourth stage of meiotic prophase, showing chiasmata. C: Normal metaphase I consisting of 12 bivalents. D: Abnormal metaphase I configuration (translocation heterogyote) with bridges (arrowed) forming quadrivalents.

Embryos

Chromosome damage sustained by the gametes during their development can be scored in the first few cleavage divisions of the embryo. Alternatively, embryos can be exposed directly to a toxicant in a bioassay procedure. The following method is used routinely in our laboratory:

1. Pool the oocytes from several female worms and make up to 20 ml with freshly filtered seawater in a clean Universal bottle. After introducing a few drops of sperm suspension, close the bottle and invert a few times to mix the contents. Place in an incubator at 10°C for 1 h.
2. Transfer the fertilised oocytes to a clean 10-ml tube, and centrifuge for 2 min at 180 g. Discard the supernatant seawater, and resuspend in clean seawater. Repeat the rinsing procedure three times to remove excess sperms. (Omit the next step when developmental effects are being investigated.)
3. Separate the oocyte suspension into three equal volumes in clean Universal bottles and treat as follows:
   (a) Negative control: make up to 20 ml with clean seawater,
   (b) Positive control: make up to 20 ml with seawater containing a known amount of a reference mutagen (see below).
   (c) Experimental group: suspend in 20 ml either of seawater to be tested or filtered seawater containing a known amount of toxicant.
4. Return to the incubator and sample after 2.5 h (and 6.5 h when step 3 is being followed (Fig. 9-3). Assay for the conditions discussed below.

Metaphase Analysis

Metaphase analysis, which is attributable to Sax (1938), is the most comprehensive method available for chromosome aberration detection. Usually the cells are treated with a spindle poison, generally colchicine or a less-toxic analogue (e.g. Colcemid), to prevent the sister chromatids from separating at anaphase. The other main feature of this method is the use of a hypotonic medium which causes the nuclei to swell so that the chromosomes are individually separated in the fixed slide preparation. Several alternative hypotonic treatments are described in the literature,

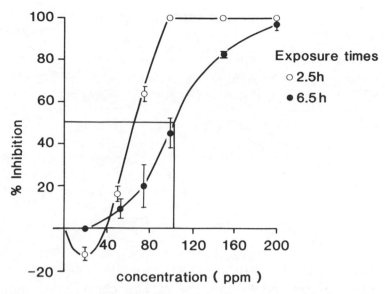

FIG. 9-3. Dose-response curves for *Pomatoceros* embryos exposed to toluene for two time periods. The results for 2.5 h show a transitory delay in cell division (inhibition = number ≥ 2-cells expressed as % of control) which could lead to an artificially low estimate of the toxic levels; anaphase scoring is carried out at the 50% inhibition level. The vertical lines depict the range above and below each mean, based on a replicated experiment.

including distilled water and dilute salt solutions (Makino and Nishimura, 1952; Darlington and La Cour, 1976; Kligerman, 1979; Sharma and Sharma, 1980), but the most successful medium has proved to be diluted seawater. The technique for metaphase analysis using seawater is as follows:

1. Place the embryos in a 0.04% solution of colchicine (Sigma) in seawater (10 ml) and leave for 3-5 h (longer exposure times will increase the level of chromosome condensation, making analysis difficult).
2. Transfer to a 10-ml centrifuge tube and spin for 1.5 min at 180 *g*. Resuspend in 50% seawater. Leave for 30 min.
3. Repeat centrifugation, but this time replace the medium with 25% seawater. Leave for 15 min.
4. Centrifuge and resuspend in cold, freshly made Carnoy's fixative (3 parts alcohol : 1 part glacial acetic acid : 1% chloroform). Change the fixative three times over the course of the next hour; material can then be stored in fixative for many months.

Since the following method of slide preparation produces temporary mounts only, it should be carried out immediately before analysis.

5. Pipette about 100 embryos onto a clean slide and rotate this so that they spread across the surface. Allow to air dry (this takes 3-5 min).
6. Add 1 or 2 drops of freshly filtered aceto-orcein stain (La Cour, 1941) and cover with a cover-glass. Leave for 5 min. If the slide is warmed (e.g. by holding in contact with a 60-W light bulb), this enhances the staining of the chromosomes and reduces the amount of background colouration.
7. Carefully express the excess stain between two pieces of absorbent card, and seal the cover-glass edges with warm glycerol-gelatin (Sigma).

The slide should then be scanned at low power ($\times$ 16 objective) to determine the positions of suitable chromosome spreads (e.g. see Tsytsugina, 1979); these should be recorded in a notebook, using the coordinates on the microscope stage for reference. Suitable spreads should then be re-examined using a good oil immersion lens, ideally with a phase-contrast capability, and the types of aberration recorded. Scoring should be carried out using coded slides. Written records are the simplest—and cheapest—way of recording results, but ideally a photographic or televised video record should also be kept. A minimum of 100 metaphases should be scored for each treatment.

The minimal categories that should be scored when evaluating metaphase preparations are chromosome number, achromatic gaps, chromatid deletions (open chromatid breaks), chromatid exchange, chromosome deletion (open chromosome break), chromosome exchange and one category for "other" aberrations (Report of the Ad Hoc Committee of The Environmental Mutagen Society and The Institute for Medical Research, 1972; Nichols et al., 1977). The most recent classification of the different types of induced chromosomal structural aberrations is by Savage (1975); further information is available in Evans and O'Riordan (1977).

In carrying out this procedure, ensure that only a minimum amount of seawater contacts the fixative, otherwise precipitated salts will seriously reduce the quality of the slide preparations. Also avoid placing too much pressure on the cover-glass when removing excess stain, since this ruptures the cell membranes and leads to disruption and mixing of the cell contents. Over-condensation of the chromosomes can be prevented by reducing the length, or concentration, of the colchicine treatment.

Anaphase Analysis

Metaphase analysis can prove very cumbersome and time consuming, especially for inexperienced investigators. This has lead some investigators to go for the less comprehensive and much simpler anaphase method (Nichols et al., 1977):

1. Allow embyros to develop to not more than the 8-cell stage. To allow for the phenomenon of mitotic inhibition (a transient delay in cell division caused by toxic substances and which generally accompanies genetic damage), two sampling times are recommended, 2.5 and 6.5 h, at $10°C$ (Fig. 9-4).
2. Harvest and fix in Carnoy's fixative, with three changes of fixative over a period of 1 h.
3. Prepare slides as described above, taking great care to avoid disrupting the cells. Stain with aceto-orcein and examine immediately.

Coded slides should be used, and a minimum of 200 anaphases should be analysed per treatment. Two classes of cellular abnormality are detectable in anaphase material, namely chromosomal aberrations—bridges (dicentric chromosomes), acentric fragments, and side-arm bridges (sub-chromatid phenomena)—and spindle abnormalities (lagging chromosomes and multipolar spindles) (Fig. 9-4).

Chromosome bridges are very fragile and may be destroyed in squash preparations. Squashing will also produce spindle artifacts, so care must be taken to avoid exerting too much pressure during slide preparation. Stickiness, which is not recognised as a true chromosomal aberration, can mimic the appearance of side-arm bridges.

Controls

It is very important when designing experiments to include adequate controls; and it is good practice to have both positive and negative controls. In a positive control, the cells are exposed to a

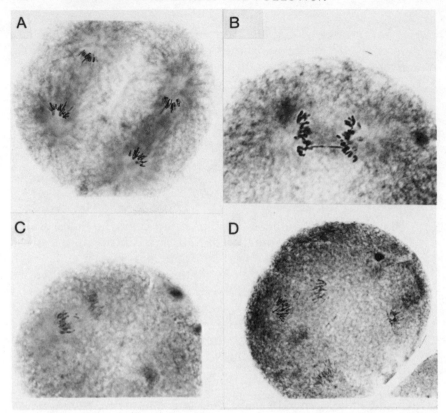

FIG. 9-4. Some types of chromosomal aberration commonly encountered in anaphase (post-metaphase) analysis. *A*: Normal 2-cell late anaphase stage embryo. *B*: chromosome bridge (dicentric chromosome). *C*: Acentric fragments. *D*: Lagging or late-separating chromatids. (See also tri-polar anaphase in Chapter 3, Fig. 3-3.)

predetermined level of a standard mutagen to provide a reference response for comparison with the experimental results. Types of chemicals used as positive controls are: (1) those that produce chromosome damage without metabolic activation, such as triethylene melamine (TEM), triethylene phosphoramide (TEPA), methylmethane sulphonate (MMS), ethylmethane sulphonate (EMS), and trimethyl phosphate (TMP) and (2) those that require metabolism for mutagenic activity, such as mitomycin, 4-nitrosoquinoline or cytoxan. Ideally both types should be used, but most investigators opt for either MMS or EMS. When first setting up a test system, a dose-response curve should be constructed using one of these agents (see Dixon and Clarke, 1982).

10

Biochemical Procedures

AMINO ACIDS:
DETERMINATION OF THE TAURINE:GLYCINE RATIO
AND THE SUM OF THREONINE AND SERINE

The determination of the T : G ratio and (thr + ser) of the whole tissues of *Mytilus edulis* involves the collection of mussels, the dissection and storage of the tissues, the extraction of the free amino acids, the analysis of the extracted fraction for taurine, glycine, threonine and serine and the calculation of the indices. The methods can most likely be used for other bivalve species and for marine invertebrates in general, although some preliminary studies may be necessary (see below).

Collection of Mussels,
Dissection and Storage of Tissues

Equipment and chemicals: Dissection equipment, plastic scintillation vials or other containers, filter paper (Whatman No. 1), Dewar flask or other insulation flask containing liquid nitrogen, Dewar flask containing dry ice (solid CO_2), freeze-drier.

TABLE 10–1. T:G Ratio and (thr + ser) of the Whole Tissues (Less Digestive Gland) of *M. edulis* Collected While Submerged or Exposed on the Shore

Population	Exposure time (h)	T:G ratio[a]		(thr + ser)[a]	
		Submerged	Exposed	Submerged	Exposed
Teignmouth	1.5	1.9 ± 0.1	1.9 ± 0.2	99 ± 2	81 ± 6[b]
Minehead	2	2.0 ± 0.3	2.3 ± 0.1	50 ± 3	39 ± 2[b]
Lynher	3	2.5 ± 0.2	2.1 ± 0.2	64 ± 4	68 ± 10
Atlantic					
College	3	3.0 ± 0.1	2.7 ± 0.2	27 ± 2	37 ± 3[b]
Swale	3.5	3.5 ± 0.3	3.8 ± 0.3	35 ± 3	34 ± 1
Mumbles	4	1.9 ± 0.03	2.2 ± 0.2	106 ± 8	75 ± 6[b]

[a]Mean ± S.E. ($n = 5$); (thr + ser) in μmol g^{-1} dry weight.
[b]$P < 0.05$ (submerged vs. exposed).

Collect a minimum of five but preferably ten mussels (4-6 cm length) preferably while they are still immersed in water. Comparisons of immersed mussels with those that have been exposed for several hours on the shore showed no change in T:G ratio but some alterations in (thr + ser) (Table 10-1). Although it is thought that glycine does not accumulate in bivalve molluscs during anaerobiosis (De Zwaan et al., 1976), under certain conditions—namely a rapid decrease in salinity followed by valve closure of the animal—marked increases in glycine (and to a lesser extent of threonine, serine and occasionally taurine) have been observed (Shumway et al., 1977; Shumway and Youngson, 1979). Immediately dissect out the whole tissues and separate and discard the byssus and the digestive gland (hepatopancreas); the latter contains ingested food. Damp-dry the whole tissues on filter paper, place the tissues of an individual mussel in a plastic vial and freeze in liquid nitrogen. Transport the frozen tissues to the laboratory in liquid nitrogen or on dry ice, remove the water from the tissues by lyophilization overnight (freeze-drying) and store the samples, preferably dessicated, at $-20\,^{\circ}$C or below. The amino acids of such samples should remain unchanged for several months or more (Barnes and Blackstock, 1974).

Extraction and Analysis of Amino Acids,
Calculation of Indices

Equipment and chemicals: Agate ball-mill, balance (to weigh to 1 mg), shaker or vortex tube mixer, test tubes or centrifuge tubes (approximately 15-ml volume), centrifuge (maximum g required, 1,000–3,000; preferably refrigerated), pipettes (100 μl to 1 ml), 5-ml volumetric flasks, amino acid analyser, 12% w:v trichloro-acetic acid (dissolve 120 gm in distilled water and make up to 1 litre; store at 6°C), 0.2 N pH 2.2 sodium citrate buffer [19.6 gm $Na_3C_6H_5O_7 \cdot 2H_2O$, 16.5 ml conc. HCl, 20 ml thiodiglycol, 2 ml Brij 35 solution (50% w:v), 0.1 caprylic acid (n-octanoic acid); make up to 1 litre with distilled water], internal standard [0.625 mM L-norleucine or β-(2-thienyl)-DL-serine; store at 6°C].

Extraction

Re-lyophilize the samples if they have been stored for any length of time. Grind the whole dried tissues into a fine powder using an agate ball-mill or other equipment. Weigh approximately 0.5 gm of the ground tissue into a centrifuge tube and add 5 ml of 12% trichloroacetic acid. Mix on a tube-mixer or shake for 5–15 min on a shaker (stopper the tube). Add a second 5 ml of trichloroacetic acid and leave to stand for about 2 h in the cold. Centrifuge the sample (3,000 g for 15 min) and decant and retain the supernatant. Repeat the extraction procedure on the pellet, recentrifuge and add the second supernatant to the first. Store the pooled supernatants at 6°C or frozen before amino acid analysis. The trichloracetic acid technique extracts free amino acids and probably also amino acids that are loosely bound (by secondary bonds, e.g. electrostatic attraction) to proteins and other high molecular weight substances. It will not remove amino acids that are covalently bound by peptide bonds to form proteins and polypeptides. Different extraction techniques will remove differing amounts of amino acids, and the same technique should be routinely used. For example, 12% trichloroacetic acid extracted greater concentrations of amino acids than did 70% ethanol (Table 10-2). Heat does not increase the amount extracted by trichloroacetic acid and in fact should be avoided as it results in a loss of material in the threonine peak (Table 10-2). Alternative methods for tissue amino

TABLE 10-2. Comparison of the Extraction of Total NPS (Ninhydrin-Positive Substances), Taurine, Glycine, Threonine and Serine from Whole Tissues by the 70% Ethanol and 12% Trichloroacetic Acid Techniques

Extraction method[a]	Total NPS	Taurine	Glycine	Threonine	Serine
(1) TCA	662 ± 6	369 ± 5	131 ± 2	12 ± 1	11 ± 0.4
(2) TCA/80°C	740 ± 10[b]	374 ± 8	133 ± 1	5 ± 0.4	13 ± 0.2
(3) EtOH	570 ± 19	327 ± 12	115 ± 4	9 ± 0.4	9 ± 0.4
(4) EtOH/80°C	565 ± 16	330 ± 11	114 ± 3	8 ± 0.8	9 ± 0.7

[a] A standard ground freeze-dried sample was extracted using (1) 12% trichloroacetic acid as described in the text (TCA); (2) 12% trichloroacetic acid and heating the homogenate at 80°C for 30 min (TCA/80°C); (3) 70% ethanol and rotary evaporation (EtOH) (Barnes and Blackstock, 1974); and (4), as for (3) but with heating of the homogenate at 80°C for 30 min before rotary evaporation. Concentrations of NPS and individual amino acids in μmol g^{-1} dry weight; mean ± S.E. (5 samples extracted).
[b] Increase in total NPS due to increase in ammonia (29 ± 3 → 104 ± 2).

acid extraction include picric acid deproteinization, sulphosalicyclic acid deproteinization and ultrafiltration techniques.

Amino Acid Analysis

The analysis of the extracted fraction can be carried out on an amino acid analyser. The sample is first diluted and an internal standard may be added. The conditions required for the separation of the amino acids are described for one particular commercial analyser (L.K.B. 4101) and may be different for other analysers with different columns, resins, etc.

Sample Preparation. Dilute sample 1 : 50, i.e. 100 μl trichloroacetic acid extracted fraction and 500 μl of 0.625 mM L-norleucine or β-(2-thienyl)-DL-serine made up to 5 ml in a volumetric flask with 0.2 N pH 2.2 sodium citrate buffer. The internal standard is added to monitor the amount of colour reaction (see the particular amino acid analyser handbook for the determination of calibration factors). Both internal standards are suitable for use with extracts of *M. edulis* (diluted as described); L-norleucine requires the longer elution time (Fig. 10-1) but β-(2-thienyl)-DL-serine is less stable and should be checked periodically. Different internal standards may be required for the samples of other organisms if endogenous amino acids co-elute. Alternatively, the internal standard can be omitted and standard amino acid mixtures run at regular intervals in between sample runs.

Analysis. Analyser: L.K.B. 4101, 9×725 mm column, Aminex A-5 resin (Bio-Rad), ninhydrin-methoxyethanol reaction system (see analyser handbook for the preparation of all solutions); temperature of run: $55\,^{\circ}$C; total (buffer plus ninhydrin) flow rate: 1.5 ml min^{-1}; elution system: for β-(2-thienyl)-DL-serine run 95 min of 0.2 N pH 3.25 sodium citrate buffer, 45 min of 0.4 M NaOH (regeneration step) and 45 min of 0.2 N pH 3.25 sodium citrate buffer (re-equilibration step); for L-norleucine run 95 min of 0.2 N pH 3.25 sodium citrate buffer, 90 min of 0.2 N pH 4.25 sodium citrate buffer, 45 min of 0.4 M NaOH and 45 min of 0.2 N pH 3.25 sodium citrate buffer.

A typical amino acid chromatogram is shown in Fig. 10-1. The concentrations of amino acids in the sample applied to the analyser are calculated from the peak areas and the calibration factors (see amino acid analyser handbook). The concentration of amino acids in tissue is given by:

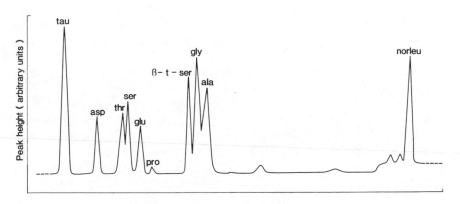

Retention time (arbitrary units)

FIG. 10-1. Amino acid chromatogram of the whole tissues of *M. edulis* showing the main peaks (for a complete analysis see Livingstone et al., 1979); tau: taurine; asp: aspartate; thr: threonine; ser: serine; glu: glutamate; pro: proline; β-t-ser: β-(2-thienyl)-DL-serine; gly: glycine; ala: alanine; norleu: L-norleucine.

Concentration (μmol g^{-1} dry wt)

$$= \frac{\text{concentration in sample } (\mu\text{mol ml}^{-1}) \times 50 \times 20}{\text{weight of tissue (g)}}$$

The indices are given by:

1. T : G ratio $= \dfrac{\text{taurine } (\mu\text{mol g}^{-1} \text{ dry wt})}{\text{glycine } (\mu\text{mol g}^{-1} \text{ dry wt})}$

2. (thr + ser) = threonine + serine (μmol g^{-1} dry wt)

It should be noted that a sodium citrate buffer system does not fully resolve minor components from threonine and serine, and contained within these peaks will be small amounts of asparagine and glutamine.

ADENYLATE ENERGY CHARGE

The adenylate energy charge (AEC; Atkinson, 1972) is calculated from measured concentrations of ATP, ADP and AMP by the formula: (ATP + $\frac{1}{2}$ADP)/(ATP + ADP + AMP). This section describes procedures for extraction and analysis of the above nucleotides from tissues of estuarine invertebrates. These procedures have been used successfully with gastropods and bivalves (Ivanovici, 1977, 1980a, 1980b) and other invertebrates (Beis and Newsholme, 1975).

Various methods for extraction and analysis of adenine nucleotides are available (Jaworek et al., 1974; Rabinowitz, 1974; Strehler, 1974; Wijsman, 1976); however, those described below are recommended because of their high level of precision (Ivanovici, 1980a), relative simplicity and ease of application. These methods, modified from those described by Hess and Brand (1974), Newsholme and Start (1973), Lamprecht and Trautschold (1974) and Jaworek et al. (1974), are suitable for samples with no less than 10^{-9} M of nucleotide.

Abbreviations

ADP   adenosine-5'-diphosphate
AMP   adenosine-5'-monophosphate

ATP   adenosine-5'-triphosphate
EDTA   ethylenediaminetetracetic acid
G6P   glucose-6-phosphate
G6PDH   glucose-6-phosphate dehydrogenase
           (D-glucose-6-phosphate:NADP 1-oxidoreductase,
           EC1.1.1.49)
HK   hexokinase (D-hexose 6-phosphotransferase, EC2.7.1.1)
LDH   lactate dehydrogenase (L-lactate:NAD oxidoreductase,
           EC1.1.1.27)
MK   myokinase (ATP:AMP phosphotransferase, EC2.7.4.3)
NAD β-nicotinamide-adenine dinucleotide, oxidized form
NADH β-nicotinamide-adenine dinucleotide, reduced form
NADP β-nicotinamide-adenine dinucleotide phosphate,
           oxidized form
NADPH β-nicotinamide-adenine dinucleotide phosphate,
           reduced form
PCA   perchloric acid
PEP   phosphoenolpyruvate
PK   pyruvate kinase
           (ATP:pyruvate 2-O-phosphotransferase, EC2.7.1.40)
TEA   triethanolamine hydrochloride buffer

Extraction of Adenine Nucleotides

Apparatus: (1) Dewar flasks and sample carriers (for details see
Fig. 10-2) for collection and storage of samples and liquid N_2. (2)
Freeze-clamps (for details see Fig. 10-3) to ensure that metabolic
reactions, which may result in changes of the concentrations of the
nucleotides, are stopped in less than 0.5 s (Hess and Brand, 1974).
(3) Small bench vice for breaking shells if gastropod is used as the
experimental animal. (4) Labelled strips of polythene food wrap,
approximately 20×5 cm. (5) Dissecting equipment. (6) Stainless
steel forceps (length 30 cm) are recommended for handling the
samples once they are in liquid N_2. (7) Thin leather gloves to protect the hands from the low temperatures. (8) Homogenizers, hand-
operated, stainless steel (for details see Fig. 10-4). (9) Several
blocks of insulating material (e.g. polystyrene or polyurethane)
approximately 4×4 cm (length of homogenizer $+ 1$ cm). A hole
should be drilled down the center of the block so that the
homogenizer will fit snugly inside it. The depth of the hole should
be 5 mm less than that of the homogenizer. (10) Balance, rapid-

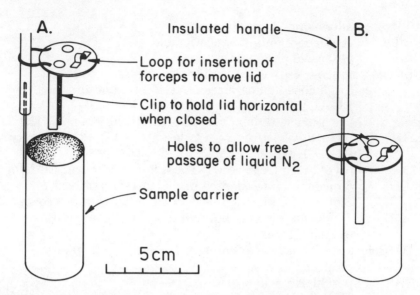

FIG. 10-2. Suggested design for a sample carrier with lid. The lid prevents samples from floating out of the carrier into body of the dewar flask. (From Ivanovici, 1977.) *A*: Lid in open position. *B*: Lid in closed position.

weighing, to three decimal places. (11) Centrifuge, refrigerated, capable of 10,000 *g*. (12) Graduated centrifuge tubes, 15-ml capacity, accurate to 0.1 ml. (13) Polyethylene centrifuge tubes, 15-ml capacity. (14) Spatulas with insulated handles. (15) Several leakproof polystryrene or polyurethane boxes, internal dimensions approximately $15 \times 10 \times 10$ cm. (16) Vortex mixer, variable speed. (17) Pipettes, graduated, 1, 5 and 10 ml. (18) Pasteur pipettes. (19) Pipetman pipette (adjustable volume), 5 ml and tips.

Reagents:
(1) PCA, 6% (v:v). Add 8.6 ml to 100 ml distilled water.
(2) 5 $M\,K_2CO_3$. Add 345.5 g to 500 ml distilled water.
(3) Universal indicator.

Sampling of Tissue

Remove animals from medium after exposure to the selected experimental treatment. Blot excess water from the body surface quickly, and measure body weight, length, etc., if required. Dissect out selected tissue, blot dry, place on labelled polythene strip and freeze clamp. After approximately 20 s remove sample from clamp, hold sample with forceps cooled in liquid N_2, wrap the film quickly

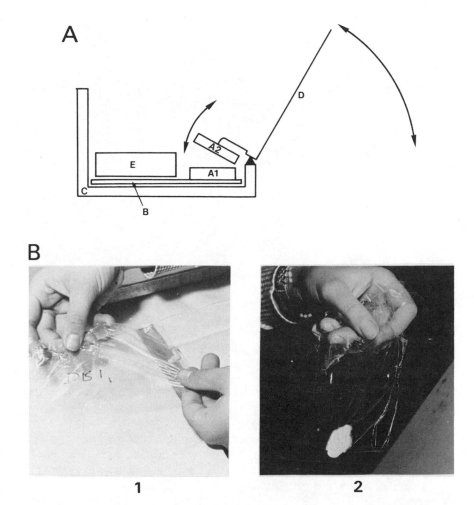

FIG. 10-3. *A*. Diagrammatic cross-section of freeze-clamp which can be operated by one person. (From Ivanovici, 1977.) One 10-cm^2 × 2.5-cm aluminium block (A1) is fixed to an aluminium plate (B), which in turn is fixed to the bottom of a polystyrene box (C). An identical aluminium block (A2) is attached to a toggle lever (D). A polystyrene block (E) is fixed inside the box to reduce its internal volume. The blocks are cooled by frequent additions of liquid N$_2$ during the sampling procedure. To operate, move Block A2 to a vertical position as the sample is brought into position on block A1, then move the lever to a vertical position quickly. This procedure compresses the sample between the cold blocks into a thin layer of 1–2 mm (Fig. 10-3*B*). The 2.5-cm thickness for the aluminium blocks is recommended because the low temperature is retained better than by thinner blocks. *B*: A sample of molluscan tissue before (1) and after (2) freeze clamping. (From Ivanovici, 1977.)

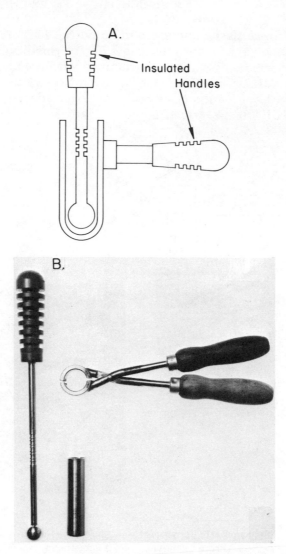

FIG. 10-4. Two types of homogenizers that are suitable for pulverizing tissue at very low temperatures. (From Ivanovici, 1977.) The recommended material is stainless steel that is resistant to corrosion and extremes of temperature, e.g. type 316. A lower grade is unsuitable, as the metal oxidizes. Joints may be silver soldered. The internal diameter of the homogenizer should not exceed 1.9 cm; a larger diameter is not as efficient, because the tissue is not pulverized as finely. *A*: Homogenizer with attached handle. Handles made of wood or plastic are suitable for protection against low temperature. Two or three are adequate if this style is made. Samples need to be transferred to centrifuge tubes rapidly after pulverizing, and should not be allowed to thaw. *B*: Homogenizer with detachable handle. If an adequate number of tubes are made (e.g. 20-30), samples can be centrifuged directly in the homogenizer and do not need to be transferred to other tubes until the neutralization step.

around the frozen tissue and store in liquid N_2. It is important to ensure that the sample does not thaw out at this stage.

Mussels can be dissected and clamped within 40 s (Ivanovici, unpublished data). Variations in dissection time of up to 90 s do not, however, have significant effects on either adenine nucleotide pools or AEC of gastropods and bivalves studied to date (Ivanovici, 1980a, 1980b).

Extraction of Adenine Nucleotides

Place homogenizers, a spatula and forceps in a bath of liquid N_2 to cool, leaving the handles out of the bath. When items have cooled sufficiently, N_2 will stop bubbling. Partly unwrap sample and place on surface of N_2 in bath. Remove homogenizer, empty N_2 from it and place inside insulation block. Transfer to balance and tare as fast as possible. With the cooled forceps, immediately transfer the tissue from its wrapping to the homogenizer, and note tissue weight. Remove the homogenizer from the insulation block and transfer it to the bath for a few seconds to recool. Remove homogenizer from bath, prop it on the bench and grind sample until it is fine powder. Periodically place homogenizer and pestle in cooling bath. The efficiency and speed of homogenizing are considerably improved by keeping the equipment as cold as possible.

Pipette 1 ml ice-cold PCA into the homogenizer, allow to freeze, loosen with spatula, then grind to a medium powder. This mixes the PCA with the tissue, and ensures that enzymes in the tissues are inactivated as the sample thaws (Newsholme and Start, 1973). If the homogenizer with the fixed handle is used (Fig. 10-4A), the contents should be quickly transferred to a plastic centrifuge tube at this point. If the other type of homogenizer is used (Fig. 10-4B), the stainless steel tube is transferred directly to the ice. Keep samples on ice until thawed, then add PCA for a ratio of tissue to PCA of 1:10 (w:v). Mix thoroughly with a clean spatula. Centrifuge the samples in a refrigerated centrifuge at $0°C$ and 6,000 g for 40 min. Transfer each supernatant to a clean centrifuge tube containing 5-10μl of Universal indicator (British Drug House). Adjust pH to 6.5 (pale yellow to colourless) by dropwise addition of K_2CO_3 (either 5 M or solid). Allow CO_2 evolution to cease between additions of the base. Leave tubes on ice for approximately 15 min, then centrifuge as before. Transfer supernatant to a graduated glass centrifuge tube and record the volume. Either assay the sample immediately or store at $-30°C$.

Analysis of the Adenine Nucleotides

The following spectrophotometric methods, which are modified from those of Lamprecht and Trautschold (1974) and Jaworek et al. (1974), are recommended for the analysis of ATP, ADP and AMP, containing 10^{-9} M or more adenylates. While the more sensitive luciferase assay (reported range, 10^{-13} M) is considered a rapid analytical method by some workers (Strehler, 1974; Wiebe and Bancroft, 1975), its sensitivity requires many more controls than the spectrophotometric method, especially for the ADP and AMP conversions. Therefore, fewer samples can be processed in a given period of time than with the spectrophotometric methods.

Enzymatic reactions which are coupled to reduction and oxidation of NADP and NADH, respectively, are used for determination of ATP, ADP and AMP. NADPH and NADH absorb maximally at 340 nm. Their extinction coefficient at this wavelength (6.22 cm^2 μmol^{-1}) is used to calculate the concentrations of ATP, ADP and AMP.

The principle of the assay for ATP is as follows. Glucose is phosphorylated by ATP to G6P with HK [reaction (1)]. G6P then reacts with NADP$^+$ to form 6-phosphoglucono-δ-lactone and NADPH. This reaction is catalyzed by G6PDH [reaction (2)]. Thus, for every μmole of ATP, one μmole of NADPH is formed and causes an increase in absorbance at 340 nm.

$$\text{ATP} + \text{glucose} \xrightarrow[\text{Mg}^{2+}]{\text{HK}} \text{G6P} + \text{ADP} \qquad (1)$$

$$\text{G6P} + \text{NADP}^+ \xrightarrow{\text{G6PDH}} \text{6-phosphoglucono-}\delta\text{-lactone} + \text{NADPH} + \text{H}^+ \qquad (2)$$

The principle of the assay for ADP and AMP is as follows. PK catalyzes the phosphorylation of one μmole of ADP by PEP to form one μmole of ATP and pyruvate [reaction (4)]. Pyruvate in turn is converted to lactate by LDH. Thus, one μmole of ADP results in the formation of one μmole of NAD$^+$ [reaction (5)]. The decrease in absorbance at 340 nm caused by the formation of NAD$^+$ from NADH is, therefore, proportional to the amount of ADP present in the sample. After this absorbance change (ΔAb$_{\text{ADP}}$) has been measured in a sample, MK is added. This enzyme catalyzes the formation of two μmoles of ADP from one μmole each of AMP and ATP [reaction (3)]. In turn, two μmoles of NAD^+ are formed [reactions (4) and (5)]:

$$AMP + ATP \xrightarrow{MK} 2\ ADP \qquad (3)$$

$$2\ ADP + 2\ PEP \xrightarrow{PK} 2\ ATP + 2\ pyruvate \qquad (4)$$

$$2\ pyruvate + 2\ NADH + 2H^+ \xrightarrow{LDH} 2\ lactate + 2\ NAD^+ \qquad (5)$$

Apparatus: (1) Dual-beam spectrophotometer (e.g. Varian model 365) with recorder. Use a wavelength of 340 nm with a visible light source. If a dual-beam spectrophotometer is not available, a single-beam machine is adequate, as long as several reference blanks are analysed. (2) Sarstedt plastic cuvettes, light path 1 cm. (3) Plastic stirring rods to mix enzymes in the cuvettes. (4) Pipetman pipettes, variable volume (20-μl, 200-μl, 1,000-μl and 5,000-μl sizes) and disposable tips. (5) Dispenser, adjustable volume, 1-5 ml. (6) Amber coloured bottles, 500-ml capacity, to be used for the buffer mixes which are light sensitive. (7) Glass pipettes, 1, 2, 5 and 10 ml.

Reagents: Make up reagents (analytical grade) in double distilled water. Dilute enzymes with 3.2 M ammonium sulphate. The procedures described below were developed using enzymes and biochemical reagents purchased from Boehringer Mannheim.

The solutions that are stored at 2-4°C are stable for at least 4 months, whereas solutions stored at -20°C or at room temperature (RT) are stable indefinitely, as are the diluted enzymes. Storage temperatures are indicated in square brackets. The aliquot sizes indicated for several solutions below are sufficient for a batch of 100 assays.

A. 0.5 M TEA, pH 7.6. Add 93 g to about 400 ml water, adjust pH with 1.N NaOH (approximately 11 ml), then add water to 1,000 ml. This is a stock solution. Dilute $\times$ 10 before use to 0.05 M [2-4°C]

B. 1 N NaOH. 20.00 g, make up to 500 ml with water. [RT]

C. 0.5 M MgCl$_2$ · 6H$_2$O. 10.17 g, make up to 100 ml with water. [2-4°C]

D. 0.5 M MgSO$_4$ · 7H$_2$O. 12.32 g, make up to 100 ml with water [2-4°C]

E. 2 M KCl. 29.82 g, make up to 200 ml with water. [2-4°C]

F. EDTA, 100 mg ml^{-1}. Weigh 5 g and make up to 50 ml with water. [2-4°C]. The crystals will not dissolve as this is a saturated solution.

G. 5% NaHCO$_3$. 5 g, make up to 100 ml with water. [2-4°C]

H. 10 mM NADH-Na$_2$ (Grade II). 7.09 mg ml^{-1}. Make up 30-40 ml with solution G, divide into 3-ml aliquots and freeze. Wrap containers in aluminium foil or use containers made of dark glass, as this compound is sensitive to light. [−20°C]

I. 10 mM NADP-Na$_2$H. 15.75 mg ml^{-1}. Make up 30-40 ml with water, divide into 3.0-ml aliquots, freeze, then as for solution H.

J. 0.4 M D-glucose. 7.21 g, make up to 100 ml. Dispense 10-20 aliquots of 1 ml, freeze these and the remaining glucose. [−20°C]]

K. 40 mM PEP-Na · H$_2$O. 8.32 mg ml^{-1}. Make up 30-40 ml, divide into 4-ml aliquots and freeze. [−20°C]

L. 20 mM ATP-Na$_2$H$_2$ · 3H$_2$O. 12.10 mg ml^{-1}. Make up between 20 and 30 ml, divide into 0.5-ml aliquots and freeze. Do not thaw same aliquot more than twice. [−20°C]

M. 10 mM ATP. Dilute solution L with water (1:1).

N. 20 mM ADP-Na$_2$. 9.42 mg ml^{-1}. Since ADP is more stable in solution than as a dry powder, the entire contents of a 500-mg bottle should be dissolved. Dispense some 0.5-ml aliquots, and freeze. The remaining solution should also be frozen until further aliquots are needed. [−20°C]

O. 20 mM AMP-Na$_2$ · 6H$_2$O. 9.98 mg ml^{-1}. Make up 20-30 ml, dispense 0.5-ml aliquots and freeze. [−20°C]

P. 3.2 M (NH$_4$)$_2$SO$_4$. 211.42 g, make up to 500 ml with water. [RT]

Q. 0.6 mg ml^{-1} G6PDH [from yeast, Grade II, 5 mg ml^{-1} suspension in 3.2 M (NH$_4$)$_2$SO$_4$]. 60 μl of enzyme plus 440 μl solution P. Do not freeze. [2-4°C]

R. 2.0 mg ml^{-1} HK [from yeast, 10 mg ml^{-1} suspension in 3.2 M (NH$_4$)$_2$SO$_4$]. 200 μl of enzyme plus 800 μl of solution P, as for Q.

S. 1 mg ml^{-1} [from rabbit muscle, 5 mg ml^{-1} suspension in 3.2 M (NH$_4$)$_2$SO$_4$]. 60 μl of enzyme plus 240 μl of solution P, as for Q.

T. 2 mg ml^{-1} PK [from rabbit muscle, 10 mg ml^{-1} suspension in 3.2 M (NH$_4$)$_2$SO$_4$]. 60 μl of enzyme plus 240 μl of solution P, as for Q.

U. 1.25 mg ml^{-1} MK [from rabbit muscle, 5 mg ml^{-1} suspension in 3.2 M (NH$_4$)$_2$SO$_4$]. 75 μl of enzyme plus 225 μl of solution P, as for Q.

Solutions for Analysis of the Adenine Nucleotides

Assay Buffers

The following assay buffers should be made up immediately prior to analysis of a batch of samples and stored at 2-4°C in the dark. The buffers are stable for 7 days but may deteriorate rapidly thereafter. The volumes given below are for 100 analyses and may be adjusted if fewer or more analyses are required.

ATP Assay Buffer. Thaw an aliquot of solution I, then mix with solutions A and C using the volumes indicated below; bring to room temperature before use:

Reagent	ml
A. TEA	285.0
C. MgCl	3.0
I. NADP	3.0

ADP-AMP Assay Buffer. Thaw aliquots of H, K and L. Make solution M. Then mix with A, D, E and F as indicated below; bring to room temperature before use:

Reagent	ml
A.TEA	260.0
D. MgSO₄	3.5
E. KCl	7.5
F. EDTA	0.5
H. NADH	3.0
K. PEP	4.0
M. ATP	1.0

Enzymes

The following volumes of enzymes are needed for approximately 100 analyses: for the ATP assay, 1.1 ml G6PDH(Q), 2.1 ml glucose (J), and 2.1 ml HK(R); for the ADP-AMP assay, LDH(S), PK(T) and MK(U), all 0.6 ml each.

Standard Mixture

0.05 mM ATP + ADP + AMP: Take 0.1 ml of each nucleotide, ATP(L), ADP(N) and AMP(O), add 3.7 ml water, mix, place on ice. Make up on day of use. Do not refreeze. Individual standards can also be made up if required in the proportion 1:39 (20 mM standard:water). 0.1 ml of the standard mixture in a cuvette with an assay volume of 3.0 ml should give the following changes in absorbance at 340 nm: ΔAb_{ATP}: 0.096 ± 0.003 (S.E.): ΔAb_{ADP}: 0.081 ± 0.005 (ADP from Boehringer is only 80% active and thus gives lower absorbancies than either ATP or AMP); ΔAb_{AMP}: 0.194 ± 0.003.

Procedure for Analyses

The analytical procedures for ATP, ADP and AMP are summarised in Fig. 10-5. ATP is analysed by itself in one set of cuvettes, while ADP and AMP are analysed sequentially in a separate set of cuvettes. The cuvettes with samples and standards are read against a reagent blank for each of the analyses. This corrects for any changes in absorbance that might be caused by the various additions of enzymes.

Thaw samples, make up standards and store on ice. Label an appropriate number of cuvettes. Allow sufficient cuvettes for a pair of standards (0.1 ml of standard mix per cuvette) and blanks, and duplicate samples. If a dual-beam spectrophotometer is available, one blank is sufficient and is placed in the reference beam. The readings thus obtained from sample cuvettes are corrected automatically for changes in the blank, and need no further adjustment.

ATP Assay

Dispense 2.85 ml of ATP assay buffer into each cuvette. Dispense 0.1-ml portions of samples and standard mixture in duplicate and one or two blanks. Add 10 μl of G6PDH to each cuvette, stir well, ensuring that there are no air bubbles inside cuvette on transparent surfaces, and then read the absorbance (A1) after 5-10 min. This allows sufficient time for oxidation of any endogenous G6P that may be in the sample. Add 20 μl of glucose, 20 μl of HK and mix well. Allow 10-20 min at room temperature for the reaction to reach completion (i.e. observe that there are no further changes in absorbance on the recorder), then read A2.

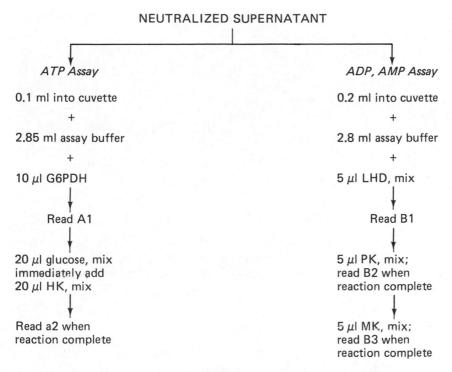

FIG. 10-5. Flow chart of summary of procedures for analysis of ATP, ADP and AMP. (From Ivanovici, 1977.)

ADP-AMP Assay

Dispense 2.8 ml of ADP-AMP assay buffer into each cuvette. Add 0.2 of sample, 0.1 ml of standard mixture plus 0.1 ml water, and 0.2 ml of water for the blank. Then add 5 μl LHD to all cuvettes, mix well, remove bubbles, and read absorbance (B1) after 5-10 min. Add 5 μl PK and read B2 after the reaction is complete (5 min). Finally, add 5 μl MK, and read B3 after 15-10 min. Since this last reaction is the slowest of the three, a check with the recorder for the reaction's completion is necessary.

Check for Enzyme Activities

New enzymes for both assays should be checked for activity before embarking on a series of assays. For enzymes used in the ATP assay, make a standard mixture of 0.05 mM G6P and ATP, and add 0.1 ml of this to cuvette with 2.85 ml of ATP assay buffer.

Read absorbance before adding G6PDH (A0), add G6PDH, wait until reaction stops, then read A1.

The difference (A1 − A0; G6P) should be approximately 0.100 if the G6PDH is active. Continue with assay as described earlier. The difference (A2 − A1; ATP) should also be 0.100 if the HK is active. For enzymes used in the assay for ADP and AMP, make a mixture containing 0.05 mM pyruvate, ADP and AMP. Read B0 before adding LDH. The difference (B1 − B0; pyruvate) should be approximately 0.100 if LDH is active for a volume of 0.1 ml of standard mixture. Similarly (B2 − B1; ADP) and (B3 − B2; AMP) should be approximately 0.080-0.100 and 0.200, respectively.

Low Concentrations of Nucleotide

If the concentrations of ATP, ADP and AMP are low in the samples, the sample volume may be increased up to 0.5 ml. If this is done, the standards are made up with 0.1 ml standard mixture and up to 0.4 ml water, and the blank cuvette has up to 0.5 ml water added to it. The assay volume (i.e. sample and assay buffer) may remain 3.0 ml by using less buffer.

Calculation of Results and Use of Statistics

Nucleotide Concentrations

The concentrations of ATP, ADP and AMP are calculated as follows:

$$\text{ATP } (\mu\text{mol g}^{-1} \text{ wet wt tissue}) = \frac{\Delta\text{Ab}_{\text{ATP}} \times \text{AV} \times \text{EV}}{6.22 \times \text{SV} \times \text{TW} \times 1.0}$$

$$\text{ADP } (\mu\text{mol g}^{-1} \text{ wet wt tissue}) = \frac{\Delta\text{Ab}_{\text{ADP}} \times \text{AV} \times \text{EV}}{6.22 \times \text{SV} \times \text{TW} \times 1.0}$$

$$\text{AMP } (\mu\text{mol g}^{-1} \text{ wet wt tissue}) = \frac{\Delta\text{Ab}_{\text{AMP}} \times \text{AV} \times \text{EV}}{6.22 \times \text{SV} \times \text{TW} \times 2 \times 1.0}$$

where:

$$\Delta\text{Ab}_{\text{ATP}} = \text{A2} - \text{A1}$$
$$\Delta\text{Ab}_{\text{ADP}} = \text{B2} - \text{B1}$$
$$\Delta\text{Ab}_{\text{AMP}} = \text{B3} - \text{B2}$$

If $\Delta\text{Ab} < 0$, use 0, not the negative number.

AV = assay volume (ml), i.e. volume of solution (buffer and sample) in cuvette.

EV = extract volume (ml), i.e. volume of neutralized supernatant measured after extraction procedure.

6.22 = extinction coefficient, i.e. absorbancy at 340 nm and pH 7.6 of a solution of NADPH or NADH containing 1 μmol ml^{-1}.

SV = volume of sample supernatant used in cuvette (ml).

TW = tissue weight (g).

1.0 = length of light path inside cuvette (cm); usually 1.0 cm.

Nucleotide ratios

Following the determination of concentrations of ATP, ADP and AMP for individual organisms, the averages of the replicates are calculated. The following variables can then be calculated from these mean values:

adenylate pool =
(ATP + ADP + AMP) μmol g^{-1} wet wt tissue

adenylate energy charge =
(ATP + $\frac{1}{2}$ADP)/(ATP + ADP + AMP)

ratio of ATP : ADP

ratio of ATP : AMP

adenylate kinase equilibrium = [ATP] [AMP]/[ADP]^2

Statistical Analyses

Means and coefficients of variation (CV) should be calculated for each nucleotide. The CV indicates the level of analytical precision and is calculated by: (standard deviation/mean) $\times$ 100 (Snedecor and Cochran, 1967).

If the CV exceeds 20% for ATP and ADP, the samples should be re-analysed, perhaps with a larger sample volume. If the CV for AMP exceeds 40%, extra analyses should be done. The higher value of CV for AMP has been set because, often, the concentrations of AMP are so low that readings are at the limit of sensitivity for the method. The higher variability for low readings can be overcome partly by increasing the volume of sample added to the cuvette, or by increasing the amount of material extracted.

A Worked Example

The data in Tables 10-3 and 10-4 are presented as an example to illustrate the procedures outlined above. The data are from 10

TABLE 10–3.   Raw Data for Gastropods (*Pyrazus ebeninus*) Collected at High and Low Tides from an Intertidal Area*

Sample					ATP assay					ADP-AMP assay				
Animal No.	Size (mm)	Clamp time (s)	EV	TW		Rep I	ΔA1	Rep II	ΔA2		Rep I	ΔB1	Rep II	ΔB2
High tide														
1	85	41	2.1	.199	G6PDH (A1)	.046		.062		LDH (B1)	.394	.040	.390	.038
					HK (A2)	.147	.101	.198	.136	PK (B2)	.354	.006	.352	−.002
										MK (B3)	.348		.354	
2	87	46	2.1	.176	G6PDH	.034		.036		LDH	.383	.033	.393	.031
					HK	.134	.100	.130	.094	PK	.350	.002	.362	0
										MK	.348		.362	
3	81	41	2.5	.239	G6PDH	.046		.033		LDH	.389	.043	.385	.044
					HK	.170	.124	.189	.156	PK	.346	.008	.341	−.001
										MK	.338		.342	
4	80	63	2.1	.081	G6PDH	.040		.036		LDH	.385	.035	.390	.031
					HK	.115	.075	.117	.081	PK	.350	.002	.359	.001
										MK	.348		.358	
5	79	36	2.3	.216	G6PDH	.028		.035		LDH	.383	.045	.393	.047
					HK	.114	.086	.100	.065	PK	.338	.001	.346	−.002
										MK	.337		.348	

STD MIX (100 μl)					G6PDH	.040		.036		LDH	.443		.376	
					HK	.148	.108	.134	.098	PK	.358	.085	.295	.081
										MK	.158	.200	.089	.206
Low tide														
1	85	41	3.0	.278	G6PDH	.045		.046		LDH	.371		.379	
					HK	.160	.115	.170	.124	PK	.277	.094	.287	.092
										MK	.247	.030	.257	.030
2	82	46	2.1	.203	G6PDH	.037		.040		LDH	.375		.383	
					HK	.140	.103	.150	.110	PK	.323	.052	.329	.054
										MK	.320	.003	.323	.006
3	86	73	2.9	.279	G6PDH	.039		.060		LDH	.388		.391	
					HK	.163	.124	.175	.115	PK	.283	.105	.286	.105
										MK	.244	.039	.252	.034
4	90	61	3.2	.298	G6PDH	.032		.100		LDH	.374		.384	
					HK	.145	.113	.258	.158	PK	.245	.129	.246	.138
										MK	.180	.065	.197	.049
5	90	60	2.4	.230	G6PDH	.057		.037		LDH	.393		.401	
					HK	.076	.019	.070	.033	PK	.331	.062	.343	.058
										MK	.255	.076	.273	.070
STD MIX (100 μl)					G6PDH	.025		.039		LDH	.443		.391	
					HK	.124	.099	.143	.104	PK	.358	.085	.315	.076
										MK	.158	.200	.130	.185

*Animals were freeze-clamped in the field. AV(ATP) = AV (ADP & AMP) = 3.0 ml; SV(ATP) = 0.21; SV(ADP & AMP) = 0.5 ml. EV = Volume of neutralized supernatant. TW = Tissue weight (g).

TABLE 10-4.   Adenine Nucleotide Variables Calculated from Data in Table 10-3

Animal No.	ATP				ADP			
	1	2	$\overline{X}$	CV	1	2	$\overline{X}$	CV
High tide								
1	2.57	3.46	3.02	20.9	0.36	0.34	0.35	4.7
2	2.88	2.71	2.80	4.4	0.38	0.36	0.37	4.4
3	3.13	3.94	3.54	16.2	0.43	0.44	0.44	1.6
4	4.69	5.07	4.88	5.5	0.88	0.78	0.83	8.6
5	2.21	1.67	1.94	19.7	0.46	0.48	0.47	3.1
Group mean ± S.E.		3.23 ± 0.49				0.49 ± 0.087		
Low tide								
1	2.99	3.23	3.11	5.5	0.84	0.82	0.83	1.4
2	2.57	2.75	2.66	4.6	0.52	0.54	0.53	2.5
3	3.11	2.89	3.00	5.4	1.05	1.05	1.05	0
4	2.93	4.09	3.51	23.5	1.34	1.43	1.38	4.8
5	0.49	0.83	0.66	38.1	0.62	0.58	0.60	5.1
Group mean ± S.E.		2.59 ± 0.49				0.88 ± 016		
t-test[a]		0.93 n.s.				−2.17*		
Overall CV		37.6%				48.8%		

[a]n.s $p > 0.05$; *$p < 0.05$; **$p < 0.01$.

gastropod molluscs (*Pyrazus ebeninus*) that were collected from their estuary at low and high tides (5 at each tide). Samples were freeze-clamped in the field.

Interpretation

Once the concentrations of all the adenine nucleotides, the AEC's and nucleotide totals for the individual animals have been calculated, group means can be calculated and significance tests carried out. In the example above, a *t*-test is adequate and indicates that differences between high- and low-tide groups are

AMP					Adenylate energy charge
1	2	$\bar{X}$	CV	(ATP+ ADP+ AMP)	
0.031	0	0.015	141.4	3.39	0.94
0.012	0	0.006	141.4	3.18	0.94
0.04	0	0.02	141.14	4.0	0.94
0.025	0.013	0.019	45.1	5.73	0.93
0.005	0	0.003	141.4	2.41	0.90
		0.013 ± 0.003		3.74 ± 0.56	0.93 ± 0.008
0.16	0.16	0.16	0	3.86	0.86
0.015	0.03	0.023	47%	3.21	0.910
0.20	0.17	0.19	11.3	4.24	0.83
0.34	0.25	0.30	20.5	5.19	0.81
0.38	0.35	0.37	5.8	1.57	0.61
		0.21 ± 0.061		3.61 ± 0.60	0.80 ± 0.051
		−3.27**		0.16 n.s.	2.32*
		123.5%		33.4%	11.8%

significant for ADP, AMP and energy charge. Of these three, energy charge shows the least between-individual variability (lowest overall CV).

The general response of AEC to stressed and non-stressed environments has been described earlier in this manual. In summary, the values that are expected are as follows:

1. For unstressed/control organisms, 0.8–0.9.
2. For stressed organisms, a *reduction* (increases in response to stress have not been reported to date) to values between 0.7 and 0.5. Within this range, organisms usually remain viable and recover if the stress is removed. Reductions below 0.5 may indicate lethal stress or onset of dormancy.

In the worked example above, AEC in *P. ebeninus* was significantly greater at high tide than at low tide, indicating that the potential for metabolic activity is higher during the former part of the tidal cycle. This correlates with the activity of this species over the tidal cycle, namely greater at high tide when it is immersed than at low tide. The adenylate pool was constant, indicating that the changes in AEC occurred because of a redistribution of nucleotides within a constant pool. Laboratory and field studies are described in detail elsewhere (Ivanovici 1980a, 1980b; Rainer et al., 1979).

Procedures for Optimization of Estimates

Due to the highly labile nature of ATP and the high activity of ATPases in biological samples (Newsholme and Start, 1973; Jaworek et al., 1974), it is essential to determine the influence of various steps of the methodology on the determinations of the adenine nucleotides. In this way, a fairly close approximation of *in vivo* levels may be obtained. If this is not done, results may be misinterpreted. In this section, three procedures are suggested as aids to the optimization of determinations of adenylate energy charge. It is further suggested that these should be carried out early in an experimental programme, to allow correction factors to be estimated and applied as necessary, and that they should be applied to each species studied.

1. The efficiency of extraction of nucleotides from sample tissue may be determined as follows: A known amount of ATP (ADP or AMP) is added to subsamples of tissues to be studied. Tissue samples with and without added nucleotide, as well as several samples consisting of standard alone, are then extracted as described previously. Efficiency of extraction of added nucleotide is then calculated by

$$\frac{ATP_{sample + standard} - ATP_{sample}}{ATP_{standard}} \times 100$$

The added standard may be either the pure nucleotide, or biological material whose nucleotide concentration has been previously determined. This method estimates the efficiency of extraction of nucleotides that are not bound to membranes and other cellular structures. Estimates for bound nucleotides are as yet unavailable, but their concentrations are thought to be low compared to the acid-extractable nucleotides (Newsholme, pers. comm.).

2. The extracted supernatants may have inhibitory or stimulatory effects on the enzymatic analyses, leading to under- or over-estimates, respectively, of ATP, ADP and AMP. These effects are determined by adding known amounts of the nucleotides to the samples. For example, 5 μl of 20 mM ATP can be added to several cuvettes with samples whose HK reactions have stabilized, and absorbances read when the reactions due to the added ATP have stopped. Samples of standards only (i.e. 5μl 20 mM ATP in x ml sample volume of water) should also be assayed. Sample concentrations can then be multiplied by the following factor:

$$CF = 1 + \left(1 - \frac{\Delta Ab_{sample + standard} - \Delta Ab_{samples}}{\Delta Ab_{standard}}\right)$$

where ΔAb is the difference in absorbances between the last and penultimate additions to the cuvette.

Correction factors need be used only when their values are less than 0.94 or more than 1.06. Once correction factors have been determined for a particular type of sample, they need only be redetermined periodically or if the samples change markedly, e.g. if animals are exposed to toxic chemicals which may be extracted along with the nucleotides.

3. The handling and dissection procedures may have effects on the nucleotides, especially if the species is very active or if the dissection is complex or prolonged. A suggested procedure here is to sample animals that have been handled for increasing periods of time, then test the data for correlations between time and nucleotide concentrations. For example, groups, of four *P. ebeninus* were dissected and handled for periods ranging from approximately 40 s to 4 min. Significant changes did not occur within the first 90 s (Ivanovici, 1977).

MAXIMAL ENZYME ACTIVITIES

A number of enzymes from the tissues of *M. edulis* have been studied in some detail, and the assay conditions are given in Table 10-5. The procedures used for the preparation of homogenates and subcellular fractions vary for different studies, but useful references include Addink and Veenhof (1975) and Zaba et al. (1978).

TABLE 10–5. Optimal Assay Conditions for a Number of Enzymes of *M. edulis*[a]

	Enzyme	Assay step[b]	Assay conditions[c]	References[d]
1.	Lactate dehydrogenase (E.C.1.1.1.27)	NADH↓	50 mM trie pH 7.6, 5 mM pyruvate, 0.12 mM NADH	4
2.	3-Hydroxyacyl CoA dehydrogenase (E.C.1.1.1.30)	NADH↑	50 mM tris pH 8.1, 3% ethanol, 2 mM NAD$^+$, 20 mM DL-β-hydroxybutyrate, 10 μg ml^{-1} antimycin A	1
3.	L-malate dehydrogenase (E.C.1.1.1.37)	NADH↓	100 mM Hepes pH 8, 1 mM oxaloacetate, 0.2 mM NAD	11
4.	Malate dehydrogenase (decarboxylating) (E.C.1.1.1.38)	NADPH↑	100 mM Hepes pH 8, 2.5 mM malate, 0.5 mM NADP$^+$, 1 mM MnCl$_2$	17, Livingstone (unpub. data)
5.	NAD$^+$-isocitrate dehydrogenase (E.C.1.1.1.41)	NADH↑	80 mM trie pH 7.5, 3.7 mM DL-isocitrate, 42 mM NaCl, 0.32 mM NAD$^+$, 3.9 mM MnSO$_4$, 3 mM ADP	1
6.	NADP$^+$-isocitrate dehydrogenase (E.C.1.1.1.42)	NADPH↑	50 mM Mops pH 7.5, 5 mM MgCl$_2$, 1 mM EDTA, 1 mM DTT, 1 mM NADP$^+$, 4 mM D,L-isocitrate	6, 8
7.	6-Phosphogluconate dehydrogenase (E.C.1.1.1.43)	NADPH↑	100 mM Hepes pH 8, 10 mM MgCl$_2$, 2 mM 6-phosphogluconate, 0.5 mM NADP$^+$	2, 6
8.	Glucose dehydrogenase (E.C.1.1.1.47)	NADPH↑	100 mM Hepes pH 8, 10 mM MgCl$_2$, 60 mM glucose, 0.5 mM NADP$^+$	Livingstone (unpub. data)
9.	Glucose-6-phosphate dehydrogenase (E.C.1.1.1.49)	NADPH↑	100 mM Hepes pH 8, 10 mM MgCl$_2$, 2 mM glucose-6-phosphate, 0.5 mM NADP$^+$	12, 6

10.	Glyceraldehyde-phosphate dehydrogenase (E.C.1.2.1.12)	NADH↓	50 mM trie pH 7.6, 12.5 mM glycerate 3-phosphate, 1 mM ATP, 0.12 mM NADH, 1 mM MgCl$_2$, 1 mM EDTA, excess phosphoglycerate kinase (E.C.2.7.2.3)	4
11.	Pyruvate dehydrogenase	NADH↑	200 mM potassium phosphate buffer pH 7.0, 0.3 mM MgCl$_2$, 0.1 mM coenzyme-A, 0.4 mM NAD$^+$, 10 mM glutathione, 0.2 mM thiamine pyrophosphate, 5 mM potassium pyruvate	1
12.	Succinate dehydrogenase (E.C.1.3.99.1)	DCIP↓	250 mM tris pH 7.4, 100 mM succinate, 2 mM ATP, 0.05 mM DCIP, 1 mM PMS	7

(continued)

[a]The assay conditions have only been partly optimized for enzymes 2, 5, 11, 13, 14, 15, 30. For details of tissues, subcellular fractions, etc. see references.

[b]NAD(P)H ↑ or ↓ : increase or decrease in absorbance measured spectrophotometrically at 334, 340 or 365 nm; DCIP (dichloro-phenolindophenol): decrease in absorbance measured spectrophotometrically at 600 nm; H$^+$↑ : rate of H$^+$ release measured by pH-stat; assay of glycogen synthetase performed in two steps; fumarate ↓ : decrease in absorbance measured at 240 nm.

[c]Assay temperature : 20 or 25° C; trie, triethanolamine-HC1; Hepes, 2-(N-2-hydroxyethylpiperazin-N^1-yl) ethanesulphonic acid; Mops, morpholinopropane sulphonic acid; EDTA, ethylenediaminetetra-acetic acid; DTT, dithiothreitol; PMS, phenazine methosulphate; IDP, inosine-5-diphosphate, UDP, uridine diphosphate.

[d]The first reference is that from which the assay conditions are taken.

1. Addink & Veenhoff (1975).
2. Bayne et al. (1979).
3. Cook & Gabbott (1978).
4. Ebberink & De Zwaan (1980).
5. Gabbot et al. (1979).
6. Gabbott & Head (1980).
7. Hammen (1975).
8. Head & Gabbott (1980).
9. Holwerda & De Zwaan (1973).
10. De Zwaan & Holwerda (1972).
11. Livingstone (1976).
12. Livingstone (1981).
13. Livingstone & Bayne (1974).
14. Livingstone & Bayne (1977).
15. Livingstone & Clarke (1983).
16. De Zwaan (1972).
17. De Zwaan (1977).
18. De Zwaan & de Bont (1975).
19. De Zwaan et al. (1975).
20. De Zwaan & Van Marrewijk (1973).

TABLE 10-5. (Continued)

Enzyme	Assay step	Assay conditions	References
13. NAD$^+$-Glutamate dehydrogenase (E.C.1.4.1.2)	NADH↓	50 mM trie pH 8.0, 0.2 mM NADH, 3 mM ADP, 2.5 mM EDTA, 100 mM ammonium acetate, 7 mM 2-oxoglutarate	1
14. Glutamate dehydrogenase (E.C.1.4.1.4)	NADPH↓	50 mM trie pH 8.0, 0.2 mM NADPH, 3 mM ADP, 2.5 mM EDTA, 100 mM ammonium acetate, 7 mM 2-oxoglutarate	1
15. 2-Oxoglutarate dehydrogenase	NADH↑	45 mM potassium phosphate buffer pH 6.5, 0.9 mM MgCl$_2$, 0.45 mM EDTA, 0.25 mM glutathione, 1 mM 2-oxoglutarate, 0.9 mM NAD$^+$	1
16. Glycogen phosphorylase (E.C.2.4.1.1)	NADPH↑	50 mM trie pH 7.6, 10 mg ml^{-1} glycogen, 80 mM KH$_2$PO$_4$, 0.6 mM NADP$^+$, 5 mM Mg acetate, 2.5 mM EDTA, 2 mM DTT, 5 mM imidazole, 0.8 mM AMP, 0.004 mM glucose-1, 6-biphosphate, excess glucose-6-phosphate dehydrogenase (E.C.1.1.1.49) and phosphoglucomutase (E.C.2.7.5.1)	4
17. Glycogen synthetase (E.C.2.4.1.11)	NADH↓	Step 1. 50 mM tris pH 7.5, 20 mM Na$_2$SO$_3$, 5 mM EDTA, 25 mM KF, 10 mM UDP-glucose, 5 mM glucose-	

242

No.	Enzyme		Conditions	References
			6-phosphate, glycogen (10 mM anhydroglucosyl units) Step 2. 50 mM potassium phosphate buffer pH 7.5, 5 mM MgCl$_2$, 10 mM hydrazine-HCl pH 7.5, 0.1 mM phosphoenolpyruvate, 0.15 mM NADH, excess pyruvate kinase (E.C. 2.7.1.40) and lactate dehydrogenase (E.C.1.1.1.27)	3, 5
18.	Hexokinase (E.C.2.7.1.1)	NADH↑	100 mM tris pH 8, 10 mM MgCl$_2$, 1 mM glutathione, 0.25 mM NAD$^+$, 20 mM glucose, 2 mM ATP, excess NAD-glucose-6-phosphate dehydrogenase (E.C.1.1.1.49)	15
19.	Phosphofructokinase (E.C.2.7.1.11)	NADH↓	50 mM tris pH 7.6, 1 mM fructose-6-phosphate, 1 mM ATP, 0.12 mM NADH, 5 mM MgCl$_2$, excess aldolase (E.C.4.2.1.13), glycerol-3-phosphate dehydrogenase (E.C.1.1.1.8) and triosephosphate isomerase (E.C. 5.3.1.1)	4
20.	Pyruvate kinase (E.C.2.7.1.40)	NADH↓	100 mM tris pH 7.7, 2.5 mM phosphoenolpyruvate, 2 mM ADP, 67 mM KCl, 6.7 mM MgCl$_2$, 0.1 mM fructose-1, 6-biphosphate, 0.15 mM NADH, excess lactate dehydrogenase (E.C.1.1.1.27)	13, 9, 10, 16, 19

(continued)

TABLE 10-5. (Continued)

Enzyme	Assay step	Assay conditions	References
21. Phosphoglycerate kinase (E.C.2.7.2.3)	NADH↓	50 mM trie pH 7.6, 12.5 mM glycerate 3-phosphate, 1 mM ATP, 0.12 mM NADH, 1 mM MgCl$_2$, 1 mM EDTA, excess glyceraldehyde-phosphate dehydrogenase (E.C.1.2.1.12)	4
22. Arginine kinase (E.C.2.7.3.3)	NADH↓	50 mM trie pH 7.6, 5 mM phosphoarginine, 0.4 mM ADP, 12.5 mM glycerate 3-phosphate, 0.2 mM NADH, 1 mM MgCl$_2$, excess phosphoglycerate kinase (E.C.2.7.2.3) and glyceraldehyde-phosphate dehydrogenase (E.C.1.2.1.12)	4
23. Adenylate kinase (E.C.2.7.4.3)	NADH↓	50 mM trie pH 7.6, 1 mM ATP, 1 mM AMP, 1 mM phosphoenol pyruvate, 0.12 mM NADH, 2 mM MgCl$_2$, 100 mM KC1, excess lactate dehydrogenase (E.C.1.1.1.27) and pyruvate kinase (E.C.2.7.1.40)	4
24. Phosphoglucomutase (E.C.2.7.5.1)	NADPH↑	50 mM trie pH 7.6, 2 mM glucose-1-phosphate, 0.6 mM NADP$^+$, 1.7 mM MgCl$_2$, 0.004 mM glucose-1.6-biphosphate, 0.9 mM EDTA, excess glucose-6-phosphate dehydrogenase (E.C.1.1.1.49)	4

244

25.	Phosphoglyceromutase (E.C.2.7.5.3)	NADH↓	50 mM trie pH 7.6, 12.5 mM glycerate 3-phosphate, 0.4 mM ADP, 0.12 mM NADH, 1 mM MgCl$_2$, excess enolase (E.C.4.2.1.11) pyruvate kinase (E.C.2.7.1.40) and lactate dehydrogenase (E.C.1.1.1.27)	4
26.	Hexosebiphosphatase (E.C.3.1.3.11)	NADPH↑	50 mM trie pH 7.6, 1.2 mM fructose-1,6-biphosphate, 0.6 mM NADP$^+$, 10 mM MgCl$_2$, 2 mM DTT, excess glucose-6-phosphate dehydrogenase (E.C.1.1.1.49) and glucose-phosphate isomerase (E.C.5.3.1.9)	4
27.	ATPase (E.C.3.6.1.3)	H$^+$↑	50 mM trie pH 7.6, 30 mM KCl, 0.1 mM CaCl$_2$, 0.5 mM MgCl$_2$, 1 mM ATP	4
28.	Phosphoenolpyruvate carboxykinase (E.C.4.1.1.32)	NADH↓	100 mM sodium cacodylate-HCl pH 6.5, 8.3 mM KCl, 2.5 mM MnCl$_2$, 1 mM glutathione, 1 mM IDP, 1.3 mM phosphoenolpyruvate, 0.15 mM NADH, excess malate dehydrogenase (E.C.1.1.1.37)	14, 18, 20
29.	Fructosebiphosphate aldolase (E.C.4.1.2.13)	NADH↓	50 mM trie pH 7.6, 1.2 mM fructose-1,-6-biphosphate, 0.12 mM NADH, excess glycerol-3-phosphate dehydrogenase (E.C.1.1.1.8) and triosephosphate isomerase (E.C.5.3.1.1)	4

(continued)

TABLE 10-5. (Continued)

Enzyme	Assay step	Assay conditions	References
30. Fumarase (E.C.4.2.1.2)	fumarate↓	33 mM phosphate buffer pH 7.3, 17 mM sodium fumarate	1
31. Enolase (E.C.4.2.1.11)	NADH↓	50 mM trie pH 7.6, 2.5 mM glycerate-3-phosphate, 0.4 mM ADP 0.12 mM NADH, 1 mM MgCl$_2$, excess pyruvate kinase (E.C.2.7.1.40) and lactate dehydrogenase (E.C.1.1.1.27)	4
32. Triosephosphate isomerase (E.C.5.3.1.1)	NADH↓	50 mM trie pH 7.6, 0.5 mM glycer-aldehyde-3-phosphate, 0.12 mM NADH, excess glycerol-3-phosphate dehydrogenase (E.C.1.1.1.8)	4
33. Glucosephosphate isomerase (E.C.5.3.1.9)	NADPH↑	50 mM trie pH 7.6, 1.5 mM fructose-6-phosphate, 0.6 mM NADP$^+$ 6.8 mM MgCl$_2$, excess glucose-6-phosphate dehydrogenase (E.C.1.1.1.49)	4

NADPH-PRODUCING ENZYMES: DETERMINATION OF THE SPECIFIC ACTIVITY OF G6PDH OF THE BLOOD CELLS OF *M. EDULIS*

The determination of the specific activity (S.A.) of glucose-6-phosphate dehydrogenase (G6PDH; E. C. 1. 1. 1. 49) involves the collection of mussels, the preparation of a blood cell homogenate and the assay of the homegenate for enzyme activity and protein.

Collection of Mussels, Preparation of Blood Cell Homogenate

Equipment and chemicals: Hypodermic syringe, 1- or 2-ml, with 23-gauge needle; stoppered glass containers (2-ml minimum volume); centrifuge tubes (2-ml minimum volume); centrifuge (maximum required g: 1,000 to 3,000; refrigerated); ultrasonic disintegrator; pipettes (500 μl to 1 ml); ice-box and ice; sterilised filtered ambient seawater; 10 mM tris-HCL pH 7.7 containing 1 mM ethylene-diaminetetra-acetic acid (EDTA) and 1 mM dithiothreitol (DTT) (dissolve 1.211 g of tris, 0.372 g of EDTA and 0.154 g of DTT in 500 ml of distilled water, cool to 4°C, adjust the pH to 7.7 with concentrated HCl and make up to 1 litre with distilled water; store at 4°C).

Collect five to ten mussels (4-5 cm length), remove a blood sample (0.5-1 ml) from each by a hypodermic syringe inserted into the posterior adductor muscle blood sinus, and place the sample in a stoppered container on ice. All subsequent procedures are performed at 4°C. Centrifuge the blood sample at 1,000-3,000 g for 10 min, decant and collect the supernant (serum), resuspend the pellet (blood cells) in 1 ml of sterilised seawater and recentrifuge as before. Decant the second supernant, add it to the first and keep the pooled sample (the "washings") on ice. Resuspend the blood cells in 1 ml of 10 mM tris-HCl pH 7.7 (4°C) containing 1 mM EDTA and 1 mM DTT. Sonicate the sample to break up the blood cells and store at 4°C. The blood cell homogenate will settle out on standing and should be shaken gently before removing aliquots for the determination of enzyme activity and protein.

G6PDH Assay

Equipment and chemicals: Visible-wavelength spectrophotometer, semi-micro cuvettes (1 cm path length), pipettes (100-500 μl), 200 mM 4-(-2-hydroxyethyl)-1-piperazine-sulphonic acid (Hepes) buffer pH 8 containing 20 mM MgCl$_2$ (dissolve 23.83 g of Hepes and 2.03 g of MgCl$_2$ in 400 ml of distilled water, adjust the pH to 8 with concentrated NaOH and make up to 500 ml with distilled water), 20 mM D-glucose-6-phosphate, disodium salt (G6P) (dissolve 36 mg in 5 ml distilled water, store frozen), 5mM nicotinamide adenine dinucleotide phosphate (NADP$^+$) (dissolve approximately 20 mg in 5 ml distilled water, store frozen or at 4°C).

Reaction:

$$G6P + NADP^+ \rightleftharpoons 6\text{-phosphogluconate} + NADPH + H^+$$

The rate of formation of NADPH is a measure of the enzyme activity, and it can be followed by means of the increase in absorbance at 340, 334, or 365 nm (Löhr and Waller, 1974).

Pipette 500 μl of 200 mM Hepes buffer pH 8 containing 20 mM MgCl$_2$, 100 μl 5 mM NADP$^+$ and 100-300 μl of sample (sonicated blood cells or washings) into a semi-micro cuvette and make up to 900 μl with distilled water. Preincubate at 25°C (or room temperature) for 10 min and start the reaction by the addition of 100 μl of 20 mM G6P. Record the increase in absorbance over several minutes; this should be linear. The enzyme activity in the sample is given by the relationship

$$\text{Activity } (\mu\text{mol min}^{-1}\text{ml}^{-1}) = \frac{\Delta Ab \times \text{dilution factor}}{6.22}$$

where ΔAb is the change in absorbance per minute, 6.22 is the extinction coefficient ϵ (cm^2 μmol^{-1}) at 340 nm (ϵ = 6.1 for 334 nm and 3.4 for 354 nm) and the dilution factor is given by 1,000 divided by the volume of sample in μl.

Protein Assay and the Determination of the S.A. of Blood Cell G6PDH

Equipment and chemicals: Visible-wavelength spectrophotometer, 50°C reaction bath, reaction tubes (2 ml), pipettes (25-750 μl), vortex tube mixer, semi-micro cuvettes (1 cm path length), solution

A (dissolve 2 g of sodium potassium tartrate and 10 g of sodium carbonate in 500 ml of 1 M NaOH and make up to 1 litre with distilled water), solution B (dissolve 2 g of sodium potassium tartrate and 1 g of copper sulphate in 90 ml of distilled water and make up to 100 ml with 1 M NaOH), solution C (prepare fresh; mix 1 volume of Folin and Ciocalteau's phenol reagent with 15 volumes of distilled water), bovine serum albumen fraction V (BSA) standards (dissolve 5 mg in 5 ml of distilled water and dilute to give concentrations of 0.4, 0.2, 0.1, 0.06, 0.04, 0.02 and 0.01 mg ml^{-1}).

The protein assay is a modification of the method of Lowry et al. (1951) (see also Peterson, 1979). Pipette an aliquot of blood cell homogenate into a reaction tube and add distilled water to make up to 250 μl. Also prepare tubes containing either 250μl of the BSA standards, a volume of 10 mM tris-HCl pH 7.7 containing 1 mM EDTA and 1 mM DTT equal to that of the sample volume (buffer blank) and 250 μl of distilled water (water blank). Add 230 μl of solution A to each tube and heat at 50°C for 10 min. Add 25 μl of solution B, mix and leave for 10 min at room temperature. Add 750 μl of solution C, mix and heat at 50°C for 10 min. Read the absorbance at 650 nm after zeroing the spectrophotometer on the water blank. Plot a log-log standard curve of protein concentration vs. absorbance and read off the protein concentration of the sample after first subtracting the absorbance due to the buffer, i.e. absorbance for sample $= Ab_1 - Ab_2$ where Ab_1 is absorbance of sample and Ab_2 is absorbance of buffer blank. The concentration of protein in the blood cell homogenate is given by the relationship:

$$\text{Protein (mg ml}^{-1}) = \frac{\text{protein (mg)} \times 250}{\text{sample volume } (\mu l)}$$

The S.A. of blood cell G6PDH is given by the relationship:

$$\text{S.A. } (\mu\text{mol min}^{-1}\text{mg}^{-1} \text{ protein})$$

$$= \frac{\text{enzyme activity of blood cells } (\mu\text{mol ml}^{-1})}{\text{protein conc. of blood cells (mg ml}^{-1})}$$

It should be noted that G6PDH activity is also present in the serum (washings), but it is usually less than 5% of the total blood G6PDH activity. As the origin of the serum activity is unknown it is not included in the calculation of S.A. However, if removal of blood from the mussel is difficult then some break-up of blood cells can occur and the activity in the washings can increase to 50%. Much of the protein from the broken cells will be spun down into the cell fraction, resulting in an erroneous S.A. Ideally such procedures should be repeated on fresh mussels. If this is not possible, then a good estimate of S.A. will be given by using total G6PDH activity in the above calculation.

MIXED-FUNCTION OXIDASE SYSTEMS

The study of mixed-function oxidase systems (MFO) as a possible detoxification mechanism requires investigation of a whole system of enzymes with many components. Thus, several approaches to measuring the capacity of this system in aquatic organisms have been developed. *In vivo* studies have focused on the administration of particular substrates, followed by measurement of the distribution of substrates and their metabolites in various body tissues and their elimination over time. Subcellular preparations from metabolically active tissues have been used in spectral studies of the key cytochrome (P-450) and to determine *in vitro* substrate conversion rates. To understand the physiological dynamics and toxic qualities of many chemical stressors, both whole organism and cellular approaches are necessary.

Methods for measuring MFO rates were derived from the study of mammalian systems, and a large literature is available, especially with regard to hepatic drug metabolism. Yet even in mammal systems the study of MFO components, requirements, substrate conversions, capacities, mechanisms and related physiological responses is still in the research stage. Some progress has been made in invertebrates—particularly insects, where high MFO rates can confer resistance to certain pesticides—but knowledge of detoxification and metabolic capacities in aquatic organisms is still rudimentary. Mammalian methodology has been fruitfully applied and modified for use with other organisms, and the methods described in this section are examples taken from such studies on fish and aquatic invertebrates. However, to reduce variability in measurements, assay conditions must be tested and optimized for each species measured. Population and seasonal differences may be minimized by choosing animals of similar size, sex and reproductive state. Normal population variations have not been large enough to mask differences in MFO rates between fish from heavily polluted and clean habitats, but they may be a problem in establishing dose-relationships of chronic low-level pollutants, especially in invertebrates. However, it is possible that, with more sensitive assay procedures and reduced errors in measuring MFO rates (e.g. MFO preparations can be unstable), a variety of invertebrates may be shown to possess an inducible detoxification system.

In Vivo Studies

There have been several studies in which marine animals were exposed to particular lipid-soluble toxicants either in food or water, or by direct injection into blood. After varying time periods the animals were killed and individual tissues analysed for the presence of the toxicant and possible metabolites (e.g. Khan et al., 1972a; Lee et al., 1972a, 1972b, 1976; Sheridan, 1975; Guarino et al., 1971; Dvorchik et al., 1970; Pritchard and Kinter, 1970; Premdas and Anderson, 1963). In other experiments the concentrations of substrates and metabolites in whole animals or urine were measured (e.g. Lee, 1975; Darrow and Harding, 1975; Corner et al., 1973, 1976). Results of these studies indicate considerable variation not only in the ability of different species to metabolize and excrete toxicants, but also in the ability of a single species to handle different chemical stressors.

Lee et al. (1972b) used in vivo techniques to study the uptake, metabolism and discharge of radio-labelled naphthalene and benzopyrene in three species of marine fish. They showed that, as in mammals, uptake was followed by accumulation of the hydrocarbons and oxygenated metabolites in the liver, gut and flesh, with the gall bladder as the final storage site before excretion. The rate of metabolism in the liver was fast enough to produce a steady state so that the amount of hydrocarbon entering the liver was balanced by the amount of hydrocarbon and metabolites leaving the liver. The major route of excretion appeared to be via urine, and the types of metabolites produced were similar to those seen in mammalian studies. They also showed faster rates of metabolizing naphthalene than benzopyrene and that halogenated hydrocarbons may not be metabolized at all in fish.

These and other in vivo studies demonstrate that at least some fish have a toxicant metabolizing system efficient enough to be used as a mechanism for clearing body tissues of certain lipid soluble contaminants. Crustaceans appear to produce similar metabolites but at rates orders of magnitude lower than most fish (Lee et al., 1976; Burns, 1976b).

In Vitro Studies

Concurrent with the *in vivo* studies, several groups of researchers began examining aquatic animals for the presence of the microsomal MFO system of enzymes. Cellular preparations from tissues of aquatic animals contained cytochrome P-450 (as measured by spectral studies) and were able to convert model substrates to polar metabolites *in vitro* (e.g. Ahokas, 1976; Ahokas et al., 1975, 1976b; Bend et al., 1976b; Burns, 1976a, 1976b; Buhler and Rasmusson, 1968; Carlson, 1972, 1973, 1974; Chan et al., 1967; Creaven et al., 1965; Elmamlouk and Gessner, 1976a, 1976b; Ludke et al., 1972; Khan et al., 1972a, 1972b; Kurelec et al., 1977; Payne, 1977; Payne and Penrose, 1975; Pedersen et al., 1976; Pohl et al., 1974; Stanton and Khan, 1973. Vink, 1975). Methods of assay were adapted from mammalian studies, but attempts to optimize conversion rates of model substrates such as aniline (hydroxylation), aminopyrine (N-demethylation) and penenacetin (O-dealkylation) showed species differences in temperature and pH optima.

The MFO system was shown to be inducible in fish both in response to drugs such as phenylbutazone and to environmental contaminants such as petroleum oils and chlorinated hydrocarbons, and many of the assay procedures employed were not sensitive enough to measure the low enzyme rates present in crustacea or molluscs (Carlson, 1972, 1973). Improved methods suggest that the MFO system is present in many phyla of marine animals (Payne, 1977), but the capacity of this basic metabolic system to process environmental toxicants is highly variable, confirming the results obtained from *in vivo* studies.

For the MFO system to be useful in detoxification, the speed with which oxygenated intermediates can be conjugated and excreted is crucial. Oxygenation in a number of instances results in the production of highly toxic metabolites (Yang et al., 1977; Kinoshita and Gelboin, 1978). James et al. (1977) measured epoxide hydrase activity, glutathione-S-transferase activity and amino acid conjugation in marine teleosts, elasmobranchs and crustaceans. They concluded that all the species tested had sufficient activity to detoxify oxygenated intermediates produced by the MFO system. Corner et al. (1960) studied the distribution of β-glucuronidase and arylsulphatase in nine marine invertebrate phyla, showing that these two detoxification pathways are probably universal. Khan et al. (1974) concluded in their review of invertebrate detoxification mechanisms that the conjugation of activated metabolites normally occurs faster than the MFO reactions. Thus the limiting factor in how fast aquatic organisms can detoxify contaminants or accumulate activated intermediates may rest on the initial oxidation steps.

Estimation of Cytochrome P-450

Studies of drug metabolism catalyzed by the MFO systems in mammalian liver have established the requirements of NADPH (reduced nicotinamide adenine dinucleotide phosphate), molecular oxygen and a carbon monoxide-binding pigment named cytochrome P-450 localized in the microsomal fraction of cell extracts. Drugs and other compounds that are substrates or inhibitors react with the reduced form of P-450 to form an enzyme-substrate complex.

The cytochrome derives its name from the difference spectrum caused by the interaction of carbon monoxide (CO) with the reduced cytochrome to produce a single peak at 450 nm. The methods for estimating P-450 in microsomal preparations are detailed in Omura and Sato (1964a, 1964b) and have been adapted for use in invertebrate as well as vertebrate systems. Optical-difference spectroscopy has been used to circumvent the light-scattering problems associated with the spectroscopy of particulate enzyme preparations such as microsomes. By placing the microsomal suspension in both sample and reference cuvettes of a split-beam spectrophotometer, the light-scattering effect is balanced and a flat base-line can be recorded. Since only a small amount of light reaches the phototube, a sensitive spectrophotometer is required. According to Omura and Sato's original method, microsomal suspensions are placed in both cuvettes and the sample is saturated with CO gas. Both sample and reference are then reduced by the addition of a few mg of solid sodium dithionite and the difference spectrum recorded from about 350 to 600 nm. Relatively pure suspensions will show a single maximum at 450 nm with a molar extinction value of 91 cm^{-1} mM^{-1}. P-450 is enzymatically degraded to a more soluble and inactive form with a difference spectral maximum at 420 nm and a molar extinction value of 110 cm^{-1} mM^{-1}. Some enzyme preparations and especially whole tissue suspensions contain other hemoproteins which interfere with P-450 estimations. Matsubara et al. (1976) described variations of the difference spectroscopy methods for eliminating such interference.

The CO difference spectrum of the reduced microsomal preparations is the basis for estimating amounts of P-450. However, the appearance of maxima at 448 nm in microsomes from animals subjected to MFO-inducing drugs suggests the existence of multiple forms of the cytochrome and has led to studies on the relationship between structure and the binding of ligands. Different forms of P-450 may be responsible for catalyzing different oxidation reactions. To date, however, it has not been possible to establish a quantitative relationship between the concentrations of various spectral forms of P-450 and the rates of substrate conversions *in vitro*. Generally, when substrates interact with the oxidized form of P-450, two characteristic types of absorption spectra occur. Type I spectra are obtained with many compounds, including drugs, pesticides and steroid hormones, and are characterized by a peak in the range of 385 to 390 nm and a trough between 418 and 427 nm. Type II spectra have been reported from aromatic and aliphatic amines and are characterized by a peak between 425 and 435 nm and a trough between 390 and 405 nm. Some variations on these types also exist (Schenkman et al., 1967; Imai and Sato, 1966; Schenkman, 1970; Mailman and Hodgson, 1972).

Work on marine organisms is fairly recent. Elmamlouk et al. (1974) used difference spectral methods to measure P-450 in lobster (*Homarus americanus*) hepatopancreas. Levels were lower than mammalian preparations, but the suspensions displayed spectral characteristics of both Type I and II interactions. However, these interactions occurred at higher substrate concentrations than those with mammalian preparations. Thus the K_s values (the concentration at 50% saturation of the cytochrome binding sites) were generally higher than those reported for mammalian P-450. Whether lobster P-450 exhibited a low affinity for the substrates tested or whether endogenous substrates were bound and limiting the interactions could not be established.

Ahokas et al. (1976b) used difference spectroscopy to study P-450 in trout (*Salmo trutta lacustris*) and showed that the trout MFO system exhibited many similarities to mammalian systems. Bend et al. (1977b) reported progress in separating and purifying components of the MFO system in skate (*Raja erinacea*) and subsequently reported the isolation of spectrally distinct cytochromes with absorption maxima at 448 and 451 nm (Bend et al., 1977a). Although MFO activity can be induced in fish, it is still unclear whether induction causes an increase in the amount of P-450 in marine animals or any shift in spectral maxima toward a P-448 type cytochrome as in mammals, or whether induction simply represents a more efficient substrate turnover mechanism.

Measurement of Substrate Conversion Rates

In vitro rates of conversion of substrates to oxidised metabolites have been used to characterise MFO systems in marine animals. Assay techniques developed for mammalian systems were applied to fish studies with reasonable success (Ahokas et al., 1975; Bend et al., 1977a; Buhler and Rasmusson, 1968; Burns, 1976a; Creaven et al., 1965; Dewaide, 1971; James et al., 1977; Kurelec et al., 1977; Payne and Penrose, 1975; Pedersen et al., 1974; Pohl et al., 1974; Stanton and Khan, 1973; Stegeman, 1978). Invertebrates, however, show much slower rates of MFO activity, and more sensitive assays such as aldrin epoxidation and benzopyrene hydroxylation are needed to measure the pmol mg^{-1} min^{-1} seen in crustacea and other aquatic invertebrates (Burns, 1976b; Carlson, 1972, 1973, 1974; Elmamlouk and Gessner, 1976a, 1976b; Khan et al., 1972a, 1972b; Bend et al., 1977a; James et al., 1977; Payne, 1977; Philpot et al., 1976). Examples of such assays from the literature are given below, but it is important to realise that modifications may be required for samples from other sources:

1. *Benzopyrene monooxygenase fluorometric assay,* as used for tissues of Blue crab *Callinectes sapidus* (Singer and Lee, 1977). The assay mixture contained, in a final volume of 1 ml, sample (0-4 mg protein; cell debris and nuclei removed by centrifugation), 0.6 μmol NADPH, 3 μmol $MgCl_2$ and 0.01 μmol benzo(a)-pyrene. The mixture was incubated at $28°C$ for 30 min and the reaction stopped by the addition of 1 ml cold acetone and 3 ml hexane. Two-ml portions of the resulting organic phase were extracted with 4 ml 1 N NaOH, and the fluorescence of the products recorded with activation of 396 nm and emission at 522 nm (Turner model 430). Assays were done in triplicate with a blank containing homogenate boiled for 30 sec prior to addition of substrates. The assay was determined to be linear with both time

and protein under these conditions in green gland homogenates. One unit of enzyme activity was defined as the fluorescence produced in a 60-min incubation at 28°C equivalent to the fluorescence of 1×10^{-12} mol of 3-hydroxybenzo(a)pyrene.

2. *Benzopyrene monooxygenase radiometric assay,* as used for eggs of the Killifish *Fundulus heteroclitus* (Binder and Stegeman, 1980). The reaction mixture contained, in a final volume of 25 μl (microscale), 5-170 μg of embryonic protein (depending on fraction assayed), 0.1 M tris-HCl pH 7, 0.4 mM NADPH, 0.06 mM [^{3}H]-benzo(a)pyrene (about 300 μCi/μmol) and 2 mg ml^{-1} of bovine serum albumen. Blanks consisted of the complete reaction mixture without NADPH. The reaction was initiated by adding benzopyrene in 1 μl of acetone, incubated at 25°C for 30 min, stopped with 50 μl of 0.15 M KOH in 85% dimethylsulphoxide, and then extracted three times with 0.375 ml of hexane. Polar metabolites were quantitated by counting 30 μl of the aqueous phase acidified with 10 μl of 0.6 N HCl, in 3 ml of scintillation mixture. The liquid scintillation counting efficiency was determined by internal standardization.

3. *Aldrin epoxidation,* as used for tissues of the mussel *Mytilus edulis* (Moore et al., 1980). The reaction mixture contained, in a final volume of 4 ml, sample, 100 mM HEPES buffer pH 7.6, 10 mM MgSO$_4$, 0.5 M NaCl, 0.3 mM NADPH, 1.8 mM glucose-6-phosphate and 0.23 μmol aldrin added in 10 μl methanol. The mixtures were incubated aerobically at 25°C for 1 h with frequent shaking. Blanks were run without cofactors, without sample, and with all components but stopped at zero time. The incubations were stopped by extraction with 4 ml of 15% (v:v) diethyl ether in hexane followed by cooling. Extraction was completed with a further two 4-ml volumes of ether/hexane, and the bulked extracts were concentrated to 2 ml and analysed for dieldrin by electron-capture detector gas chromatography.

Methods for measuring MFO activity in marine animals are still in the research stage. Any species used for stress measurements must be studied for enzyme stability, the presence of endogenous inhibitors, tissue activity, and optimum assay conditions such as protein concentration, temperature and pH. MFO enzymes tend to be unstable and subject to inactivation by storage and freezing. No agreement even exists as to whether activity can be preserved by quick freezing and storage in liquid nitrogen. Most workers have prepared enzymes at ice temperatures (2-4°C) and assayed substrate conversion rates the same day. Carlson (1974) added 1 mM dithiothretol to enzyme preparations to prevent breakdown of P-450 to P-420. Burns (1976a, 1976b) used a carefully timed procedure so that all assays were done with microsomal suspensions prepared in identical manner in order to minimize variability due to instability.

Assay of various tissues from fish have shown that, as in mammals, the liver is the major site of MFO conversions. Bend et al. (1977a) reported bile as a potent inhibitor of MFO activity in fish and advised that gall bladders be carefully excluded from fish liver preparations. Pohl et al. (1974) and James et al. (1977) noted that extracts from crustacean hepatopancreas inhibited substrate turnover by fish enzymes, and they advised research on the presence of endogenous inhibitors. Initially, the concept of functional similarity was generalised to crustaceans and the hepatopancreas was assumed to be the major site for MFO activity (Carlson, 1973; Elmamlouk and Gessner, 1976a, 1976b). However, tissue distribution studies in crayfish (Khan et al., 1972b), fiddler crabs (Burns, 1976b) and blue crabs (Singer and Lee, 1977) have shown the green gland and other tissues to contain higher MFO activity than the hepatopancreas, which the latter authors suggest may be due to hormonal influences during molt cycles. Bayne et al. (1979) observed maximum activity in the blood cells of *M. edulis*.

Optimum assay conditions vary with species, and marine organisms tend to require lower incubation temperatures than mammals. Uncertainty also exists on the requirements of the incubation mixture. For example, Creaven et al. (1965) argued that nicotinamide is necessary to prevent inactivation of MFO enzymes by proteases, while Buhler and Rasmusson (1968) and Dewaide and Henderson (1968) reported inhibition of MFO activity by the same compound. James et al. (1977) substituted cumene hydroperoxide and sodium periodate in place of the NADPH-generating system and found each supported MFO activity at different levels in different species.

These reports demonstrate the requirement to research optimum enzyme preparations and assay conditions in test species. After standardizing procedures, populations should be studied for variations in enzyme activity due to sex and size (Stegeman, 1980), racial differences (Pedersen et al., 1974), influence of environmental temperature (Dewaide, 1971), seasonal effects due to reproductive cycles (Singer and Lee, 1977) and possible dietary effects.

Interpretation of Results

The use of MFO activities as measurements of response to chemical pollutants requires a quantitative change to be measurable above the normal variability in populations. Evidence of induction or depression of the system is found in different enzyme kinetics (change in V_{max} or K_m) or substrate turnover rates. MFO induction in fish has been demonstrated to result from exposure to specific drugs like phenylbutazone (Burns, 1976a) and 5,6-benzo-flavone (Chevion et al., 1977) and organic pollutants such as aromatic hydrocarbons (Bend et al., 1977b; Pedersen et al., 1976; Chevion et al., 1977), some halogenated hydrocarbons (Poland and Glover, 1977; Gruger et al., 1977), and some complex mixtures of petroleum hydrocarbons (Payne and Penrose, 1975; Burns, 1976a; Kurelec et al., 1977). Conversely, Ahokas et al. (1976a) showed a depression of MFO activity in fish exposed to pulp mill effluents. Thus, at least for fish populations, changes in MFO activity may be useful as a semi-specific indicator of stress from certain classes of organic pollutants. However, to date there is little evidence of induction of MFO activity in marine invertebrates exposed to organic xenobiotics, and therefore the techniques can only be recommended at present for use with fish.

METALLOTHIONEINS

Many reports of trace metal levels in organisms from polluted areas exist in the literature, but little can be inferred from these data as to the actual biological significance to the exposed organism. The following procedures describe a biochemically meaningful assay based upon the actual toxicology of the trace metals; it measures the levels of those metals that are bound by the trace metal detoxifying protein metallothionein, and those that are free to exert toxic effects by binding enzymes in the high molecular weight protein pool. These procedures are modifications of these described by Webb (1972), Shaikh and Lucis (1971) and Olafson and Thompson (1974) and were used in studies by Brown et al. (1977), Brown (1977), Brown and Chatel (1978), Brown and Parsons (1978), and Brown (1978).

Sample Preparation and Measurement

Equipment and Chemicals: Dissection instruments, motorised homogeniser with teflon pestle, centrifuge (maximum g required: 27,000), heater waterbath (70°C), ultracentrifuge (not essential), Pharmacia columns packed with Sephadex G-75 gel, fraction collector, UV spectrophotometer, atomic absorption spectrophotometer; 0.9% NaCl, 0.01 M NH$_4$HCO$_3$.

Liver (digestive gland), kidney and gills should be excised and analysed where possible, since metallothionein is particularly concentrated in these tissues (Nordberg, 1972; Bouquegneau et al., 1975; Roesijadi, 1979). Whole tissue of phytoplankton, zooplankton or bivalves can also be processed with elution of significant metallothionein peaks (Noël-Lambert, 1976; Talbot and Magee, 1978; Brown, 1978; Brown and Parsons, 1978).

A cytosolic extract is prepared by homogenizing tissue in 0.9% NaCl for exactly 3 min at a standard speed on a laboratory motor equipped with a teflon pestle (Fig. 10-6, steps 1-3). Sample sizes and volumes of sodium chloride used for different tissue types are given in Table 10-6. Homogenates are centrifuged at 27,000 g for exactly 10 min and the supernatant is collected (steps 4-5). An extraction of pellet can be done to increase the portion of metallothionein and other proteins extracted from tissue (steps 6-9). The homogenization and centrifugation settings are the same as for the first extraction. Volumes of sodium chloride used for different sample sizes and types are given in Table 10-6. For phytoplankton, zooplankton and smaller bivalves, minimal sample size may be available; in order that readily measurable levels of metals are eluted (step 15) a second extraction of pellet is not done (steps 6-9) as this would result in a dilution of tissue metal levels with resultant dilution of metal levels in fractions collected (step 16). Similar procedures are followed for very small samples of liver, kidney or gill tissue (Table 10-6).

Supernatants are heated in a 70°C water bath for 5 min (step 11, Fig 10-6) and then centrifuged to clear the tissue extract of cellular debris (step 12). The supernatant is collected (step 13) and the pellet discarded. An alternative to heating supernatants to remove cellular debris (step 11) is to centrifuge the supernatant at 105,000 g for 60 min. This latter procedure avoids losses of heat-coagulable enzymes from the high molecular weight protein pool. The ultracentrifugation procedure is particularly preferable if enzyme activities are to be measured in the high molecular weight

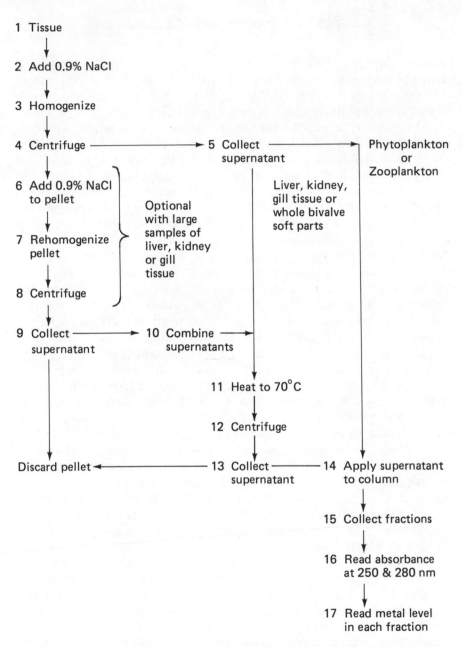

1 Tissue

2 Add 0.9% NaCl

3 Homogenize

4 Centrifuge ⟶ 5 Collect supernatant ⟶ Phytoplankton or Zooplankton

6 Add 0.9% NaCl to pellet

7 Rehomogenize pellet

8 Centrifuge

Optional with large samples of liver, kidney or gill tissue

Liver, kidney, gill tissue or whole bivalve soft parts

9 Collect supernatant ⟶ 10 Combine supernatants

11 Heat to 70°C

12 Centrifuge

Discard pellet ⟵ 13 Collect supernatant ⟶ 14 Apply supernatant to column

15 Collect fractions

16 Read absorbance at 250 & 280 nm

17 Read metal level in each fraction

FIG. 10-6. A flow diagram of the steps involved in the extraction of metallothionein and the high and low molecular weight pools from tissue. See text for details.

TABLE 10–6.   Recommended Procedures for Various Tissue Types

Tissue type	Sample size (1)[a] (g)	First homogenization (3) 0.9% NaCl volume (ml)	Second homogenization (7) 0.9% NaCl volume (ml)	Time to heat at 70°C (11) (min)	Volume to apply to column (14) (ml)	Column type[b] and size used	Fraction size[c] to collect (15) (ml)
Phytoplankton (whole tissue)	1	3	not done	not done	2	K.9/60	1.5
Zooplankton (whole tissue)	1	3	not done	not done	2	K.9/60	1.5
Bivalves (soft parts)	1	3	not done	5	2	K.9/60	1.5
Liver, kidney or gill tissue	0.1	1.5	not done	5	1.0	K.9/60	0.8
	0.5	2.0	not done	5	1.5	K.9/60	1.0
	1	2.5	1.5	5	2	K.9/60	1.5
	2	4.5	2.5	5	5	K1.6/100	6
	3	9	6	5	14	K2.5/100	15

[a]Number in brackets refers to the step number in Fig. 10–6.
[b]Pharmacia brand; column type (K) and diameter/length (cm).
[c]To produce about 30 fractions per profile.

261

TABLE 10–7. The Specifications for Various Sizes of Pharmacia Columns when Packed with Sephadex G-75 Gel

Column type, diameter/length (cm)	Bed volume (ml)	Min/max sample size (ml)	Maximum flow rate (ml)	Void volume (ml)	Time for first macromolecules to elute (h)
K.9/60	38	0.4/10	17	13	0.8
K1.6/100	200	2/50	44	70	1.6
K2.5/100	485	5/120	114	168	1.5

From Pharmacia technical literature.

pool, as many enzymes are irreversibly denatured by heat. It is not necessary to heat phytoplankton and zooplankton supernatants (Table 10-6) as these appear clear (free of cellular debris) after one extraction and centrifugation (steps 1–5) Resulting supernatants are applied to a column packed with Sephadex G-75 gel (step 14) and eluted with 0.01 M NH$_4$HCO$_3$; maximal flow rates are given in Table 10-7.

The size of the column employed (Table 10-7) will depend mainly upon the sample size used (Table 10-6). A narrower column is used for smaller sample sizes to prevent sample dilution. A longer column is preferable to a shorter column as it provides a better resolution of peaks. Better resolution of peaks can also be obtained by collecting smaller fraction sizes as eluant from the column (step 15). Resolution also improves with reductions of sample size down down 1–2% of the bed volume (Table 10-7). Sample sizes up to 25–40% of the bed volume give less-diluted cytoplasmic pools, but with less resolution.

The elutant will be collected as fractions using a standard fraction collector. The high molecular weight protein pool will be eluted as the first peak, with a shoulder or separate peak following due to the presence of haemoglobin, if applicable (Fig. 10-7). The metallothionein peak will elute next, followed by a double-peaked low molecular weight cytoplasmic pool (Shaikh and Lucis, 1971; Olafson and Thompson, 1974; Irons and Smith, 1976; Marafante, 1976; Noël-Lambert, 1976; Talbot and Magee, 1978). The position of peaks is determined initially by reading absorbances at 250 and 280 nm (step 16). The high and low molecular weight pools have high absorbance at 250 and 280 nm (Brown et al., 1977) whereas metallothionein absorbance is usually very low at 280 nm due to the absence of aromatic amino acids (Kagi and Vallee, 1961);

metallothionein may have a high absorbance at 250 nm due to the presence of sulfhydryl-Cd bonds (Kagi and Vallee, 1961). Each absorbance peak will correspond to a peak of various metals (Fig. 10-7). The high molecular weight protein pool usually contains Cu and Zn due to the presence of metalloenzymes (Brown et al., 1977). Metallothionein binds and thereby detoxifies the metals Hg, Cd, Ag and Sn, and also stores and/or detoxifies excesses of Cu and Zn above levels required for metalloenzymes (Brown and Parsons, 1978; Brown and Chatel, 1978). The low molecular weight cytoplasmic pools bind a small portion of metals in most organisms, but very high portions in phytoplankton and zooplankton (Brown, 1978).

In a gel elution profile comprising 45 fractions, the peaks will be tentatively identified as the high molecular weight protein pool (tubes 1–15), metallothionein (tubes 16–25), and the low molecular

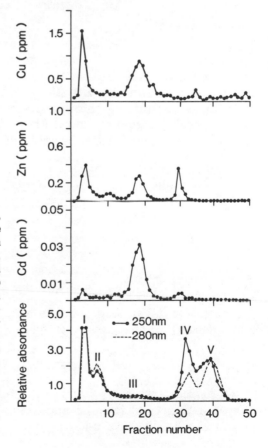

FIG. 10-7. Amounts of copper, zinc and cadmium in five cytoplasmic pools isolated from the liver of a Greater Scaup duck, using a Sephadex column and absorbance at 250 and 280 nm to identify the positions of the main protein peaks. Peak I corresponds to the high molecular weight protein pool which includes enzymes, peak II to haemoglobin, peak III to metallothionein, and peaks IV and V to low molecular weight cytoplasmic materials, such as amino acids, nucleic acids, and ATP. (After Brown et al., 1977.)

weight cytoplasmic pool (tubes 26–45) on the basis of elution position (Fig. 10-7). In other gel elution profiles from a variety of organisms, the high molecular weight protein pool consistently comprised the first 15/45 (0.33) tubes of the profile, metallothionein the next 11/45 (0.24) tubes of the profile, and the low molecular weight cytoplasmic pool the last 20/45 (0.44) tubes of the profile (Brown, 1978). The composition of the high molecular weight pool and metallothionein pool may be confirmed by procedures described later.

Metal levels in each fraction are then analysed using an atomic absorption spectrophotometer equipped with deuterium arc background correction and flame burner or graphite furnace as necessitated by the concentration of metal.

Calculation of results

Once metal levels have been determined in each fraction (step 17, Fig. 10-6), these can be added in each cytoplasmic pool and then expressed as a concentration of metal in each cytoplasmic pool per gram of tissue (wet weight). For instance, in a high molecular weight pool comprising 15 fractions (Fig. 10-7), the concentrations of Zn in each fraction (as mg Zn liter^{-1}) are added, correcting for the volume of each fraction (in this case, 10.2 ml):

$$\left(\frac{X_1 \text{ mg Zn}}{1{,}000 \text{ ml}} \times 10.2 \text{ ml}\right) + \left(\frac{X_2 \text{ mg Zn}}{1{,}000 \text{ ml}} \times 10.2 \text{ ml}\right) + \cdots$$

$$+ \left(\frac{X_{15} \text{ mg Zn}}{1{,}000 \text{ ml}} \times 10.2 \text{ ml}\right)$$

or

$$\frac{X_1 + X_2 + \cdots + X_{15} \text{ mg Zn}}{1{,}000 \text{ ml}} \times 10.2 \text{ ml}$$

A correction is applied for the wet weight of tissue initially homogenized (in this case, 3 g liver, wet weight):

$$\times \frac{1}{3 \text{ g liver (wet wt)}}$$

A further correction is made for the fact that not all supernatant (step 13, Fig. 10-6) may be applied to the column (step 14). For instance, a 3-g liver sample comprised of approximately 2.4 ml of water and soluble substances is homogenized initially in 9 ml of 0.9% NaCl, and the pellet extracted in 6 ml of solution. Of this 17.4 ml of tissue extract, 14 ml are applied to the column (Table 10-6). Therefore a correction factor is needed for discarded tissue extract:

$$\times \frac{17.4}{14}$$

A further correction is made since data is converted into μmol so that competition between metals can be evaluated in terms of the relative numbers of molecules of each metal present:

$$\times \frac{1 \text{ mmol Zn}}{65.4 \text{ mg Zn}} \times \frac{1,000 \ \mu\text{mol}}{\text{mmol}}$$

The complete calculation is:

$$\frac{(X_1 + X_2 + \cdots + X_{15}) \text{ mg Zn}}{1,000 \text{ ml}} \times 10.2 \text{ ml}$$

$$\times \frac{1}{3 \text{ g liver (wet wt)}} \times \frac{17.4}{14}$$

$$\times \frac{1 \text{ mmol Zn}}{65.4 \text{ mg Zn}} \times \frac{1,000 \ \mu\text{mol}}{\text{mmol}}$$

Calculations from a typical gel elution profile (Fig. 10-7) are:

$X_1 + X_2 + \cdots + X_{15} = 1.515$ mg Zn $= 0.098$ μmol Zn g^{-1} liver (wet wt) in the high molecular weight protein pool

$X_{16} + \cdots + X_{25}$ $= 1.035$ mg Zn $= 0.067$ μmol Zn g^{-1} liver (wet wt) bound to metallothionein

$X_{26} + \cdots + X_{45}$ $= 0.690$ mg Zn $= 0.045$ μmol Zn in the low molecular weight cytoplasmic pool

These procedures and calculations have been used in studies to determine the loading capacity of metallothionein (Brown and Parsons, 1978); spillover from metallothionein to the enzyme-containing pool (Brown and Parsons, 1978; Roesijadi, 1979); the normal metal component of the enzyme-containing pool (Brown and Chatel, 1978); displacement interactions between metals in, and between, cytoplasmic pools (Brown and Chatel, 1978); reductions in metallothionein synthesis as a result of exposure to organic carcinogens (Brown 1977, 1978); and reductions in the metal components of the enzyme pool as a result of exposure to organic carcinogens (Brown, 1978).

Confirmation of Metallothionein

The fractions corresponding to the usual elution position for metallothionein are pooled, and metallothionein, if present, is separated into its two charge separable forms on a diethylaminoethyl (DEAE) A25 Sephadex column (40 × 1.5 cm). All fractions are then analysed for Cd, Cu and Zn content. If the metal-binding proteins are metallothionein, they will separate out into at least two forms: MT1 and MT2.

The various forms can then be analyzed for their amino acid content. Metallothionein is confirmed if approximately one-third of the amino acids of MT1 and MT2 are cysteine and if no aromatic amino acids are present (Kagi and Vallee, 1960, 1961).

In addition, a technique using isolectric focusing followed by gel electrophoresis can be used to determine the number of different proteins that occur in the partially purified metallothionein pool eluted from the Sephadex G-75 column. The proteins can then be analyzed for metal content and, where possible, isolates should be subjected to amino acid analysis. This procedure may be necessary because there is some evidence to suggest that metal-binding proteins other than metallothionein, which also may have detoxification capabilities, occur in the same molecular weight pool as metallothionein. For example, Premakumar et al. (1975) have described a copper-binding protein called Cu-chelatin which is distinct in properties from metallothionein.

11

The Use of Hydroids in Toxicology

METHODOLOGY

Introduction

Hydroids have been used in experimental studies by many people since the work of Rees and Russell (1937), but it was not until *Artemia salina* eggs became commercially available that the large-scale culture of hydroids became feasible for those without access to freshly caught plankton. Since then, many have used hydroids for studies of regeneration (Tardent, 1963), morphogenesis (Braverman, 1974) and other fundamental processes. Their size, sessile habit, tolerance and mode of asexual reproduction make them ideal experimental organisms for many purposes. As they generally reproduce by budding, a laboratory population can be built up from a single explant, providing a genetically homogenous source of experimental material. This is one of the main reasons for using hydroids for toxicology, because the use of a single genotype reduces variability and improves precision.

Culture Technique

When beginning this work several different hydroid species were isolated and cultured, but for a number of reasons none proved as suitable as *Campanularia flexuosa* (Fig. 11-1). For two of the species, *Artemia* nauplii were not suitable food; others were difficult to subculture easily, or grew too slowly (Stebbing, 1976). Even within the population of clones from which the one now used was chosen, there was considerable variation in some important characteristics.

The easiest way to grow hydroids is on microscope slides in staining racks, but larger surfaces are needed for growth of colonies in toxicological or bioassay experiments: in nearly all experiments 10-cm^2 plates, which are large enough for colonies to grow to about 200 colony members, have been used. When fed daily the colonies reach this size in about two weeks. Seven such plates are held in a perspex rack which fits comfortably in a 2-litre tank. Occasionally a scaled-up system in which ten plates 15 × 20 cm are held in 5-litre tanks has been used. This makes three-week experiments possible, but by this time the colonies may have 1,000 members each, making the work of counting them prohibitive. Hydroids, like other colonial species, grow exponentially (Stebbing, 1971) and the number of colony members doubles every 2-3 days.

The techniques involved in maintaining *Campanularia* and its use in toxicological experiments will be considered in detail. Much of the rationale and methodology also applies to the freshwater counterpart of this bioassay using *Hydra littoralis*, but for a full account the reader is refered elsewhere (Stebbing and Pomroy, 1978). At an early stage it was decided to carry out experiments in a static rather than a flow-through system. The chief criticism of static systems is that the levels of toxicants added, or the biological characteristics of natural waters, do not remain constant when isolated in small experimental vessels. It has been repeatedly shown that significant amounts of mercury (Corner and Rigler, 1957; Baier et al., 1975; Topping, 1977) and other metals such as copper (Brown et al., 1974) are lost from experimental solutions in a matter of hours. The problem is obviously even more serious when dealing with highly volatile toxicants like the aromatic hydrocarbons. Bacteria play a key role in such processes (Saxena and Howard, 1977), so it must be assumed that, unless axenic conditions are maintained, contaminant levels are unlikely to remain stable. However, the complexity and cost of flow-through systems inevitably restricts the number of treatments or concentrations that can be included in a single experiment. Therefore, small static systems are used here, and the water, or experimental solution, is replaced daily to maintain approximately

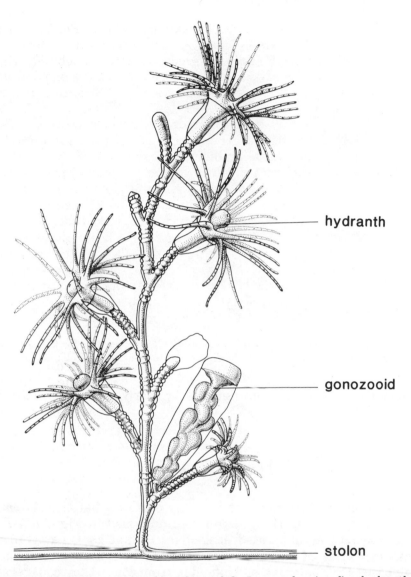

hydranth

gonozooid

stolon

FIG. 11-1. A single upright of a colony of *C. flexuosa* bearing five hydranths; there are two empty positions where hydranths have degenerated. The proximal hydranth is smaller than the others, indicating that it is about to degenerate, or is regenerating. As in this case, the gonozooids typically arise in the axils between hydranths and the upright. The height of the upright is 10 mm.

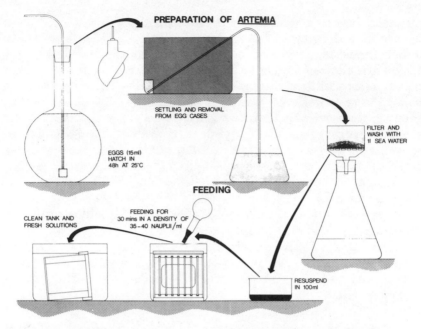

FIG. 11-2. A schematic diagram to summarise the procedure for hatching and preparing *Artemia* nauplii before feeding them to the hydroid colonies.

nominal concentrations of toxicants, or nearly constant conditions of water quality.

Feeding Procedure

All experimental cultures are fed daily on newly hatched *Artemia salina* nauplii using the procedure summarised in Fig. 11-2. The eggs are hatched in aerated flasks over 48 h at 25°C using 15 ml eggs in 5 litres of seawater. The nauplii are separated from their egg cases after hatching by siphoning from where they congregate at the illuminated corner of a blackened tank. Then, because the seawater in which the nauplii hatch tends to be slightly toxic to hydroids, they are filtered from the seawater and then washed on the filter with at least a litre of clean seawater. They are resuspended in about 100 ml seawater, and 10 ml is pipetted into each tank. Hydroids are impingement feeders and, as the nauplii are positively phototactic, it is essential to agitate the colonies or aerate the water during feeding. Typically, *Campanularia* hydranths ingest a maximum of 10-15 nauplii in 30 min when they are at a density of 30-40 nauplii ml^{-1}. At this density, the number ingested does not become significantly greater if the colonies are allowed longer to feed. Clearly the object is to ensure that variations in food availability do not cause differences in the growth or responses of the hydroid colonies. If there is any difficulty, the minimum time to satiate colonies for any new regime can easily be determined. Uprights from a feeding colony can be removed at intervals, and when slightly compressed under a cover slip the eyes of the nauplii can be counted, even when well digested.

For a number of years *Artemia* eggs from San Francisco Bay were used, because work by Wickens (1972) had shown that they were least contaminated by metals and pesticides. Although these eggs have become difficult to obtain, others originating from China have given similar colonial growth rates.

After feeding, the seawater or experimental solutions, together with the nauplii that are not ingested, are discarded and the experimental solutions replaced. In experiments with specific toxicants this involves making up fresh solutions from stock, and in bioassay experiments a further 2 litres is drawn from a 20-litre aspirator holding the original sample.

Hydroids do not need to be fed daily; in fact, they are remarkable for their ability to remain viable for long periods without food. This is an advantage during holiday periods, since the stock colonies can be kept for weeks at 5-10°C without food. However, during experiments and for a week beforehand the stock colonies are fed daily. It seems that there is a lag of several days between increasing the frequency of feeding and the stabilisation of growth at the new, higher rate.

Subculturing

Stock colonies prepared as above provide material for subculturing new colonies (Fig. 11-3). The stolons can be peeled from the plates using fine forceps. The ease with which this can be done depends on the thickness of the perisarc, which is a genetically variable trait and should be borne in mind when selecting a clone. Uprights with three or more hydranths are cut from the detached lengths of stolon, ensuring that sufficient stolon remains to tuck under a nylon thread. Uprights with fewer hydranths do not attach to the glass as rapidly, and sometimes fail to attach at all. As gonozooid

SUBCULTURING

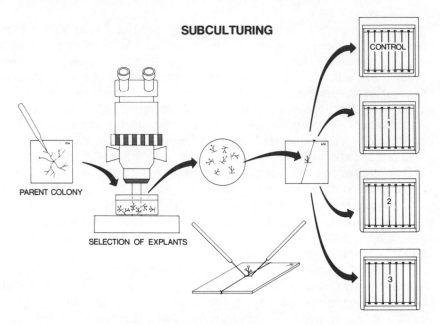

PARENT COLONY

SELECTION OF EXPLANTS

CONTROL

1

2

3

FIG. 11-3. A schematic diagram to summarise the procedure for subculturing new colonies of *C. flexuosa* from stock colonies for an experiment.

production is one of the indices of unfavourable conditions (see below), it is also necessary to exclude explants that already bear gonozooids.

Before subculturing, a monofilament nylon thread is tied tightly round each plate and then further tensioned by sliding the thread sideways a little (Fig. 11-3). If the parent colony is growing rapidly, firm attachment by new stolon growth takes no more than 3 days, when the threads can be cut off and an experiment started. To exclude the effects of unintended selection of explants that might bias the results, the plates are then randomised and subcultures that fail (typically < 5%) are replaced from a rack of spare subcultures.

Duration of Experiments

The optimum duration of experiments depends upon a number of factors that relate, to some extent, to the constraints of the technique itself. The account here refers exclusively to 14-day experiments; the explants take 3 days to become established, leaving 11 days for the experiment itself. By this time colonies consist of about 200 members; because the colonies grow exponentially, the work involved in assessing the responses of colonies older than these becomes too great.

It was often assumed that sensitivity to toxicants increases as a function of time, due partly to the formal expression of the idea as Haber's Rule for equitoxic doses or more recent elaborations of it (Herbert, 1952; Hayes, 1975). However, Haber's Rule applies to lethal effects and does not take account of detoxification mechanisms and acquired resistance to the effects of toxicants. The conclusion to be drawn is that if maximum sensitivity is required, as is the case here, the development of responses should be monitored as they develop. It will be shown that in some cases acquired resistance may result in *increases* in threshold concentrations towards the end of experiments (Fig. 11-8).

Some Possible Difficulties

If the purpose of a test is to detect the effects of low levels of toxicants, or small differences in water quality, the responses of hydroid colonies to small changes in their laboratory environment must also be considered. Most of these changes will impinge on control and experimental organisms alike, so if the responses of the experimental organisms are expressed as percentages of those of the controls, such extraneous effects can be filtered out. For example, the effects of variations in hatching of *Artemia* nauplii can be effectively excluded from the results in this way.

It is also important to consider the various likely sources of extraneous toxic laboratory contaminants and how the problems they create can be avoided. The most frequent causes of difficulty in the use of *Campanularia* have been air-borne toxicants, which find their way into the cultures through the aeration system. In our laboratory all tanks are now covered to exclude dust and aerated to maintain dissolved oxygen levels. At an early stage in the work, oil-lubricated piston pumps were replaced by reciprocating membrane air pumps. Paint fumes were also suspected of having a harmful effect on the cultures, and on another occasion an entire population in one laboratory was killed by fumes from fibre glass resin. All air to the cultures is now passed through activated charcoal and a 2-μm filter before entering the cultures.

The choice and treatment of vessels in which to conduct experiments is important because quite marked deleterious effects may sometimes arise from the use of new vessels. It is important that vessels for culturing hydroids or for keeping water for bioassay experiments should be retained solely for that purpose. It used to be thought necessary to use the most rigorous procedures —some even involving treatment with boiling acids—for cleaning glassware for maintaining sensitive organisms. While rinsing in 2 N hydrochloric acid and several rinses in deionised water has been our usual practice for cleaning new vessels, the most import-ant requirement is to allow the vessels to stand for some months filled with seawater. Any surface not previously exposed to seawater may be regarded as an ion exchange surface which will not only remove ions, but also release potentially toxic ions into the water. It is important, therefore, to allow several weeks for new vessels to reach a chemical equilibrium with seawater. Hard glass usually provides no problem after the initial cleaning procedure, but polyethylene and other plastics can give variable results until they have been in use for some time.

All cultures are held in a constant temperature room at 18°C, (which is higher than the temperature that gives maximum growth of *Campanularia*), but it is important that the water temperature should not be too different from the ambient laboratory temper-ature to minimise the possible effects of changes while handling and counting cultures in the laboratory.

The levels of toxic substances added to seawater rarely remain stable and typically concentrations in solution decrease. The concentrations given here are nominal concentrations, in that they indicate amounts added to seawater and do not include whatever ambient levels that might be present. No attempt is made to keep the nominal levels constant other than to replace experimental solutions daily. For all experiments, seawater col-lected 16 miles off shore has been used, which is the cleanest water of most consistent quality that can be conveniently procured.

RESPONSES

Introduction

A number of responses of *C. flexuosa* have been identified which are suitable as generalised indices of stress, in that they are non-specific effects of, or responses to, stress of different kinds. Unlike some of the other indices described in this manual, nothing can be

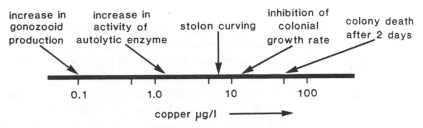

FIG. 11-4. Relative sensitivities of the different indices of *C. flexuosa* in relation to copper concentration.

said about the nature of the stressor from the response of the hydroid. For example, the effects of metals using these indices are similar not only to one another, but also to those of reduced salinity. The descriptions of the responses that follow are derived from experiments using the range of metals with which we have most experience.

The relative sensitivities of these responses in relation to exposure levels of copper are shown in Fig. 11-4. The different responses, their assessment, the handling of data and presentation of results will be described for each in turn. Lethality is shown in the figure simply to indicate the lowest concentration at which it occurs, but for our purposes, it is too insensitive as an index and will not be considered further.

One of the reasons that hydroids are good experimental organisms is that they are robust and adaptable, capable of tolerating a wide range of conditions. *Campanularia* often occurs in physiologically demanding environments like the littoral region of estuaries. Nevertheless, in our experiments *Campanularia* has responded to extremely low concentrations of copper (Fig. 11-4) and other toxic agents, some indices showing much greater sensitivity than the hydroids' apparent hardiness would suggest. The point to be made here is that tolerance and sensitivity are not, as is often supposed, mutually exclusive traits. This paradox can best be explained by describing the way growth is affected by sublethal levels of toxic agents, and how hydroids respond adaptively to the toxic challenge they present. At very low levels of inhibition, the growth regulatory mechanism detects inhibition and responds to counteract it, with the result that growth inhibition does not actually occur until the counteractive capacity is exceeded (Stebbing, 1981a). In this case, it is the sensitivity of the control mechanism that mobilises homeorhetic resistance to toxic inhibition, which ultimately confers tolerance. It would appear that sensitivity is more closely related to the choice of index or response (Fig. 11-4) than is often supposed. In this example, the growth control mechanism responds adaptively to concentrations of copper as low as 1 μg litre^{-1}, but mean colonial growth rate is not inhibited by concentrations below 15 μg litre^{-1}.

Colonial Growth

The primary response used in the hydroid bioassay has been growth, because it is probably the most fundamental organismic response, providing an integration of many key physiological processes. Increase in colony size can be determined by counting the numbers of colony members (hydranths, buds and gonozooids). Estimates of biomass can be made from these data as numbers are linearly related to biomass (Fig. 11-5a). If one is concerned with changes of growth rates with time, it is obviously an advantage to be able to estimate biomass in a non-sacrificial way. The colonies grow exponentially, so numbers of colony members are about 40 after 1 week, 200 after 2 weeks and 600 after 3 weeks. Counts are therefore time-consuming, but, as the number of uprights is linearly related to the number of colony members (Fig. 11-5b), they provide a much more rapid means of estimating biomass.

Growth is usually interpreted in a cumulative sense, and the inhibitory effects of toxicants on growth are expressed as

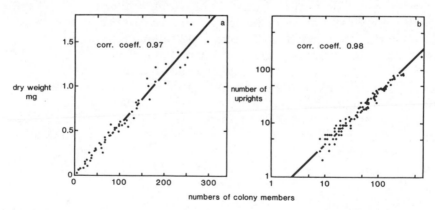

FIG. 11-5. Relationships between the number of colony members of *C. flexuosa* and (*a*) dry weight and (*b*) number of uprights. These linear relationships are used to estimate dry weights from colony members, and numbers of colony members from numbers of uprights.

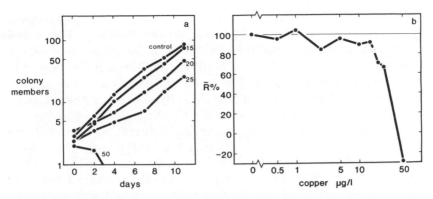

FIG. 11-6. The effect of copper at different concentrations on the growth of *C. flexuosa* colonies over 11 days. The data are presented in two ways to show (a) cumulative colony growth at various concentrations against time and (b) the same data replotted as mean specific colonial growth rate expressed as a percentage of that of the controls ($\bar{R}\%$) against copper concentration. For clarity some of the data included in (b) are omitted from (a). The point at which $\bar{R}\%$ is significantly inhibited in relation to the controls is the threshold concentration (17 μg litre^{-1}) and is marked with an open circle.

differences in growth curves relating biomass to time (Fig. 11-6a). For two reasons this is rather unsatisfactory. First, from the physiological point of view, toxicants impinge on the rate at which new tissue is being formed, rather than directly affecting an organism's size. It is more appropriate, therefore, to consider the effect of toxicants on the growth process, rather than the cumulative product of that process. However, growth rates vary due to differences in colony size alone, because growth increments depend on the amount of biomass capable of growth. It is therefore necessary to exclude the effects of size on growth rates by considering increase in biomass per unit time per unit biomass. This is the specific growth rate (R) and is more likely than any other index to reflect the rate of biosynthesis (Stebbing, 1981a). It also has the practical advantage that it makes it possible to relate the growth rates of organisms or cultures of different sizes, thus avoiding the complications of having to start experiments with same-size colonies.

The second reason that the cumulative presentation of data (Fig. 11-6a) is not ideal is the difficulty of deriving from the data the lowest concentrations of toxicant that causes a significant inhibition of growth. However, if the mean specific growth rates, as a percentage of that of the control colonies ($\overline{R}\%$), are calculated from the cumulative data and plotted against toxicant concentrations (Fig. 11-6b), it is possible by linear interpolation to determine threshold concentrations at which inhibition of the specific growth rate becomes significant. If the null hypothesis is that specific growth rate is not expected to deviate from that of the controls, it is possible, using some measure of the variability of the data, to determine the point at which a significant deviation occurs. Here, standard errors of $\overline{R}\%$ are calculated for each group of replicate colonies (Fig. 11-6a) and Bartlett's test for the homogeneity of variance is used to determine whether a pooled standard error can be used. (Only rarely has significant heterogeneity been found; these instances can usually be related to obvious causes). Multiples of the pooled standard error can be plotted as probability parallels below the 100% line, depending on the value of P chosen to indicate a significant departure from $\overline{R}\%$ of the control colonies. In this work, three times the pooled standard error ($P < 0.001$) has been taken as the level at which any deviation becomes significantly different from the controls, so a line at this level of probability is plotted below and parallel to the 100% or control line. The point at which this line intercepts the concentration vs. response curve is where inhibition becomes significant, and a perpendicular to the x-axis gives the threshold concentration (Fig. 11-6b).

Threshold concentrations determined in this way decrease with duration of exposure, due mainly to the improved precision of $\overline{R}\%$ as the colonies grow (Fig. 11-7). If it is intended to maximise sensitivity, then the experiment should last long enough for the curve to become asymptotic. From the examples given, it can be seen that the time required may vary and that the second half of some experiments adds little to the sensitivity of response. Furthermore, in some experiments effective adaptation to low levels of toxicants can be seen in that threshold concentrations derived from colonial growth rates ($\overline{R}\%$) for successive 2-day periods may increase significantly, as in the example for copper given in Fig. 11-8. Clearly, if the intention is to maximise sensitivity there is an optimum duration of exposure.

Precision is an essential feature of any bioassay technique, and here variability of responses due to genetic heterogeneity has been eliminated by using a clone of the hydroid. Typically, experiments incorporate seven replicates per treatment, and standard errors of $\overline{R}\%$ for 0–11 days for each treatment are usually less than 5%; if necessary, this can be further reduced by increased replication, but at a considerable cost in work load (10 replicate colonies, S.E. < 3%; 20 replicate colonies, S.E. < 2%). These values refer primarily to the growth of unstressed or control colonies, as there is a tendency for standard errors to be larger when colonies are exposed to inhibitory levels of toxicants. Typical concentration vs. response curves for a number of substances are given in Fig. 11-9, and mean threshold concentrations derived from such curves are given in Table 11-1.

In experiments with *Campanularia* (Stebbing, 1981c), and in other toxicological work on growth (Stebbing, 1982), otherwise inhibitory agents are often found to stimulate growth when

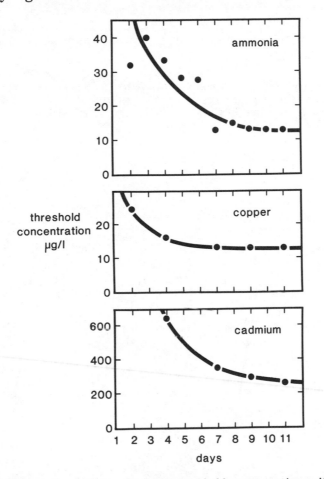

FIG. 11-7. Curves showing changes in the threshold concentrations with increasing periods of exposure of colonies of *C. flexuosa* to ammonia, copper and cadmium. Curves for ammonia and copper have become asymptotic, but the threshold concentration for cadmium might become lower still in longer experiments.

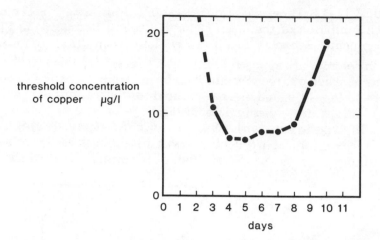

threshold concentration
of copper   µg/l

FIG. 11-8. Threshold concentrations derived from plots of $\bar{R}\%$ against copper concentrations for successive overlapping 2-day periods. When considered in this way, it can be seen that inhibition is becoming less marked, indicating that the colonies are becoming more resistant to the copper.

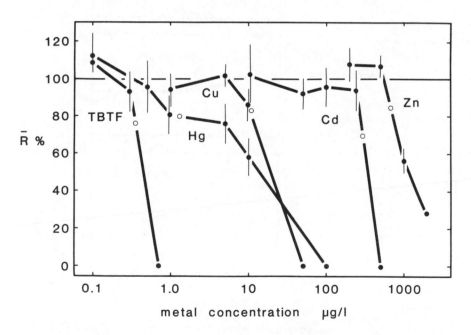

FIG. 11-9. Concentration vs. response curves showing the effect of a number of metals (tributyl tin fluoride, mercury, copper, cadmium and zinc) on the growth ($\bar{R}\%$) of *C. flexuosa* colonies in 11-day experiments. Vertical bars indicate two standard errors of the means, and open circles give the thresholds for each metal.

280

TABLE 11-1. Threshold Concentrations Indicating the Point at which Inhibition of the Mean Colonial Growth Rate ($\bar{R}\%$) in 11-day Experiments Becomes Significantly Less than That of Control Colonies, and the Concentrations at which the Cytochemical Index Becomes Significantly Greater than the Controls

Substance	Mean growth threshold concentration (μg litre^{-1})	Mean cytochemical threshold concentration (μg litre^{-1})
Ammonia	17.0 (1)	—
Cadmium	195 (2)	57.5 (2)
Copper	14.3 (9)	1.4 (4)
Mercury	1.6 (2)	0.2 (1)
Tributyl tin fluoride	0.2 (2)	—
Zinc	740 (1)	—

Note: The number experiments from which the mean threshold values are derived are indicated in parentheses.

organisms are exposed to very low concentrations. This phenomenon is called hormesis, and it has been suggested that in hydroids at least it is due to the behaviour of a growth regulatory mechanism that normally maintains growth at a constant specific rate. When growth is disturbed, the control mechanism works to neutralise or counteract any tendency to be deviated from its preferred rate. Over a narrow range of subthreshold concentrations it seems that the overcorrections of this rate-sensitive control mechanism may cumulatively produce a significant increase in size. Hormesis is interesting, both in its own right and because of its possible association with growth regulation. Here it is useful as an indication that the hydroids are responding effectively to low levels of inhibitory challenge, but it is often absent when the levels of a substance being tested span the narrow range of concentrations in which hormesis typically occurs.

Cytochemical Index

In the early stages of this work a cytochemical index of stress was adapted for use with *Campanularia* and tested in a series of experiments with metals (Moore and Stebbing, 1976). The response proved to be more sensitive than the growth index, and it was hoped to be of use as an index of the quality of samples from polluted waters. Before discussing some results, the nature of the response will be considered.

The usual response of hydroids to unfavourable conditions is to degenerate, whatever the cause. Before this occurs, there is increased activity of those enzymes responsible for autolytic degeneration. The cytochemical index used is a measure of the activity of the lysosomal enzyme, N-acetyl-β-D-glucosaminidase (see Chapter 4).

The form of the relationship between enzyme activity and concentration of the metals tested is consistent. The enzyme activity data from an experiment with mercury are typical and are given in Fig. 11-10 with those for $\overline{R}\%$ from the same experiment for comparison. At levels of mercury below those which inhibit colonial growth, there is an increase in enzyme activity. Activity is at a peak at about the threshold concentrations for growth inhibition, and at higher levels both enzyme activity and growth become increasingly inhibited with further increases in mercury concentration.

Thresholds of sensitivity are determined in the same way as before, but here the threshold concentration is the lowest at which there is a significant *increase* relative to the controls ($P < 0.001$). Threshold concentrations for three different metals are given in Table 11-1, and reproducibility is indicated by comparing threshold concentrations from four separate experiments with copper given in Table 11-2.

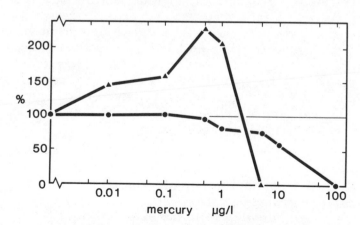

FIG. 11-10. Concentration vs. response curves showing the effect of mercury on glucosaminidase reactivity (triangles), in relation to the inhibition of $\overline{R}\%$ (circles) of *C. flexuosa* colonies.

TABLE 11-2. Reproducibility of Thresholds of Sensitivity of *C. flexuosa* to Copper Using Mean Specific Colonial Growth Rate ($\bar{R}\%$) over 11 days and the Cytochemical Index

Experiment number	Threshold of $\bar{R}\%$ (μg litre^{-1})	Cytochemical threshold (μg litre^{-1})
1	2.4* (5)	1.20 (5)
2	13.0 (5)	1.39 (5)
3	10.0 (6)	1.90 (6)
4	12.0 (3)	1.24 (3)
5	18.0 (3)	—
6	12.0 (5)	—
7	12.0 (4)	—
8	18.5 (5)	—
9	17.0 (9)	—
10	17.0 (2)	—
	mean 14.39, S.E. ± 3.2	mean 1.43, S.E. ± 0.32

Note: The numbers of copper concentrations used are given in parentheses.

*A different subculturing technique was used in this experiment which invalidates the $\bar{R}\%$ threshold.

Stolon Curling

Another growth response observed in *Campanularia* when conditions are unfavourable is the curling of stolons (Stebbing 1979). The typical form of cultured colonies grown on glass plates is that the stolons radiate outwards from the position of the explant more or less linearly (Fig. 11-11a). However, when stressed there is a tendency for the stolons to curve as they grow (Fig. 11-11b), although without becoming detached from the substratum. Curvature tends to increase with the severity of stress (Fig. 11-11c) and the direction of curvature is typically anti-clockwise.

The form of curves and their similarity in replicate cultures suggested that in some way the response might be adaptive, although there is no obvious explanation. However, it seems possible that *Campanularia* cannot differentiate the source of any toxic effect as originating from the substratum or the water. In which case, this seems to be an appropriate response because it allows the colony to continue to grow without venturing onto any new and possibly even more unfavourable substrata.

Whatever the reason for the response, the frequency of stolon curling provides another generalised index of stress that can be used to assess the effect of toxicants or water quality. The frequency of curling is estimated by scoring the numbers of major stolons that curl by 90° or more. A more sophisticated method for measuring the response is to compute the average curvature of stolons by calculating the curvature of triplets of upright positions by their x, y co-ordinates. Mean curvatures for complete colonies and sets of replicates gave marginal improvements in data quality, but for routine use this method was too labour-intensive. However, the simpler method was adequate and gave consistent results (Fig. 11-12). At concentrations greater than 5 μg litre^{-1} the frequency of 90° curls increases, reaching a maximum at 15 μg litre^{-1}. At higher concentrations than this, colony growth is inhibited and the numbers of curves decreases to zero at concentrations where there is no growth.

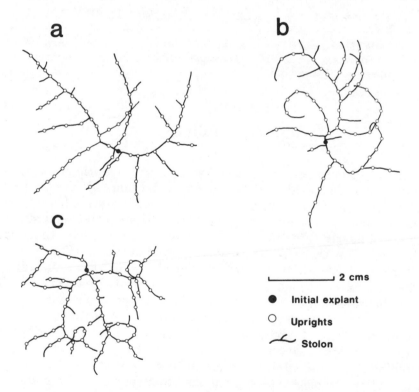

FIG. 11-11. Diagrams of 2-week-old colonies of *C. flexuosa* to show the variation in the curvature of stolons induced by stress: *a*, unstressed control; *b*, stressed colony; and *c*, severely stressed colony.

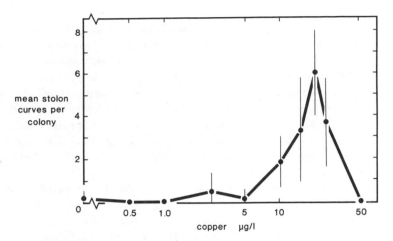

FIG. 11-12. Stolon curving frequencies of *C. flexuosa* colonies after growing for 14 days in different concentrations of copper. Bars indicate standard errors of the means.

While thresholds of sensitivity for this index can be determined in the same way as the other indices, they tend to be more variable and less sensitive than the cytochemical index and gonozooid frequency (see below). Nevertheless, the index has proved most helpful in corroborating other indices in water-quality experiments.

Gonozooid Frequency

The more sensitive indices of stress for organisms are those that measure adaptive responses that avoid or counteract the effects of stress, rather than those that simply provide a measure of the damage or deleterious effects of stress. Obviously, avoidance may not be achieved, or effective counteraction initiated, if the organism is damaged before there is a response.

In *Campanularia* when conditions are unfavourable, resources are diverted from the production of hydranths to form more gonozooids, the function of which is to produce planktonic gametes (Stebbing, 1980a, 1981b). Under natural conditions, gonozooids are formed when a colony has reached a certain size and in response to seasonal stimuli; however, when stressed, colonies produce considerably more gonozooids. A sessile organism obviously cannot escape when its environment becomes noxious, but putting additional resources into the dispersal phase, must increase the likelihood that the genotype will survive.

Hydroids like *Obelia* release male and female planktonic medusae that produce gametes, which after fertilisation form a planula larva. In *Campanularia*, however, the medusoid stage is suppressed, in that the rudimentary medusae never become detached and only their gametes are released into the plankton. Nevertheless, it is the only phase in the life cycle when the organism is not fixed to the substratum, and the increase in gonozooid frequency in unfavourable conditions is clearly a response that has survival value.

In our experiments, gonozooid frequency typically becomes maximal in the last day or so, and it is clear that more than a week is required for the response to develop fully. In an experiment where reduced salinity was used to impose stress on *Campanularia*, the response was observed at 2- or 3-day intervals (Fig. 11-13). Gonozooid frequency at 60, 70 and 80% seawater was maximal at day 9 and decreased slightly thereafter.

As an adaptive response, it is to be expected that gonozooid frequency would respond to stress in a non-specific way. In our experiments, increased frequencies have been observed in response to a variety of toxic agents, including cadmium, copper, mercury and tributyl tin fluoride (Stebbing, 1980a). Data from an experiment with copper are given in Fig. 11-14 to indicate the typical form of the response. There is a tendency for gonozooid frequencies to vary independently of any experimental factor, in a way that suggests that the age and size of colonies from which explants originate may be important. It is best, therefore, for the purposes of these experiments to express gonozooid frequencies as a percentage of those in control colonies, but it must be appreciated that small changes in the numbers of gonozooids in control colonies may have marked effects on the percentage frequencies. Thus the frequency peak may show an increase of two or three times that in the controls, as in the example given in Fig. 11-14, but occasionally colonies show a 20-fold increase due largely to very low gonozooid frequencies in control colonies.

The most useful feature of this response is its great sensitivity, and it can be seen from the experiment with copper (Fig. 11-14) that peak frequency occurs at a concentration of 0.1 μg litre^{-1} over an order of magnitude more sensitive than the cytochemical index (Tables 11-1 and 11-2). Analysis of metal concentrations of this order is difficult, whether it is hoped to check on levels in an experiment, or in environmental samples. It should

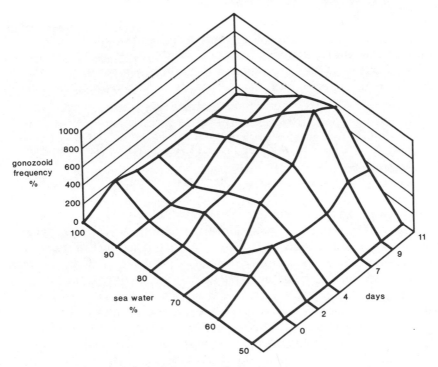

FIG. 11-13. Gonozooid frequencies in colonies of *C. flexuosa* exposed to different salinities showing the development of the response with time.

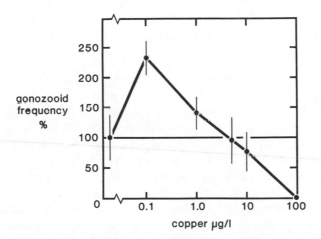

FIG. 11-14. Gonozooid frequencies in colonies of *C. flexuosa* after 11 days exposure to various copper concentrations. The ratio of gonozooids and gonozooid buds to total number of colony members is expressed as a percentage of the same ratio in the control colonies. Bars indicate standard errors of the means.

therefore be reiterated that the nominal concentrations given are those added to the ambient levels in seawater. While it is appreciated that such dilute solutions are highly unstable, no attempt has been made to monitor or maintain constant concentrations during experiments, other than to replace solutions daily.

BIOASSAY OF WATER SAMPLES

Introduction

The rationale for developing bioassay techniques with which to assess water quality is considered in Chapter 5. The hydroid bioassay technique and four different responses of *Campanularia* to stress are also described there, together with the form of these responses when colonies are exposed to a range of toxicant concentrations. In this chapter, two examples will be given of applications of the technique to the assessment of water quality of samples brought back to the laboratory. At this stage, the results will be considered in terms of the responses of the different indices in relation to their geographical distribution. The correlation of responses with the distribution of potential causal agents and their positive identification will be considered later.

Swansea Bay

The region around Swansea and Port Talbot has long been industrialised. Although most of the activity in the Swansea Valley has now stopped, there remain steelworks, refineries and an ore terminal near Port Talbot. The effluents from these industries are released into Swansea Bay, most by way of long outfalls that discharge some distance offshore (Fig. 11-15). Another major input is from an outfall sited off Mumbles Head on the west side of Swansea Bay.

On a number of occasions, near-surface water samples from Swansea Bay have been tested using the hydroid bioassay technique and significant variations in water quality have been detected. Only once has there been significant inhibition of colonial growth rate ($\bar{R}\%$, 0–11 days), suggesting that the variations in water quality detected are not sufficient to have a deleterious effect on the organism. Variations have been detected in terms of enhanced stolon curving, or gonozooid frequency, and some results are given in Fig. 11-15. It can be seen that there is an association between the discharge points and the responses in a number of cases, particularly the stolon curving index (Fig. 11-15c and d). However, it is clear that there are difficulties in interpreting gonozooid frequencies because in some cases they are enhanced, while in others they are depressed. Reference to the form of the concentration vs. response curve (Fig. 11-14) makes it clear why this is so. The form of the curve shows that for much of the range of copper concentrations, for any given gonozooid frequencies

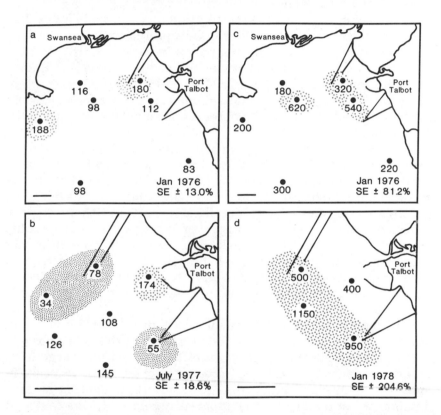

FIG. 11-15. Results of experiments with *C. flexuosa* on water samples from Swansea Bay (*a, c*) and off Port Talbot (*b, d*). Gonozooid frequencies (*a, b*) and the frequency of stolon curves (*c, d*) are scored after 11 days exposure to the water samples, and are expressed as percentages of the frequencies in control colonies. Pooled standard errors are given, and the areas from which samples were taken that elicited significant stimulation of gonozooid frequency or stolon curving is marked with light stipple, and significant inhibition of gonozooid frequency by a heavier stipple. The positions of outfalls are given, and scale bars represent 1 nautical mile (ca. 1.85 km).

there are two concentrations that might have caused it. For example, the frequency of 108% (Fig. 11-15b) represents a response equivalent to that which might be elicited by less than 0.1 μg litre^{-1} or by 3.2 μg litre^{-1} of copper (Fig. 11-14). One solution is to consider the linear relationship for copper concentration against gonozooid frequency from 0.1 to 100 μg litre^{-1} as a calibration curve and express the stress loading imposed on the hydroids in terms of equivalent concentrations of copper. However, this makes some assumptions that are not yet justified about the generality of the response and the consistency of the form of the relationship between stress and gonozooid frequency.

Stolon curving is a less sensitive and more variable index, but there are not the same difficulties in interpretation that occur with gonozooid frequency. Curling frequency increases sharply in relation to stress, and the fall in frequency at higher levels is due to the inhibition of colonial growth (Fig. 11-12). Despite large standard errors, the responses tend to corroborate those for gonozooid frequency indicating areas of poorer water quality associated with the outfalls.

Several experiments during this investigation indicated an area to the south of Swansea Bay where water samples caused significant responses in bioassay experiments even though the area was not associated with any particular outfalls. We began to investigate the bay in more detail upon realising that the area coincided with the centre of a gyre predicted by a hydrographic model of the Bristol Channel (Uncles, 1982). While we currently lack evidence to explain this phenomenon, it is instructive to consider data from sampling stations sited closely along a transect bisecting the gyre, which is centred on the Scarweather Sands (Fig. 11-16a).

As before, gonozooid frequency is high off Port Talbot and decreases to the south (stations 1–10), although the lesser peak at station 4 may indicate the effect of effluents that discharge from the offshore outfalls nearby. Of greater interest is the increase in gonozooid frequency that occurs at station 10, indicating an area of poorer water quality that is apparently related to the centre of the gyre (Fig. 11-16b).

Tamar Estuary

Hydroid bioassay has been used in the Tamar Estuary to estimate water quality in an estuary. Sampling stations are distributed

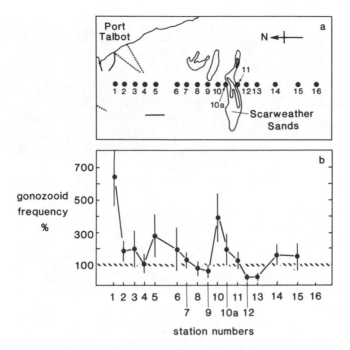

FIG. 11-16. Results of an experiment in May 1979 with *C. flexuosa* on water samples from a transect running south from Port Talbot across the Scarweather Sands (*a*). The positions of outfalls are given, and the scale bar represents 1 nautical mile (ca. 1.85 km). Gonozooid frequencies are expressed as percentages of the frequencies in control colonies, and bars indicate standard errors of the means (*b*).

axially (Fig. 11-17) both to avoid the possible effects of small localised inputs, and to see whether there is some overall trend in water quality as this river drains a highly metalliferous area. There is a significant increase in gonozooid frequency centred on station 15 and either side of it. This suggests an area of poor water quality, which is apparently due to an input in the area sampled rather than metal-rich water from further upstream. On this occasion, only gonozooid frequency shows a clear response, but in other experiments there have been significant increases in stolon curving of colonies grown in samples from the same area.

More Difficulties

The purpose of the hydroid bioassay approach is to establish a measurement of water quality that might be a more appropriate index for biological purposes than a knowledge of the types and concentrations of toxic contaminants. For the response of the organism to be a realistic indication of water quality, it is necessary that changes that occur in the water samples after collection do not invalidate extrapolation of bioassay data back to the environment from which the samples originated.

Change in the chemistry of stored water samples is inevitable. Such changes can be minimised by freezing, but where numbers of 20-litre samples are involved this is impractical. Changes in the

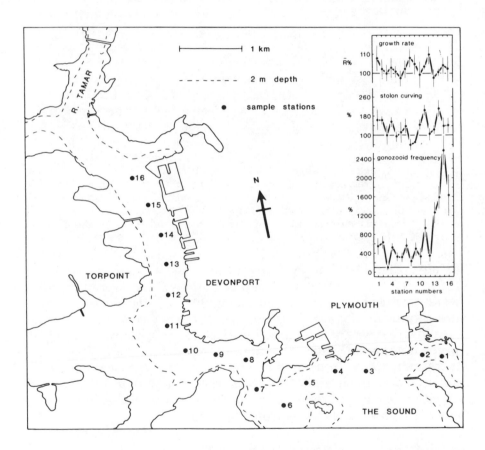

FIG. 11-17. Results of an experiment in April 1980 with *C. flexuosa* on midstream water samples from Plymouth Sound and River Tamar. The positions of sampling stations are given, and the scale bar represents 1 kilometre. Data for growth rate ($\bar{R}\%$, 0–11 days), stolon curving and gonozooid frequencies are given. Bars indicate standard errors of the means.

levels of metals can be significantly reduced by membrane filtration (0.45 μm) as soon after collection as possible. It seems that microbiota and particulates are responsible for changes in the levels of metals in solution, but membrane filtration effectively removes some pesticides (Kurtz, 1977) and possibly other contaminants. While we have carried out most experiments on either unfiltered or membrane-filtered water samples, more recently we have used glass fibre filters (Whatman GF/F) to improve filtration rates and reduce the likelihood that pesticides, or other toxic contaminants, will be removed.

The chief problem in using the hydroid bioassay in an estuary is that the indices are generalised responses to stress and can be elicited by reduced salinity as well as by chemical contaminants. This problem has been avoided by determining the sensitivity and form of the responses to reduced salinities (Stebbing, 1981b) and then limiting the samples to those with salinities above the levels ($> 30^0/_{00}$) that stimulate stress responses of the hydroid.

It is an advantage in any laboratory-based bioassay to be able to limit responses to variations in the water chemistry of samples by controlling other variables; but the most useful option is that of manipulating water samples in order to investigate the causes of the responses they elicit.

CHEMICAL MANIPULATION OF WATER SAMPLES

The Problem of Identifying Causal Agents

When an area of poor water quality has been detected using bioassay techniques, the next stage is to attempt to identify the causal agents; without that knowledge specific measures to improve water quality cannot be taken. A first step is to attempt to correlate the occurrence of bioassay responses with that of potentially toxic contaminants. In a typical system, where there are numerous inputs intermittently discharging complex and varying effluents of domestic and industrial origin, it is unlikely that correlation will reveal clear-cut associations. The responses of the organisms are an integration of the effects of all those constituents of the water sample that impinge on their physiology, or contribute to the stress loading. This is helpful in the sense that wherever or whenever there are biologically significant levels of a contaminant present, one may expect a response; but a clear association with a single compound is unlikely unless one compound is sufficiently toxic or abundant to stand out. When there is a good correlation, the distributions of factors should be definable on more than one occasion, but any water sample is likely to have a blend of contaminants that is unlikely to recur. Strictly speaking, any bioassay experiment must stand in isolation; it cannot be repeated if identical conditions cannot be recreated. While it is evident that this argument is true, it is also true that in any system effluents are discharged from the same places and tend to have the same constituents which are diluted in the same geographical area, so some success can be expected using the correlative approach.

Nevertheless, it is clear that there is a requirement for more rigorous methods to identify biologically significant contaminants. Two possibilities are, first, the use of specific indices where the biological response or index measured occurs only in response to particular toxicants or perhaps a class of toxicants (see Chapter 5); here the occurrence of the response is expected to identify the contaminant(s) responsible. Second, the measurement of some biological response to a water sample before and after the selective removal of an individual contaminant, or a group of chemically related contaminants. If a particular contaminant is responsible for eliciting a response, it can be identified if it can be removed selectively from the water sample, because if the contaminant is absent the bioassay response will not occur. The success of this approach depends on the specificity of the chemical manipulation, because it is essential that the chemistry of the water sample should be altered in no other biologically significant way.

In practice such manipulations are difficult because of the problem of processing a chemically complex medium like seawater without removing other normal constituents that might be required by organisms. It is also important not to add to the water sample anything that could have toxic effects. Despite these difficulties, sufficient progress has been made with broad-spectrum manipulations to show that the approach has some promise and can be developed further.

Ion-Exchange Resin

A number of ion-exchange resins are used by analytical chemists to extract and concentrate particular contaminants from seawater.

TABLE 11-3. The Effect of Copper (20 μg litre^{-1}) in Seawater on the Growth of Colonies of *C. flexuosa* with and without Passing the Water through Chelex 100 Ion-exchange Resin

Medium	$\bar{R}\%$	S.E. (%)
Controls	100	3.8
Treatment controls	111	4.5
Copper added	46	6.8
Copper added then water passed through resin	102	9.0

Two types in common use by marine chemists are XAD resin for the extraction of polychlorinated hydrocarbons (Osterroht, 1977) and chelex resin for the extraction of divalent metals (Riley and Taylor, 1968). In the case of chelex resin, treated seawater has been shown to be suitable for biological use (Davey et al., 1970), so possible applications of the technique in a bioassay context have been explored.

In preliminary experiments it was established that enough copper to inhibit growth could also be removed without apparently changing the water in any other biologically detectable way (Table 11-3). Experiments with samples from the area of poor water quality off Port Talbot (Figs. 11-15 and 11-16) have shown that metals are partly responsible, because resin treatment of samples significantly reduced the enhanced gonozooid frequencies (Table 11-4).

TABLE 11-4. The Effect of Water Collected off Port Talbot on Stolon-curving Frequency, with and without Passing the Water through Chelex Ion-exchange Resin

Medium	Frequency (%)	S.E. (%)
Control	100	50.3
Treatment control	60	28.3
Port Talbot water	540	120.0
Port Talbot water after passing through resin	220	73.9

TABLE 11-5. The Effect of the Photo-oxidation of Organic Matter in Seawater on the Inhibitory Effect of Copper (20 μg litre^{-1}) on Colonial Growth Rate of *C. flexuosa*

Medium	$\bar{R}\%$	S.E. (%)
Control	100	2.6
Treatment control	101	4.1
Copper added	84	6.9
Copper added to photo-oxidised seawater	53	4.7

Ultraviolet Photo-oxidation

The technique of employing UV light to photo-oxidise seawater has been widely used for chemical purposes since it was advocated by Armstrong et al. (1966). Its effect is to break up organic molecules, reducing them to their elemental constituents. The technique has been used not so much to remove toxic organic contaminants from seawater, as to destroy its capacity to chelate metals by breaking up the normal organic compounds present in seawater. Water treated in this way has been used to show the relatively greater toxicity of copper in water with no natural chelating capacity (Table 11-5).

There is no reason why this technique could not be used to manipulate water samples for bioassay experiments, as in some cases it could be useful to know whether an observed effect was due to organic or inorganic contaminants. While UV photo-oxidation might have other chemical effects on the seawater than those intended, they did not have any apparent effect on the behaviour of hydroid colonies cultured in it, so the changes that occurred are assumed to be unimportant to the hydroids.

Conclusions

There are a number of existing techniques that could be adopted for manipulating water samples in conjunction with bioassay techniques to identify biologically active contaminants (Stebbing, 1980a; Stebbing et al., 1980), but none have yet been used in this way. It has been suggested that, when there are enough, they might be used sequentially in the manner of a taxonomic key to ask increasingly specific questions about the nature of the toxicant(s) responsible for an observed bioassay response.

PART **III**

CONCLUSIONS

12

A Possible Synthesis

HOW IS THE APPROACH DIFFERENT?

The approach to the detection and measurement of the effects of toxic pollutants on individual organisms that we have developed over the last 10 years has its roots in physiology; this is important because it acknowledges at the outset that the adaptive and homeostatic responses of the organism to perturbations of physiological processes are important in ameliorating the effects of disturbance.

The indices we describe are sublethal responses, which are inevitably more sensitive than the lethal tests of traditional toxicology and offer better possibilities for extrapolation to the environment.

The concept of "stress" (Bayne, 1975, 1980; Stebbing, 1981d) is central to the approach we have developed and is discussed at greater length in the Introduction. Often "stress" is used as an experimental perturbation of a homeostatic steady state, because there is a limited amount one can expect to learn about physiological processes if only steady-state conditions are studied.

Adaptive responses and capacities (Fig. 12-1) can best be determined experimentally by disturbing those processes and observing the responses of the organism. But we have also used measurements originating from our physiological and other work

301

in a reciprocal manner to understand stress imposed by environmental contaminants (Bayne et al., 1979), its distribution in space and time and its causes (Stebbing, 1979).

While some responses to particular agents are specific—such as the activation of detoxication pathways (see Chapters 4 and 10)—the majority of the responses that we use as indices are nonspecific responses to stress. This is both the strength and the weakness of the stress concept when applied in an environmental context, because we can recognise in organisms—as Selye (1950) did—a syndrome of responses that indicate that they are stressed but tell us little or nothing about the nature of the causal agent(s). For example, the responses of *Mytilus* and *Campanularia* to reduced salinity (Chapters 1 and 11) are in many respects similar to their responses to toxic agents. Nevertheless, the problem is typically one of first establishing whether organisms are stressed, before attempting to determine whether the causes are physical or chemical, natural or anthropogenic.

Prediction of biological consequences of toxic environmental contaminants depends on understanding the processes upon which they impinge. But these predictions depend on being able to assess the extent to which an organism is already stressed, and to relate that to its innate capacity to resist stress (Fig. 12-1).

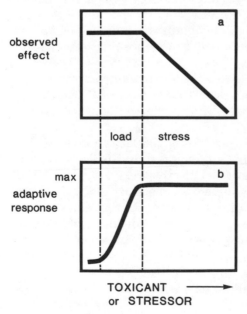

FIG. 12-1. The relationship between a curve relating the observed effect of some toxicant or stressor on a biological process (a) and a curve showing the adaptive response (b). The object is to indicate that a threshold concentration is not reached until the capacity of adaptive mechanisms is exceeded. Up to that point the effect of the toxicant can be termed load, but once it is exceeded the process is stressed and the effect upon the organism becomes deleterious, and less reversible if the toxicant is removed.

"Health" and "stress" are closely related concepts, if health is considered to be the capacity to resist stress (Frenster, 1962). "Health" is then quantified in terms of the range of concentrations, or levels of some stress-inducing factor, over which a physiological process can be maintained at its unstressed state or rate. Health of organisms from the environment can be estimated in terms of the levels of experimental load or stress required to precipitate overload, in relation to the levels for an unstressed organism. Clearly, the health of the organism in this sense is its residual capacity to withstand stress, and the more stressed it is, the less capable it is of withstanding further stress.

INTEGRATION OF RESPONSES

One feature of the approach we have developed is the use of a number of different indices spanning several levels of biological organisation: biochemical, cytological, physiological and autecological. This not only makes it possible to provide an integrated view of the organism's condition and of its responses to stress, but a marked variation in one response can be correlated with, and corroborated by, the behaviour of others. Comparisons with the responses at different levels also makes it possible to make a number of points about the way toxicants impinge upon an organism, and the homeostatic responses that may be expected to ameliorate their effects. These ideas can be better discussed by considering the organism as a hierarchically arranged system, not only in the structural sense (Woodger, 1930), but also in a functional sense (Mesarovic et al., 1970) (Fig. 12-2).

In such a system the impact of the toxicant occurs first at the lowest level of organisation and may then become apparent to the investigator making measurements at this or higher levels of organisation. For example, the effect of a metal such as mercury upon an organism at the molecular level is to block the thiol groups of enzymes (Albert, 1968) such as those that regulate biosynthesis, or the metal may destabilise lysosomal membranes and, by the release of degradative hydrolytic enzymes, lead to cell death and tissue degeneration. Any inhibition of biosynthesis is likely to become apparent in the form of reduced growth rate of a cell population, impaired cellular hypertrophy to functional overload of some tissue or organ, or perhaps a reduction in the growth of the organism as a whole. What the investigator sees depends largely on the level of biological organisation at which he chooses to observe the effect of the metal. At any particular level of organisation a measured effect is preceded by, and is a consequence of, the impact of the toxicant at a lower level of organisation. All the effects of toxicants have their origins in chemical processes at the

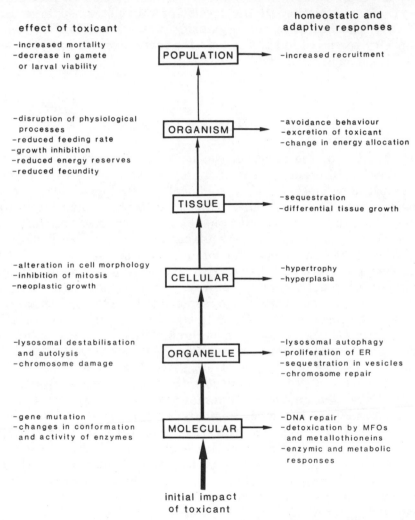

FIG. 12-2. A hypothetical scheme suggesting how the impact of a toxicant upon an organism might pass through, and be dissipated by, its hierarchical organisation. Some effects of toxicants that we have considered, and adaptive responses to counteract those effects, are listed.

molecular level. Furthermore, if the impact of the toxicant at any level is great enough to exceed the capacity of the neutralising responses at that level, then its effect passes to successively higher levels of organisation. For example, it is only when the capacity of cells to produce metallothionein to bind the influx of a non-essential metal is exceeded that free ions can poison metallo-enzymes by displacing the usual metal, and so inactivate the enzyme (Chapter 10). In such a causal sequence, molecular effects may result in cellular changes, which in turn may have an effect on the functions of tissues and organs. It follows then that there must also be a temporal succession; biochemical changes must precede cellular changes, and so on, as the impact of the toxicant reaches higher levels of organisation. (Implicit in this interpretation is the concept of threshold level, which may not apply to gene mutation.)

The temporal sequence of these effects is more or less compressed in time depending on the rate of uptake and toxicity of the agent. Nevertheless, where low levels of environmental contaminants are being considered, the temporal sequence is important in that indices at lower levels of organisation offer the means of anticipating and predicting effects that may occur later at a higher level of organisation. Such indices can provide early warning in a situation where water quality is deteriorating, and at a stage when damage to the organism or population is preventable (Moore and Bayne, 1982).

There are other consequences of viewing the organism as a multilevel system through which perturbations pass as a cascade (Fig. 12-2). At each level of organisation there are homeostatic mechanisms of various kinds that counteract and neutralise the disruptive effects of biologically active toxicants. At the same time there are various processes operating at different levels that excrete, break-down, sequester or otherwise inactivate the toxicant. Consequently, as its impact passes through the system its effect is dissipated by the activation of an increasing number of mechanisms whose function is to neutralise perturbation and maintain internal stability. The observed effect may be arrested at any level, depending on the amount of toxicant taken up, its potency and the capacity of the organism to detoxify and counteract its effects. Clearly, if the capacity of the ameliorative responses exceeds the rate of uptake of the toxicant, then the progress of the toxicant's effect through the hierarchy is arrested.

A corollary of this rationale is that the intrinsic sensitivity of indices to toxicants is likely to be greatest at the molecular level, although few techniques are available that realise that potential. It is therefore not surprising that it has proved so difficult to find good ecological indices with which to assess pollution effects (McIntyre and Pearce, 1980).

Furthermore, indices at lower levels of organisation have a degree of generality not found in responses at higher levels, in that one can expect to employ the same kind of cellular or subcellular index in different organisms and expect comparable results. For example, latency of lysosomal enzymes (Chapter 8) is used as an index of stress in many different phyla, including mammals, plants and numerous invertebrate groups. Likewise, chromosomal aberrations are similar in different taxa and often have the same causes (Chapter 9). It is to be expected, therefore, that indices depending on cellular and subcellular properties of organisms are likely to be more readily applicable in different taxa, but more important is that such indices can provide results that can be extrapolated more reliably between taxa.

Consideration of an organism as a hierarchical system through which perturbation might pass as a cascade makes it possible to identify features of the system that are not obvious from the properties of the components. Most important of these is the idea that the effect of a toxicant at one level is not likely to spill over to the next until a threshold level is reached, when the capacity of mechanisms to ameliorate its effect at that level is exceeded (Fig. 12-1).

The hierarchical organisation of organisms is in itself an adaptation, since this confers what Bronowski (1970) called "stratified stability"—its organisation provides a number of levels of resistance to the impact of exogenous factors that tend to destabilise physiological processes. This was interpreted as giving meaning to the direction of evolution toward increasing complexity, since the implication is that the more levels of organisation the more stable its physiology is likely to be, or, more important, the wider range of conditions the organism may be expected to tolerate.

We are aware that there are exceptions to this hierarchical interpretation of the responses of organisms. For example, detoxication pathways may sometimes synthesise lethal compounds from relatively innocuous parent compounds. However, the non-specific nature of homeostatic responses and the hierarchical organisation of organisms implies that this or a related interpretation is necessary.

POLLUTION CONTROL SYSTEMS

The system by which regulatory authorities control pollution has, in a number of respects, been far from ideal, often due to the absence of sensitive techniques to measure water quality in biological terms in a way that is relevant to the environment. Regulatory authorities typically make recommendations to those wishing to release toxic materials to the marine environment on the basis of existing information about their toxicity, their chemistry in seawater, the hydrography of the area, local resources that could be at risk and so on. This may sometimes be backed up by acute lethal, or sometimes longer sublethal, experiments to assess the toxicity of the particular effluent. The flow of information and action in such a system is indicated diagrammatically in Fig. 12-3a. Typically, in the U.K. data on the effluent are related to site-specific information in order to arrive at a recommendation that will safeguard local biological and other resources, by estimating the capacity of the receiving waters to dilute and disperse the effluent to give concentrations that do not put at risk the biota that it is hoped to protect. Such estimates have often tended to be by "rule of thumb" with some more than adequate safety margin incorporated in the recommendation, but there is a growing trend toward quantifying the "assimilative capacity" of the environment, and we shall consider this concept in more detail in the next section.

However, the main weakness in the system described (Fig. 12-3a) is the absence of information about water quality from the environment itself in terms that can be related to biological criteria for water quality.

The problem here is that we are concerned not with the presence of contaminants in the marine environment as such, but with their actual or potential deleterious effects on the biota, so our criteria must ultimately be biological. However, while analytic techniques are available that make it possible to analyse and monitor the levels of each contaminant in seawater, biological techniques have not been sensitive enough to measure the effects of low levels of contaminants upon organisms in the environment. If our criteria for water quality are biological, it is obviously appropriate to measure it in biological terms, besides which there are a number of practical advantages in doing so. Most important of these is the fact that the organism's response is an integration

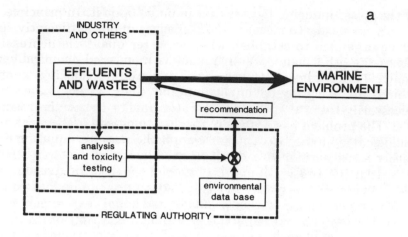

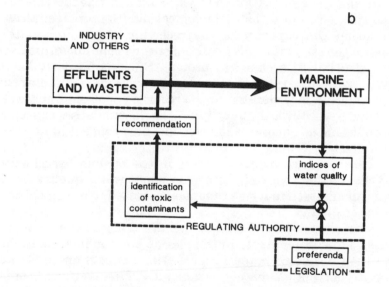

FIG. 12-3. Water quality control systems indicating the major routes of biological information in the kind of system that has operated in the past (*a*) and in a system that new techniques, such as those we describe, are making possible (*b*). The essential difference is the use of information about water quality in biological terms from the environment to regulate water quality.

of the stress-inducing factors that impinge upon it. In principle, it is only necessary to measure the responses of one sufficiently sensitive organism to establish whether water quality is depressed. If, on the other hand, water quality is monitored chemically by analysis of contaminants, the choice presupposes that it is known which are likely to be important and their absence does not necessarily mean that biological water quality is not depressed.

The problem has not been whether to choose a chemical or a biological approach to the measurement of water quality, but rather a realisation, as a result of examining the problem in this way, that the paucity of appropriate biological techniques did not allow a choice to be made. In the last 10 years a number of people have become aware of this problem, and many techniques have been developed to measure the effects of toxic contaminants on organisms in the environment (McIntyre and Pearce, 1980), making possible the kind of regulatory system indicated in Fig. 12-3b. A number of these techniques are described in this manual.

One area of research now is to solve the problem of relating a detected response to the toxicant that elicits it, because it is clearly not possible to impose control without first establishing causal relationships (Fig. 12-3b). It is not particularly helpful to know that water quality is depressed without also being able to identify the contaminant responsible, and correlations between the distribution of a response and a contaminant—however suggestive —are never conclusive.

There are several approaches to the problem of how to identify the toxicant(s) responsible for a detected effect, and a number are considered in this manual. The idea that some responses are so specific that observation of the response identifies its cause is the neatest answer, and there is some hope that work on mixed-function oxidases and metallothioneins might provide this kind of solution for some toxicants. Typically, for a contaminant to have an effect upon an organism it needs to be taken up, and, while in some cases it may be rapidly excreted, it is usual to find some kind of tissue burden. If the levels of a toxicant in the tissues that are necessary to cause a deleterious effect are known, then it must be possible to predict that effect from data on tissue burdens. Another approach that is being developed in conjunction with the hydroid bioassay technique depends on manipulating the chemistry of water samples from the environment (Chapter 11).

The combination of sensitive biological techniques together with new methods of establishing causal relationships should make it possible not simply to set limits for the toxicity of efflu-ents that safeguard the biota, but to develop a more positive kind of control (Fig. 12-3b) that could maximise the use of the natural capacity of the receiving waters to disperse, to sequester or to degrade effluents, while minimising the risk to the biota that are in part responsible.

ASSIMILATIVE CAPACITY

In recent years a new approach has been developing, the essence of which is implicit in the concept of "assimilative capacity" of ecosystems to cope with effluents. For some years the concern of biologists involved in pollution research was to detect the deleterious effects of toxic contaminants with increasingly sensi-tive systems in order to make a case for having the effluent treated to reduce its toxicity, or for the toxic components to be disposed of elsewhere. The idea of assimilative capacity indicates a willing-ness to accept the fact that marine ecosystems do have an ability to cope with certain levels of waste discharges without suffering any deleterious effects.

The concept was first formulated in this context by Cairns (1977) who argued that even for the most sensitive organisms there are concentrations of toxicants taken up that can be assimilated, and levels of toxicant-induced stress that can be tolerated.

More recently the concept has been considered in greater depth at workshops in the United States (Goldberg, 1980) and Taiwan. Assimilative capacity has been defined in a variety of ways, but a consensus definition might be the quantity of effluent that can be discharged into a body of water without producing a deleterious or irreversible biological impact.

The concept is providing a focus for research, bringing together those who work on the numerous factors that contribute to assimilative capacity. These factors are of two kinds: first, the physico-chemical variables that affect the concentrations and availability of the toxicants that organisms are exposed to, and, second, the variables that determine the response of the organism to the uptake of a toxicant. Into the first category fall the hydrographic processes that dilute and disperse, the physical pro-cesses that determine associations with suspended particulates and the chemical processes that account for changes in speciation, which play such an important part in their toxicity. However, we are more concerned here with the biological processes of excretion, detoxication and sequestration, and at higher levels with adaptation, tolerance and recovery. Nevertheless, all such processes play a part in determining the assimilative capacity of ecosystems, and the concept provides a focal point, as well as a rationale, for an interdisciplinary approach to water quality.

A STRATEGY FOR MONITORING ENVIRONMENTAL QUALITY

This manual describes a suite of techniques whose development and evolution has been continuous: some are being improved, new ones are being evolved, others discarded when they can be replaced by something better. However, it is useful to describe in some hypothetical situation how the present range of techniques and indices might be applied to detect, measure and identify the effects of unknown effluents. While the different phases of such an investigation inevitably overlap, it is helpful to define three stages, which follow approximately those identified by GESAMP (1980):

1. Detecting change in space and/or time: The first stage is one of detecting variations in water quality in biological and chemical terms and establishing the stability of their distributions in space and time. Collation of input data and other available information can quickly provide a list of the contaminants likely to be important to guide further analytical chemistry. The most helpful biological approach at this stage is the use of bioassay techniques, such as that described with colonial hydroids in Chapter 11. These techniques make it possible to look at a large number of stations on a grid or transect, or levels on depth profiles, with whatever degree of spatial discrimination seems appropriate, as we have done in the River Tamar (Stebbing et al., 1983). The relationship between the distribution of toxic effluents and bioassay responses should make it possible to detect pollution "hot spots" and delineate their spatial distribution, indicating whether they are due to constant or transient inputs.

    This kind of information can be backed up by considering the indigenous sessile or sedentary fauna. For example, the lysosomal and microsomal responses of *Mytilus* and *Littorina* (Moore, 1980a, Moore et al., 1982) and genetic and teratogenic aberrations in littorinids (Dixon, 1982; Dixon and Parry, unpublished) have been used to demonstrate pollution gradients. However, it is better not to proceed too far with indigenous populations because a number of sources of variability in such data can be significantly reduced by employing experimental populations transplanted from a single site.

2.   Establishing the degree of change: The next stage involves directing the full suite of indices to the area identified in stage 1 as a "hot spot" in order to quantify biological damage and establish its possible ecological consequences. Here we would use scope for growth (Chapter 7), lysosomal latency (Chapter 8), taurine:glycine ratios (Chapter 10) and other indices on transplanted populations of *Mytilus* kept in cages. In this way it is possible to minimise some sources of variability that contribute to poor signal-to-noise ratios and reduced sensitivity. For example, the effects of genetic heterogeneity can be minimised by using organisms from a single population. Likewise, the effects of variations in habitat such as level on the shore or the effects due to substratum or intensity of competition can be reduced, or kept constant, by using populations caged on the seashore or suspended from buoys at intervals through the water column. However, it is not possible to eliminate all such factors that are unrelated to the effects of effluents, and temperature, salinity, turbidity or the availability of food are likely to vary between sites or at different levels on a profile.

3.   Determining the cause of observed change: It is obviously not possible to impose control without establishing both the identity and source of effluents (Fig. 12-3b) whose toxic effects have been detected and measured in stages 1 and 2. The first step is to identify, among the effluents whose distribution correlates with the biological responses, those whose concentration is of the same order as that which could have caused the observed response. Clearly, contaminants that do not meet this criterion are unlikely to have contributed significantly to the observed responses. Failure to find contaminants at high enough concentrations to have caused the responses requires a return to stage 1 and a further examination of effluent data, or the need to extend the chemical data base. Often the data tend to include those contaminants whose analysis is straightforward, rather than

those that are likely to be biologically important, so some development work is sometimes required here.

Once appropriate correlations have been established it is still necessary to demonstrate a causal relationship. In marine systems this is often more difficult than in fresh water because in a linear, riverine system where water movement is unidirectional, biologically active toxicants can be identified by their source and a knowledge of the constituents of the effluent. In estuaries and coastal waters, where flow of the receiving waters reverses with each tidal cycle, the problem is more difficult and requires a different approach and new techniques.

One such technique involves specific indices, which, it is hoped, are like the immune response in that the response is specific to its cause, so that occurrence of the response can be used to identify its cause. This work is at an early stage, but it is possible to identify the effects of exposure to petroleum hydrocarbons by the activity of enzymes produced to detoxify them (Chapter 8). Likewise, the production of metallothioneins which bind and detoxify metals can be used to identify metal toxicity (Chapter 10); this concept is not unrelated to that of Luoma (1977), who suggested that tolerance of a metal provides evidence of an organism's prior exposure to the metal.

For a toxicant to have a deleterious effect upon an organism it must be taken up by crossing biological membranes. If it is known from toxicological experiments what concentration is required to cause such an effect, the converse reasoning can be used. Tissue burdens that exceed known threshold concentrations can perhaps be used to diagnose deleterious effects. Unfortunately, this does not always follow and very high concentrations may sometimes accumulate in apparently healthy animals (Bryan and Hummerstone, 1978). Nevertheless it is obviously necessary that a toxicant be present in an organism, and tissue analysis can provide evidence of its identity.

A different approach to the problem depends on chemically manipulating water samples known to be polluted, followed by bioassay experiments to establish the effect of the manipulation. Clearly, following removal of the biologically active contaminant from a water sample, the bioassay response it caused will not occur. This in itself is unimportant, but if the manipulation is specific to the contaminant its activity can be positively identified in this way (Chapter 11). The techniques available at present are not specific, although a number of possible manipulations that could be used in this way have been identified (Stebbing et al., 1980).

It would be unwise to imply that the adoption of such a strategy and the application of these techniques guarantee success; nevertheless our attempts to apply this strategy have made us aware of other problems and attempts to solve them should lead to improved techniques. For example, it is difficult to investigate the effects of transient or erratic inputs of toxic effluents, yet it may require only brief exposure to high concentrations of some toxicants to severely affect a population. There are a number of coastal and estuarine fisheries for oysters, shrimps and other species that no longer exist whose loss may be explained in this way. It is also difficult to investigate water quality in a hydrographically energetic system, because the conformation of the waters contaminated changes rapidly. Bioassay techniques provide an approach that is as nearly synoptic as any, but the answer may be to integrate with time using sentinel organisms deployed in the environment. However, there is then the problem of deciding whether depressed scope for growth, for example, is attributable to the turbidity or salinity regime, or to some aspect of water chemistry that is unrelated to anthropogenic contamination.

Techniques described in this manual are the basis of an approach to the problem of detecting, monitoring and controlling the biological quality of estuarine and coastal waters receiving noxious wastes. However, it should also be appreciated that, while the techniques are effective for the purposes for which they are intended, development of new techniques and improvement of old ones is a continuous process for the group responsible. We are also aware that environmental problems—particularly those related to marine pollution—involve a number of disciplines, and that this manual of biological techniques does not reflect the importance we attach to the physical and chemical analytical methods, synecological studies and modelling techniques that colleagues have developed and used in parallel with us (Morris, 1984). The contents were defined by practical constraints alone, as we believe that success in solving pollution problems in the marine environment depends on a willingness to bridge disciplinary boundaries, since all such problems are intrinsically multidisciplinary.

References

Abati, J. L. & Reish, D. J. 1972. The effects of lowered dissolved oxygen concentrations and salinity on the free amino acid pool of the polychaetous annelid *Neanthes arenaceodentata*. Bull. Sth. Calif. Acad. Sci. 71, 32–39.

Abel, P. D. & Skidmore, J. F. 1975. Toxic effects of an anionic detergent on the gills of rainbow trout. Water. Res. 9, 759–765.

Abraham, R., Morris, M. & Smith J. 1967. Histochemistry of lysosomes in rat heart muscle. J. Histochem. Cytochem. 15, 596–599.

Addink, A. D. F. & Veenhof, P. R. 1975. Regulation of mitochondrial matrix enzymes in *Mytilus edulis L.* In: Proc. 9th Europ. mar. biol. Symp., edited by H. Barnes, Aberdeen University Press, Aberdeen, pp. 109–119.

Addison, R. F., Zinck, M. E. & Willis, D. E. 1978. Induction of hepatic mixed-function oxidase (MFO) enzymes in trout *(Salvelinus fontinalis)* by feeding Aroclor (R) 1254 or 3-methylcholanthrene. Comp. Biochem. Physiol. 61C, 323–325.

Ade, P., Banchelli Soldiani, M. G., Castelli, M. G., Chiersara, E., Clementi, F., Fanelli, R., Funari, E., Ignesti, G., Marabani, A., Oronesu, M., Palmero, S., Pirisino, R., Ramundo Orlando, A., Silano, V., Viarengo, A. & Vittozzi, L. 1982. Comparative biochemical and morphological characterization of microsomal preparations from rat, quail, trout, mussel and *Daphnia magna*. In: Cytochrome P-450. Biochemistry, biophysics and environmental implications, edited by E. Hietanen, M. Laitinen & O. Hänninen, Elsevier, Amsterdam, pp. 387–390.

Ahmed, M. & Sparks, A. K. 1970. Chromosome number, structure and autosomal polymorphism in the marine mussels *Mytilus edulis* and *Mytilus californianus*. Biol. Bull mar. biol. Lab., Woods Hole 138, 1–13.

Ahokas, J. T. 1976. Metabolism of 2,5-diphenyloxazole (PPO) by trout liver microsomal mixed function mono-oxygenase. Res. Comm. Chem. Pathol. Pharm. 13, 439–447.

Ahokas, J. T., Kärki, N. T., Oikari, A. & Soivio, A. 1976a. Mixed function monooxygenase of fish as an indicator of pollution of aquatic environment by industrial effluent. Bull. Environ. Contam. Toxicol. 16, 270–274.

Ahokas, J. T., Pelkonen, O. & Kärki, N. T. 1975. Metabolism of polycyclic hydrocarbons by a highly active aryl hydrocarbon hydroxylase system in the liver of trout species. Biochem. biophys. Res. Commun. 63, 635–641.

Ahokas, J. T., Pelkonen, O. & Kärki, N. T. 1976b. Cytochrome P-450 and drug induced spectral interactions in the hepatic microsomes of trout, *Salmo trutta lacustris*. Acta pharmac. tox. 38, 440–449.

Albert, A. A. 1968. Selective toxicity. Methuen, London, 531 pp.

Alderdice, D. F. 1976. Some concepts and descriptions of physiological tolerance: Rate–temperature curves of poikilotherms as transects of response surfaces. J. Fish. Res. Bd. Can. 33, 299–307.

Allen, J. A. & Garrett, M. R. 1971. Taurine in marine invertebrates. In: Advances in marine biology Vol. 9, edited by F. S. Russell & M. Yonge, Academic Press, London, New York, pp. 205–253.

Allen, J. M. 1969. Lysosomes in bacterial infection. In: Lysosomes in biology and pathology, Vol. 2, edited by J. T. Dingle & H. B. Fell, North Holland/American Elsevier, Amsterdam, New York, pp. 41–68.

Allen, J. R., Carstens, L. A. & Abrahanson, L. J. 1976. Responses of rats exposed to polychlorinated biphenyls for fifty-two weeks. I. Comparison of tissue levels of PCB and biological change. Arch. Environ. Contam. Toxicol. 4, 404–419.

Allen, J. R., Carstens, L. A., Abrahanson, L. J. & Marlar, R. J. 1975. Responses of rats and nonhuman primates to 2,5,2',5'-tetrachlorobiphenyl. Environ. Res. 9, 265–273.

Allen, J. R., Carstens, L. A. & Barsotti, D. A. 1974. Residual effects of short-term, low-level exposure of non-human primates to polychlorinated biphenyls. Toxic. appl. Pharmac. 30, 440–451.

Allison, A. C. 1969. Lysosomes and cancer. In: Lysosomes in biology and pathology Vol. 2, edited by J. T. Dingle & H. B. Fell, Elsevier/North Holland, Amsterdam, pp. 178–204.

Allison, A. C. & Mallucci, L. 1964. Uptake of hydrocarbon carcinogens by lysosomes. Nature, Lond. 209, 303–304.

Altman, F. P. 1972. Quantitative dehydrogenase histochemistry with special reference to the pentose shunt dehydrogenases. Progr. Histochem. Cytochem. 4, 225–273.

Anderson, J. W. 1977. Responses to sublethal levels of petroleum hydrocarbons: Are they sensitive indicators and do they correlate with tissue contamination? In: Fate and effects of petroleum in marine organisms and ecosystems, edited by D. Wolfe, Pergamon, New York, pp. 95–114.

Anderson, K. B. & von Meyenburg, K. 1977. Charges of nicotinamide adenine nucleotides and adenylate energy charge as regulatory parameters of the metabolism in *Escherichia coli*. J. biol. Chem. 252, 4151–4156.

Anderson, R. S. 1978a. Developing an invertebrate model for chemical carcinogenesis: Metabolic activation of carcinogens. Comp. Pathobiol. 4, 11–24.

Anderson, R. S. 1978b. Benzo(a)pyrene metabolism in the American oyster *Crassostrea virginica*. EPA Ecol. Res. Ser. Monogr. (EPA–600/3–78–009).

Ansell, A. D. & Sivadas, P. 1973. Some effects of temperature and starvation on the bivalve *Donax vittatus* (da Costa) in experimental laboratory populations. J. exp. mar. Biol. Ecol. 13, 229–262.

Armstrong, F. A. J., Williams, P. M. & Strikland, J. D. H. 1966. Photooxidation of organic matter in seawater by ultraviolet radiation, analytical and other applications. Nature, Lond. 211, 481–483.

Atkinson, D. E. 1968. The energy charge of the adenylate pool as a regulatory parameter. Interaction with feedback modifiers. Biochemistry, N.Y. 7, 4030–4034.

Atkinson, D. E. 1969. Regulation of enzyme function. A. Rev. Microbiol. (Annu) 23, 47–68.

Atkinson, D. E. 1971a. Adenine nucleotides as stoichiometric coupling agents in metabolism and as regulatory modifiers: The adenylate energy charge. In: Metabolic pathways Vol. V, Metabolic regulation, edited by H. J. Vogel, Academic Press, New York, pp. 1–21.

Atkinson, D. E. 1971b. Adenine nucleotides as universal stoichiometric metabolic coupling agents. Advan. Enzyme Regul. 9, 207–219.

Atkinson, D. E. 1972. The adenylate energy charge in metabolic regulation. In: Horizons of bioenergetics, edited by A. San Pietro & H. Gest, Academic Press, New York.

Atkinson, D. E. 1976. Adaptations of enzymes for regulation of catalytic function. In: Biochemical adaptation to environmental change, edited by R. M. S. Smellie & J. F. Pennock, The Biochemical Society, London, pp. 205–223.

Atkinson, D. E. 1977. Energy metabolism and its regulation, Academic Press, New York, 293 pp.

Atkinson, D. E. & Fromm, H. 1977. Cellular energy control. Trends biochem. Sci. 1, N198–N200.

Atkinson, D. E. & Walton, G. M. 1967. Adenosine triphosphate conservation in metabolic regulation. Rat liver citrate cleavage enzyme. J. Biol. Chem. 242, 3239–3241.

Auerbach, C. 1976. Mutation research, Chapman and Hall, London, 528 pp.

Awapara, J. 1962. Free amino acids in invertebrates: A comparative study of their distribution and metabolism. In: Amino acid pool, edited by J. T. Holden, Elsevier, Amsterdam, pp. 158–175.

Baginski, R. M. & Pierce Jr. S. K. 1975. Anaerobiosis: A possible source of osmotic solute for high-salinity acclimation in marine molluscs. J. exp. Biol. 62, 589–598.

Baginski, R. M. & Pierce Jr. S. K. 1977. The time course of intracellular free amino acid accumulation in tissues of *Modiolus demissus* during high salinity adaptation. Comp. Biochem. Physiol. 57A, 407–412.

Baier, R. W., Wojnowich, J. & Petrie, L. 1975. Mercury loss from culture media. Anal. Chem. 47, 2464–2467.

Baird, R. H. 1958. Measurement of condition in mussels and oysters. J. Cons. perm. int. Explor. Mer 23, 249–257.

Baird, R. H. 1966. Factors affecting the growth and condition of mussels (*Mytilus edulis L*). M.A.F.F. Fishery Investigations Ser. II, Vol. 25, No. 2, 1–33.

Ball, W. J. & Atkinson, D. E. 1975. Adenylate energy charge in *Saccharomyces cerevisiae* during starvation. J. Bact. 121, 975–982.

Barnes, H. & Blackstock. J. 1974. The separation and estimation of free amino acids, trimethylamine oxide, and betaine in tissues and body fluids of marine invertebrates. J. exp. mar. Biol. Ecol. 16, 29–45.

Barrett, A. J. & Dingle, J. T. 1967. A lysosomal component capable of binding cations and a carcinogen. Biochem. J. 105, 20.

Barszcz, C., Yevich, P. P., Brown, L. R., Yarbrough, J. D. & Minchew, C. D. 1978. Chronic effects of three crude oils on oysters suspended in estuarine ponds. J. Environ. Pathol. Toxicol. 1, 879–996.

Battaglia, B., & Beardmore, J. A. 1978. Marine organisms: Genetics, ecology and evolution, Plenum Press, New York, 767 pp.

Battaglia, B., Bisol, P. M., Fossato, V. U. & Rodino, E. 1980. Studies on the genetic effects of pollution in the sea. Rapp. P.-v. Réun. Cons. int. Explor. Mer 179, 267–274.

Bayley, P. B. 1977. A method for finding the limits of application of the von Bertalanffy growth model and statistical estimates of the parameters. J. Fish. Res. Bd Can. 34, 1079–1084.

Bayne, B. L. 1971. Ventilation, the heart beat and oxygen uptake by *Mytilus edulis* L. in declining oxygen tension. Comp. Biochem. Physiol. 40A, 1065–1085.

Bayne, B. L. 1972. Some effects of stress in the adult on the larval development of *Mytilus edulis*. Nature, Lond. 237, 459.

Bayne, B. L. 1973a. Physiological changes in *Mytilus edulis* L. induced by temperature and nutritive stress. J. mar. biol. Ass. U.K. 53, 39–58.

Bayne, B. L. 1973b. Aspects of the metabolism of *Mytilus edulis* during starvation. Neth. J. Sea Res. 7, 399–410.

Bayne, B. L. 1975. Aspects of physiological condition in *Mytilus edulis* (L.) with special reference to the effects of oxygen tension and salinity. In: Proceedings of the 9th European marine biology symposium, edited by H. Barnes, Aberdeen University Press, Aberdeen, pp. 213–238.

Bayne, B. L. 1976. Marine mussels: Their ecology and physiology. Cambridge University Press, Cambridge, 494 pp.

Bayne, B. L. 1984. Response to environmental stress: Tolerance, resistance and adaptation. In: Proceedings 18th European marine biology symposium, Oslo, edited by J. Gray & M. Christenson, Wiley, New York (in press).

Bayne, B. L., Anderson, J., Engel, D., Gilfillan, E., Hoss, D., Lloyd R. & Thurberg, F. P. 1980a. Physiological techniques for measuring the biological effects of pollution at sea. Rapp. P.-v. Réun. Cons. int. Explor. Mer 179, 88–99.

Bayne, B. L., Brown, D. A., Harrison, F. & Yevich, P. D. 1980b. Mussel health. In: The international mussel watch, edited by National Academy of Sciences, Washington, D.C., pp. 163–235.

Bayne, B. L., Bubel, A., Gabbott, P. A., Livingstone, D. R., Lowe, D. M. & Moore, M. N. 1982. Glycogen utilisation and gametogenesis in *Mytilus edulis* L. Mar. Biol. Letts. 3, 89–105.

Bayne, B. L., Clarke, K. R. & Moore, M. N. 1981. Some practical considerations in the measurement of pollution effects on bivalve molluscs, and some possible ecological consequences. Aquat. Toxicol. 1, 159–174.

Bayne, B. L., Gabbott, P. A. & Widdows, J. 1975. Some effects of stress in the adult on the eggs and larvae of *Mytilus edulis* L. J. mar. biol. Ass. U.K. 55, 675–689.

Bayne, B. L., Holland D. L., Moore, M. N., Lowe, D. M. & Widdows, J. 1978. Further studies on the effects of stress in the adult on the eggs of *Mytilus edulis*. J. mar. biol. Ass. U.K. 58, 825–841.

Bayne, B. L. & Livingstone, D. R. 1977. Responses of *Mytilus edulis* to low oxygen tension: Acclimation of rate of oxygen consumption. J. Comp. Physiol. 114, 129–142.

Bayne, B. L., Livingstone, D. R., Moore, M. N. & Widdows, J. 1976a. A cytochemical and biochemical index of stress in *Mytilus edulis* L. Mar. Poll. Bull. 7, 221–224.

Bayne, B. L., Moore, M. N., Widdows, J., Livingstone, D. R. & Salkeld, P. 1979. Measurement of the responses of individuals to environmental stress and pollution: Studies with bivalve molluscs. Phil. Trans. R. Soc. Lond. B. 286, 563–581.

Bayne, B. L., Salkeld, P. N. & Worrall, C. M. 1983. Reproductive effort and value in different populations of the marine mussel, *Mytilus edulis* L. Oecologia (Berlin) 59, 18–26.

Bayne B. L. & Scullard, C. 1977. Rates of nitrogen excretion by species of *Mytilus* (Bivalvia: Mollusca). J. mar. biol. Ass. U.K. 57, 355–369.

Bayne, B. L. & Thompson, R. J. 1970. Some physiological consequences of keeping *Mytilus edulis* in the laboratory. Helgoländer wiss. Meeresunters. 20, 526–552.

Bayne, B. L., Thompson, R. J. & Widdows, J. 1976b. Physiology: I. In: Marine mussels: Their ecology and physiology, edited by B. L. Bayne, Cambridge University Press, Cambridge, pp. 121-206.

Bayne, B. L. & Widdows, J. 1978. The physiological ecology of two populations of *Mytilus edulis L.* Oecologia. Berl. 37, 137-162.

Bayne, B. L., Widdows, J. & Newell, R. I. E. 1977. Physiological measurements on estuarine bivalve molluscs in the field. In: Biology of benthic organisms, edited by B. K. Keegan, P. O'Ceidigh & P. J. S. Boaden, Pergamon, New York, pp. 57-68.

Bayne, B. L., Widdows, J. W. & Thompson, R. J. 1976c. Physiology: II. In: Marine mussels: Their ecology and physiology, edited by B. L. Bayne, Cambridge University Press, Cambridge, pp. 207-260.

Bayne, B. L., Widdows, J. & Thompson, R. J. 1976d. Physiological integrations. In: Marine mussels: Their physiology and ecology, edited by B. L. Bayne, Cambridge University Press, Cambridge, pp. 261-291.

Bayne, B. L. & Worrall, C. M. 1980. Growth and production of mussels *Mytilus edulis* from two populations. Mar. Ecol. Progr. Ser. 3, 317-328.

Beamish, F. W. H. & Dickie, L. M. 1967. Metabolism and biological production in fish. In: The biological basis of freshwater fish production, edited by S. D. Gerking, Wiley, New York, pp. 215-242.

Beardmore, J. A., Barker, C. J., Battaglia, B., Berry, R. J., Crosby Longwell, A., Payne, J. F. & Rosenfield, A. 1980. The use of genetical approaches to monitoring biological effects of pollution. Rapp. P.-v. Réun. Cons. int. Explor. Mer 179, 299-305.

Behm, C. A. & Bryant, C. 1975. Studies of regulatory metabolism in *Monieza expansa*: General considerations. Int. J. Parasit. 5, 209-217.

Beis, I. & Newsholme, E. A. 1975. The contents of adenine nucleotides, phosphagens and some glycolytic intermediates in resting muscles from vertebrates and invertebrates. Biochem. J. 152, 23-32.

Bell, G. R. 1968. Distribution of transaminases (Aminotransferases) in the tissues of Pacific salmon (*Oncorhynchus*), with emphasis on the properties and diagnostic use of glutamic-oxalacetic transaminase. J. Fish. Res. Bd Can. 25, 1247-1268.

Bend, J. R., James, M. O. & Dansette, P. M. 1977a. *In vitro* metabolism of xenobiotics in some marine animals. Ann. N.Y. Acad. Sci. 298, 505–521.

Bend, J. R., Pohl, R. J., Arinc, E. & Philpot, R. M. 1977b. Hepatic microsomal and solubilized mixed-function oxidase systems from the little skate, *Raja erinacea*, a marine elasmobranch. In: Proc. of 3rd int. symp. on microsomes and drug oxidations, edited by V. Ullrich, I. Roots, A. Hildebrandt, R. W. Estabrook & A. H. Conney, Pergamon, New York, pp. 160–169.

Benijts-Claus, C. & Benijts, F. 1975. The effects of low load and zinc concentrations on the larvae development of the mud crab *Rhithropanopeus harrisii* Gould. In: Sublethal effects of toxic chemicals on aquatic organisms, edited by H. Koeman & J. Strik, Elsevier, Amsterdam, pp. 43–52.

Bernard, F. R. 1974. Particle sorting and labial palp function in the Pacific oyster, *Crassostrea gigas* (Thurnberg, 1975). Biol. Bull. mar. biol. Lab. Woods Hole 146, 1–10.

Bernard, F. R. 1973. Crystalline style formation and function in the oyster *Crassostrea gigas* (Thunberg 1975). Ophelia. 12, 159–170.

Berry, R. J. 1977. Inheritance and natural history, Collins New Naturalist, London, 350 pp.

Bewley, J. D. & Gwozdz, E. A. 1975. Plant dessication and protein synthesis. III. On the relationship between endogenous adenosine triphosphate levels and protein-synthesizing capacity. Pl. Physiol. Lancaster 55, 1110–1114.

Binder, R. L. & Stegeman, J. J. 1980. Induction of aryl hydrocarbon hydroxylase activity in embryos of an estuarine fish. Biochem. Pharmac. 29, 949–951.

Bishop, S. H. 1976. Nitrogen metabolism and excretion: Regulation of intracellular amino acid concentrations. In: Estuarine processes, Vol. 1, edited by M. Wiley, Academic Press, New York, pp. 414–431.

Bitensky, L., Butcher, R. S. & Chayen, J. 1973. Quantitative cytochemistry in the study of lysosomal function. In: Lysosomes in biology and pathology, Vol. 3, edited by J. T. Dingle, North Holland/American Elsevier, Amsterdam, New York, pp. 465–510.

Blackman, R. A. A. & Law, R. J. 1980. The *Eleni V* oil Spill: Fate and effects of the oil over the first twelve months. Mar. Poll. Bull. 11, 199–204.

Blackstock, J. 1980a. A biochemical approach to assessment of effects of organic pollution on the metabolism of the non-opportunistic polychaete *Glycera alba*. Helgoländer wiss. Meeresunters. 33, 546–555.

Blackstock. J. 1980b. Phosphofructokinase in the marine polychaete worm, *Glycera alba* (Müller): Maximal activities and some properties of the enzyme in crude extracts. In: Control processes, edited by K. A. Munday, University of Southampton, Southampton, pp. 14–15.

Blackstock, J. D. 1978. Activities of some enzymes associated with energy yielding metabolism in *Glycera alba* (Müller) from three areas of Loch Eil. In: Physiology and behaviour of marine organisms, edited by D. S. McLusky & A. J. Berry, Pergamon, Oxford, pp. 11–20.

Boehm, P. D. & Quinn, J. G. 1976. The effect of dissolved organic matter in sea water on the uptake of mixed individual hydrocarbons and Number 2 fuel oil by a marine filter-feeding bivalve (*Mercenaria mercenaria*). Estuar. cstl. mar. Sci. 4, 93–105.

Bostock, C. J. & Sumner, A. T. 1977. The eukaryotic chromosome, Elsevier/North Holland, Amsterdam, New York and Oxford, 525 pp.

Bouquegneau, J. M. 1979. Evidence for the protective effect of metallothioneins against inorganic mercury injuries to fish. Bull. Environ. Contam. Toxicol. 23, 218–219.

Bouquegneau, J. M., Gerday, C. & Disteche, A. 1975. Fish mercury-binding thionein related to adaptation mechanisms. FEBS Letters 55, 173–177.

Brand, A. R. & Taylor, A. C. 1974. Pumping activity of *Arctica islandica* (L) and some other common bivalves. Mar. Behav. Physiol. 3, 1–15.

Braverman, M. 1974. The cellular basis of morphogenesis and morphostasis in hydroids. Oceanogr. Mar. Biol. Ann. Rev. 12, 129–221.

Bremner, I. & Davies, N. T. 1975. The induction of metallothionein in rat liver by Zn injection and restriction of food intake. Biochem. J. 149, 733–738.

Bresnick, E. & Yang H-Y. 1964. The influence of phenobarbital administration upon the 'soluble' NADP-requiring enzymes in liver. Biochem. Pharmac. 13, 497–505.

Brett, J. R. 1958. Implications and assessments of environmental stress. In: Investigations of fish-power problems, edited by P. A. Larkin, University of British Columbia Press, Vancouver, pp. 69–83.

Brett, J. R. 1965. The relation of size to rate of oxygen consumption and sustained swimming speed of sockeye salmon (*Oncorhynchus nerka*). J. Fish. Res. Bd Can. 22, 1491–1501.

Briarty, L. G. 1975. Stereology: Methods for quantitative light and electron microscopy. Sci. Prog. Oxf. 62, 1–32.

Bronowski, J. 1970. New concepts in the evolution of complexity. Synthese 21, 228–246.

Brown, D. A. 1977. Increases of Cd and the Cd:Zn ratio in the high molecular weight protein pool from apparently normal liver of tumor-bearing flounders (*Parophrys vetulus*). Mar. Biol. 44, 203–209.

Brown, D. A. 1978. Toxicology of trace metals: Metallothionein production and carcinogenesis. Ph. Diss., University of British Columbia. Canadian Thesis Division, National Library of Canada, Ottawa, 271 pp.

Brown, D. A., Bawden, C. A., Chatel, K. W. & Parsons, T. R. 1977. The wildlife community of Iona Island jetty, Vancouver B.C., and heavy-metal pollution effects. Environ. Conserv. 4, 213–216.

Brown, D. A. & Chatel, K. W. 1978. Interactions between cadmium and zinc in cytoplasm of duck liver and kidney. Chem. Biol. Interactions 22. 271–279.

Brown, D. A. & Parsons, T. R. 1978. Relationship between cytoplasmic distribution of mercury and toxic effects of zooplankton and churn salmon (*Oncorhynchus keta*) exposed to mercury in a controlled ecosystem. J. Fish. Res. Bd Can. 35, 880–884.

Brown, V. M., Shaw, T. L. & Shurben, D. G. 1974. Aspects of water quality and the toxicity of copper to rainbow trout. Water Res. 8, 797–803.

Bruce, W. R., Furrer, R. & Wyrobek, A. J. 1974. Abnormalities in the shape of marine sperm after acute testicular irradiation. Mutation Res. 23, 381–386.

Brun, A. & Brunk. U. 1970. Histochemical indications for lysosomal localisation of heavy metals in normal rat brain and liver. J. Histochem. Cytochem. 18, 820–827.

Bryan, G. W. 1976. Heavy metal contamination in the sea. In: Marine pollution, edited by R. Johnston, Academic Press, New York, pp. 185–302.

Bryan, G. W. & Hummerstone, L. G. 1978. Heavy metals in the burrowing bivalve *Scrobicularia plana* from contaminated and uncontaminated estuaries. J. mar. biol. Ass. U.K. 58, 401–419.

Bubel, A., Moore, M. N. & Lowe, D. 1977. Cellular responses to shell damage in *Mytilus edulis* L. J. Exp. mar. Biol. Ecol. 30, 1–27.

Buhler, D. R. & Rasmusson, M. E. 1968. The oxidation of drugs by fishes. Comp. Biochem. Physiol. 25, 223–239.

Bullock, T. H. 1955. Compensation for temperature in the metabolism and activity of poikilotherms. Biol. Rev. 30, 311–342.

Burns, K. A. 1976a. Microsomal mixed function oxidases in an estuarine fish, *Fundulus heteroclitus*, and their induction as a result of environmental contamination. Comp. Biochem. Physiol. 53B, 443–446.

Burns, K. A. 1976b. Hydrocarbon metabolism in the intertidal fiddler crab *Uca pugnax*. Mar. Biol. 36, 5–11.

Butcher, R. G. & Altman, F. P. 1973. Studies on the reduction of tetrazolium salts. II. The measurement of the half reduced and fully reduced formazans of neotetrazolium chloride in tissue sections. Histochemie 37, 351–363.

Cairns, J. 1977. Quantification of biological integrity. In: The integrity of water, edited by R. K. Ballentine and L. J. Guarraia, U.S. Government Printing Office, Washington, D.C., pp. 171–187.

Caldwell, R. S. 1974. Osmotic and ionic regulation in decapod crustacea exposed to methoxychlor. In: Pollution and physiology of marine organisms, edited by F. J. Vernberg & W. B. Vernberg, Academic Press, New York, pp. 197–223.

Calow, P. 1979. The cost of reproduction—A physiological approach. Biol. Rev. 54, 23–40.

Calow, P. & Fletcher, C. R. 1972. A new radiotracer technique involving ^{14}C and ^{51}Cr, for estimating the assimilation efficiencies of aquatic, primary consumers. Oecologia 9, 155–170.

Campbell, J. W. & Bishop, S. H. 1970. Nitrogen metabolism in molluscs. In: Comparative biochemistry of nitrogen metabolism, Vol. 1, edited by J. W. Campbell, Academic Press, New York, London, pp. 103–206.

Carlson, G. P. 1972. Detoxification of foreign organic compounds by the quahaug, *Mercenaria mercenaria*. Comp. Biochem. Physiol. 43B, 295–302.

Carlson, G. P. 1973. Comparison of the metabolism of parathion by lobsters and rats. Bull. Environ. Contam. Toxicol. 9, 296–300.

Carlson, G. P. 1974. Epoxidation of aldrin to dieldrin by lobsters. Bull. Environ. Contam. Toxicol. 11, 577–582.

Carter, C. O. 1977. The relative contribution of mutant genes and chromosome abnormality to genetic ill-health in man. In: Progress in genetic toxicology, edited by D. Scott, B. A. Bridges & F. H. Sobels, Elsevier/North Holland, Amsterdam, pp. 1–14.

Chambers, J. E., Heitz, J. R., McCorkle, F. M. & Yarbrough, J. D. 1978. The effects of crude oil on enzymes in the brown shrimp (Penaeus sp.). Comp. Biochem. Physiol. 61C, 29–32.

Chambers, J. E., Heitz, J. R., McCorkle, F. M. & Yarbrough, J. D. 1979a. Enzyme activities following chronic exposure to crude oil in a simulated ecosystem. I. American oysters and brown shrimp. Environ. Res. 20, 133–139.

Chambers, J. E., Heitz, J. R., McCorkle, F. M. & Yarbrough, J. D. 1979b. Enzyme activities following chronic exposure to crude oil in a simulated ecosystem. II. Striped mullet. Environ. Res. 20, 140–147.

Chan, T. M., Gillett, J. W. & Terriere, L. C. 1967. Interaction between microsomal electron transport systems of trout and male rat in cyclodiene epoxidation. Comp. Biochem. Physiol. 20, 731–742.

Chapman, A. G. & Atkinson, D. E. 1973. Stabilization of adenylate energy charge by the adenylate deaminase reaction. J. biol. Chem. 248, 8309–8312.

Chapman, A. G., Fall, L. & Atkinson, D. E. 1971. Adenylate energy charge in Escherichia coli during growth and starvation. J. Bact. 108, 1072–1086.

Chayen, J. 1978. Microdensitometry. In: Biochemical mechanisms of liver injury, edited by T. F. Slater, Academic Press, New York, pp. 259–291.

Cherian, M. G., Goyer, R. A. & Delaquerrier-Richardson, L. 1976. Cadmium-metallothionein-induced nephropathy. Toxic. appl. Pharmac. 38, 399–408.

Chevion, M., Stegeman, J. J., Peisach, J. & Blumberg, W. E. 1977. Electron paramagnetic resonance studies on hepatic microsomal cytochrome P-450 from a marine teleost. Life Sci. 20, 895–900.

Ching, T. M. 1976. Regulation of nitrogenase activity in soybean nodules by ATP and energy charge. Life Sci. 18, 1071–1076.

Ching, T. M., Hedtke, S., Russell, S. A. & Evans, H. J. 1975. Energy state and dinitrogen fixation in soybean nodules of dark-grown plants. Pl. Physiol. Lancaster, 55, 796–798.

Chipman, W. A. 1972. Ionizing radiation: Animals. In: Marine ecology Vol 1, Part 3, edited by O. Kinne, Wiley-Interscience, New York, pp. 1621–1643.

Chipperfield, P. N. J. 1953. Observations on the breeding and settlement of *Mytilus edulis* (L.) in British waters. J. mar. biol. Ass. U.K. 32, 449–476.

Chulavatnatol, M. & Haesungcharern, A. 1977. Stabilization of adenylate energy charge and its relation to human sperm motility. J. biol. Chem. 252, 8088–8091.

Coleman, N. 1973. Water loss from aerially exposed mussels. J. exp. mar. Biol. Ecol. 12, 145–155.

Colombatti, A., Fossato, V. U., Collavo, D., Chieco-Bianchi, L. & Battaglia B. Risultati preliminari sulla possibile azione cancerogena di estratti ottenuti da mitili eduli. VIII. Congresso Nazionale della Soc. It. di cancerologia. 301–302.

Conney, A. H. 1967. Pharmacological implications of microsomal enzyme induction. Pharmac. Rev. 19, 317–366.

Conney, A. K. & Burns, J. J. 1972. Metabolic interactions among environmental chemicals and drugs. Science, N.Y. 178, 576–586.

Connor, P. M. 1972. Acute toxicity of heavy metals to some marine larvae. Mar. Poll. Bull. 3, 190–192.

Conover, R. J. 1966. Assimilation of organic matter by zooplankton. Limnol. Oceanogr. 11, 338–354.

Conover, R. J. 1978. Transformation of organic matter. In: Marine ecology, Vol. IV. Dynamics, edited by O. Kinne, Wiley-Interscience, Chichester, pp. 221–500.

Cook, L. M. & Wood, R. J. 1976. Genetic effects of pollutants. J. Inst. Biol. 23, 129–139.

Cook, P. A. & Gabbott, P. A. 1978. Glycogen synthetase in the sea mussel *Mytilus edulis* L. I. Purification, interconversion and kinetic properties of I and D forms. Comp. Biochem. Physiol. 60B, 419–421.

Corner, E. D. S. & Cowey, C. B. 1968. Biochemical studies on the production of marine zooplankton. Biol. Bull. 43, 393–426.

Corner, E. D. S., Harris, R. P. Kilvington, C. C. & O'Hara, S. C. M. 1976. Petroleum compounds in the marine food web: Short-term experiments on the fate of naphthalene in *Calanus*. J. mar. biol. Ass. U.K. 56, 121–134.

Corner, E. D. S., Kilvington, C. C. & O'Hara, S. C. M. 1973. Qualitative studies on the metabolism of naphthalene in *Maia squinado* (spider crab). J. mar. biol. Ass. U.K. 52, 819–832.

Corner, E. D. S., Leon, Y. A. & Bulbrook, R. D. 1960. Steroid sulphatase, arylsulphatase and B-glucuronidase in marine invertebrates. J. mar. biol. Ass. U.K. 39, 51–61.

Corner, E. D. S. & Rigler, F. H. 1957. The loss of mercury from stored seawater solutions of mercuric chloride. J. mar. biol. Ass. U.K. 36, 449–458.

Coughlan, J. 1969. The estimation of filtering rate from the clearance of suspensions. Mar. Biol. 2, 356–358.

Crabtree, B. & Newsholme, E. A. 1975. Comparative aspects of fuel utilisation and metabolism by muscle. In: Insect muscle, edited by P. N. R. Usherwood, Academic Press, New York, pp. 405–500.

Creaven, P. J., Parke, D. V. & Williams, R. T. 1965. A fluorimetric study of the hydroxylation of biphenyl *in vitro* by liver preparations of various species. Biochem. J. 96, 879–885.

Crisp, D. J. 1971. Energy flow measurements. In: Methods for the study of marine benthos, edited by N. A. Holme & A. D. McIntyre, Blackwell Scientific Publications, Oxford, pp. 197–279.

Crisp, D. J. 1974. Factors influencing the settlement of marine invertebrate larvae. In: Chemoreception in marine organisms, edited by P. T. Grant & A. M. Mackie, Academic Press, New York, pp. 177–265.

Crisp, D. J. 1975. The role of the pelagic larva. In: Perspectives in experimental biology, Vol. 1, edited by P. Spencer Davies, Pergamon, London, pp. 177–285.

Dame, R. F. 1972. The ecological energies of growth respiration and assimilation in the American Oyster, *Crassostrea virginica*. Mar. Biol. 17, 243–250.

Dare, P. J. & Edwards, D. B. 1975. Seasonal changes in flesh weight and biochemical composition of mussels (*Mytilus edulis* L.) in the Conway Estuary, North Wales. J. exp. mar. Biol. Ecol. 18, 89–97.

Darlington, C. D. & La Cour. L. F. 1976. The handling of chromosomes, 6th edn., Allen and Unwin, London, 201 pp.

Darrow, D. C. & Harding, G. C. H. 1975. Accumulation and apparent absence of DDT metabolism by marine copepods, *Calanus spp.* in culture. J. Fish. Res. Bd Can. 32, 1845–1849.

Davey, E. W., Gentile, J. H., Erickson, S. J. and Betzer, P. 1970. Removal of trace metals from marine culture media. Limnol. Oceanogr. 15, 486–488.

Davies, P. Spencer-. 1966. A constant pressure respirometer for medium sized animals. Oikos 17, 108–112.

Davis, H. C. & Hidu, H. 1969. Effects of pesticides on embryonic development of clams and oysters and on survival and growth of the larvae. Fish. Bull. fish Wildl. Serv. U.S. 67, 393–404.

Dayton, P. K. 1971. Competition, disturbance and community organisation: The provision and subsequent utilisation of space in a rocky intertidal community. Ecol. Monogr. 41, 351–389.

DePierre, J. W. & Ernster, L. 1978. The metabolism of polycyclic hydrocarbons and its relationship to cancer. Biochim. biophys. Acta 473, 149–186.

DesVoigne, D. M. & Sparks, A. K. 1968. The process of wound healing in the Pacific Oyster, *Crassostrea gigas*. J. invertebr. Pathol. 12, 53–65.

Dewaide, J. H. 1971. Alterations in microsomal drug oxidation in thermally acclimated fish. Archs int. Pharmocodyn. Thér 189, 377–379.

Dewaide, J. H. & Henderson, P. T. 1968. Hepatic *n*-demethylation of aminopyrine in rat and trout. Biochem. Pharmacol. 17, 1901–1907.

De Wilde, P. A. W. J. 1975. Influence of temperature on behaviour, energy metabolism and growth of *Macoma balthica* (L). Proceedings of the ninth European marine biology symposium, edited by H. Barnes, Aberdeen University Press, Aberdeen, pp. 239–256.

De Zwaan, A. 1972. Pyruvate kinase in muscle extracts of the sea mussel *Mytilus edulis* L. Comp. Biochem. Physiol. 42B, 7–14.

De Zwaan, A. 1977. Anaerobic energy metabolism in bivalve molluscs. Oceanogr. Mar. Biol. Ann. Rev. 15, 103–187.

De Zwaan, A. & de Bont, A. M. T. 1975. Phosphoenolpyruvate carboxykinase from adductor muscle tissue of the sea mussel *Mytilus edulis* L. J. Comp. Physiol. 96, 85–94.

De Zwaan, A. & Holwerda, D. A. 1972. The effect of phosphoenolpyruvate, fructose-1,6-diphosphate and pH on allosteric pyruvate kinase in muscle tissue of the bivalve *Mytilus edulis* L. Biochim. biophys. Acta 27b, 430–433.

De Zwaan, A., Holwerda, D. A. & Addink, A. D. F. 1975. The influence of divalent cations on allosteric behaviour of muscle pyruvate kinase from the sea mussel *Mytilus edulis*. Comp. Biochem. Physiol. 52B, 469–472.

De Zwaan, A., Kluytmans, J. H. F. M. & Zandee, D. I. 1976. Facultative anaerobiosis in molluscs. In: Biochemical adaptation to environmental change, edited by R. M. S. Smellie & J. F. Pennock, The Biochemical Society, London, pp. 133–168.

De Zwaan, A., Thompson, R. J. & Livingstone, D. R. 1980. Physiological and biochemical aspects of the valve snap and valve closure response in the giant scallop *Placopecten magellanicus*. I. Biochemistry. J. Comp. Physiol. 137, 105–114.

De Zwaan, A. & Van Marrewijk, W. J. A. 1973. Intracellular localization of pyruvate carboxylase, phosphoenol pyruvate carboxy kinase and 'malic enzyme' and the absence of glyoxylate cycle enzymes in the sea mussel (*Mytilus edulis* L.). Comp. Biochem. Physiol. 44B, 1057–1066.

De Zwaan, A. & Wijsman, T. C. M. 1976. Anaerobic metabolism in Bivalvia (Molluscs) I. Characteristics of anaerobic metabolism. Comp. Biochem. Physiol. 54B, 313–324.

Dingle, J. T. & Fell, H. B. 1969a. Lysosomes in biology and pathology, Vol. 1, Elsevier/North Holland, Amsterdam, Oxford, New York, 543 pp.

Dingle, J. F. & Fell, H. B. 1969b. Lysosomes in biology and pathology, Vol. 2, Elsevier/North Holland, Amsterdam, Oxford, New York, 668 pp.

DiSalvo, L. H., Guard, H. E. & Hunter, L. 1975. Tissue hydrocarbon burden of mussels as potential monitors of environmental hydrocarbon insult. Environ. Sci. Technol. 9, 247–251.

Dixon, D. R. 1982. Aneuploidy in mussel embryos (*Mytilus edulis*) originating from a polluted dock. Mar. Biol. Letts. 3, 155–161.

Dixon, D. R. & Clarke, K. R. 1982. Sister chromatid exchange, a sensitive method for detecting damage caused by exposure to environmental mutagens in the chromosomes of adult *Mytilus edulis*. Mar. Biol. Letts. 3, 163–172.

Drake, J. W. & Flamm, W. G. 1972. The molecular basis of mutation. In: Mutagenic effects of environmental contaminants, edited by H. E. Sutton & M. I. Harris, Academic Press, New York, London, pp. 15–26.

Dvorchik, B. H. & Woodwort, R. M. 1970. Fate of ^{14}C-2,2-bis(*p*-chlorophenyl)-1,1,1-trichloroethane (*p,p'*-DDT) in *Squalus acanthias*. Bull. Mt. Desert Isl. Mar. Lab. 9, 12–15.

Ebberink. R. H. M. & De Zwaan, A. 1980. Aspects of glycolytic control and ATP utilization in the posterior adductor muscle of the sea mussel *Mytilus edulis*. J. Comp. Physiol. 137, 165–171.

Edwards, R. R. C. 1978. Effects of water-soluble oil fractions on metabolism, growth and carbon budget of the shrimp *Crangon crangon*. Mar. Biol. 46, 259–265.

Eigener, U. 1975. Adenine nucleotide pool variations in intact *Nitrobacter winogradskyi* cells. Arch. Microbiol. 102, 233–240.

Elcombe, C. R. & Lech, J. L. 1978. Induction of monooxygenation in rainbow trout by polybrominated biphenyls: A comparative study. Environ. Health Perspect. 23, 309–314.

Elias, H., Hennig, A. & Schwartz, D. E. 1971. Stereology: Application to biomedical research. Physiol. Rev. 51, 158–200.

Elliott, J. M. & Davison, W. 1975. Energy equivalents of oxygen consumption in animal energetics. Oecologia 19, 195–201.

Elmamlouk, T. H. & Gessner, T. 1976a. Mixed function oxidases and nitroreductases in hepatopancreas of *Homarus americanus*. Comp. Biochem. Physiol. 53C, 57–62.

Elmamlouk, T. H. & Gessner, T. 1976b. Species difference in metabolism of parathion: Apparent inability of hepatopancreas fractions to produce paraoxon. Comp. Biochem. Physiol. 53C, 19–24.

Elmamlouk, T. H., Gessner, T. & Brownie, A. C. 1974. Occurrence of cytochrome P-450 in hepatopancreas of *Homarus americanus*. Comp. Biochem. Physiol. 48B, 419–425.

Elmamlouk, T. H., Philpot, R. M. & Bend, J. R. 1977. Separation of two forms of cytochrome P-450 from hepatic microsomes of 1,2,3,4-dibenzanthracene (DBA) treated little skates (*Raja erinacea*). Pharmacologist 19, 160.

Emmerson, B. K. & Emmerson, J. 1976. Protein, RNA and DNA metabolism in relation to ovarian vitellogenic growth in the flounder *Platichthys flesus* (L). Comp. Biochem. Physiol. 55B, 315–321.

Engel, D. W. & Fowler, B. A. 1979. Factors influencing the accumulation and toxicity of cadmium to marine organisms. Environ. Health Perspect. 28, 81–88.

Engel, R. H., Neat, M. J. & Hillman, R. E. 1972. Sublethal chronic effects of DDT and lindane on glycolytic and gluconeogenic enzymes of the Quahog, *Mercenaria mercenaria*. In: Marine pollution and sea life, edited by M. Ruivo, Fishing News (Books) Ltd., London, pp. 257–260.

Ericsson, J. L. E. 1969. Mechanism of cellular autophagy. In: Lysosomes in biology and pathology, Vol. 2, edited by J. T. Dingle and H. B. Fell, North Holland/American Elsevier, Amsterdam, Oxford, New York, pp. 345–394.

Evans, H. J. 1962. Chromosome aberrations induced by ionizing radiation. In: International review of cytology Vol. 13, edited by G. H. Bourne & J. F. Danielli, Academic Press, New York, London, pp. 221–321.

Evans, H. J. & O'Riordan, M. L. 1977. Human peripheral blood lymphocytes for the analysis of chromosome aberrations in mutagen tests. In: Handbook of mutagenicity test procedures, edited by B. S. Kilbey, M. Legator, W. Nichols & C. Ramel, Elsevier, Oxford, pp. 261–274.

Falkowski, P. G. 1977. The adenylate energy charge in marine phytoplankton: The effect of temperature on the physiological state of *Skeletonema costatum* (Grey) Cleve. J. exp. mar. Biol. Ecol. 27, 37–45.

Farley, C. A. 1969a. Probable neoplastic disease of the haemopoietic system in oysters, *Crassostrea virginica* and *Crassostrea gigas*. Natl. Cancer. Inst. Monogr. 31, 541–555.

Farley, C. A. 1969b. Sarcomatoid proliferative disease in a wild population of blue mussels (*Mytilus edulis*). J. natn. Cancer Inst. 43, 509–516.

Farley, C. A. & Sparks, A. K. 1970. Proliferative diseases of haemocytes, endothelial cells and connective tissue cells in molluscs. Bibl. Haemat. 36, 610–617.

Farrington, J. W. & Quinn, J. G. 1973. Petroleum hydrocarbons in Narragansett bay. l. Survey of hydrocarbons in sediments and clams. Estuar. cstl. mar. Sci. 1, 71–79.

Felbeck, H. 1980. Investigations on the role of the amino acids in anaerobic metabolism of the lugworm *Arenicola marina* L. J. Comp. Physiol. 137, 183–192.

Feng, S. Y. 1965. Pinocytosis of proteins by oyster leucocytes. Biol. Bull. 129, 95–105.

Feng, S. Y., Khairallah, E. A. & Canzonier, W. J. 1970. Hemolymph-free amino acids and related nitrogenous compounds of *Crassostrea virginica* infected with *Bucephalus* sp and *Minchinia nelsoni*. Comp. Biochem. Physiol. 34, 547–556.

Finney, C. M. 1978. Isotopic labelling of taurine: Implications for its synthesis in selected tissues of *Homarus americanus*. Comp. Biochem. Physiol. 61B, 409–413.

Fong, W. C. 1976. Uptake and retention of Kuwait Crude Oil and its effects on oxygen uptake by the Soft-Shell Clam, *Mya arenaria*. J. Fish. Res. Bd Can. 33, 2774–2780.

Fossato, V. U. & Canzonier, W. J. 1976. Hydrocarbon uptake and loss by the mussel *Mytilus edulis*. Mar. Biol. 36, 243–250.

Fossato, V. U., Nasci, C. & Dolci, F. 1979. 3,4-Benzopyrene and perylene in mussels, *Mytilus* sp., from the Laguna Veneta, North-East Italy. Mar. Environ. Res. 2, 47–53.

Foster-Smith, R. L. 1975a. The effect of concentration of suspension and inert material on the assimilation of algae by three bivalves. J. mar. biol. Ass. U.K. 55, 411–418.

Foster-Smith, R. L. 1975b. The effect of concentration of suspension on filtration rates and pseudofaecal production for *Mytilus edulis* L., *Cerastoderma edule* (L) and *Venerupis pullastra* (Montagu). J. exp. mar. Biol. Ecol. 17, 1–22.

Freeman, K. R. & Dickie, L. M. 1979. Growth and mortality of the blue mussel (*Mytilus edulis*) in relation to environmental indexing. J. Fish. Res. Bd Can., 36, 1238–1249.

Freere, R. H. 1967. Stereologic techniques in microscopy. J. Roy. Micro. Soc. 87, 25–34.

Frenster, J. H. 1962. Load tolerance as a quantitive estimate of health. Ann. Int. Med. 57, 788–794.

Friedberg, F. 1974. Effects of metal binding on protein structure. Q. Rev. Biophysics 7, 1–33.

Friedrich, A. R. & Filice, F. P. 1976. Uptake and accumulation of the nickel ion by *Mytilus edulis*. Bull. Environ. Contam. Toxicol. 16, 750–755.

Froutin, G. H. 1937. Contribution a l'étude du Tissu Conjonetif des Mollusques et Plus Particulierment des Lamellibranches et des Gasteropodes. Doctor of Science Thesis, Paris.

Fry, F. E. J. 1947. Effects of the environment on animal activity. Univ. Toronto Studies Biol. Ser. 55; Publs Ont. Fish. Res. Lab. 68, 1–62.

Fry, F. E. J. 1971. The effect of environmental factors on the physiology of fish. In: Fish physiology, edited by W. S. Hoar & D. J. Randall, Academic Press, New York, pp. 1–98.

Fuji, A. & Hashizume, M. 1974. Energy budget for a Japanese common scallop, *Patinopecten yessoensis* (Jay) in Mutsu Bay. Bull. Fac. Fish. Hokkaido Univ. 25, 7–19.

Fukami, J. I., Shishido, T. & Casida, J. E. 1969. Oxidative metabolism of rotenone in mammals, fish, and insects and its relation to selective toxicity. J. agric. Fd Chem. 17, 1217–1226.

Gabbott, P. A. 1976. Energy metabolism. In: Marine mussels: Their ecology and physiology, edited by B. L. Bayne, Cambridge University Press, Cambridge, pp. 293–355.

Gabbott, P. A. & Bayne, B. L. 1973. Biochemical effects of temperature and nutritive stress on *Mytilus edulis* L. J. mar. biol. Ass. U.K. 53, 269–286.

Gabbott, P. A., Cook. P. A. & Whittle, M.A. 1979. Seasonal changes in glycogen synthase activity in the mantle tissue of the mussel *Mytilus edulis* L.: Regulation by tissue glucose. Biochem. Soc. Trans. 7, 895–896.

Gabbott, P. A. & Head, E. J. H. 1980. Seasonal changes in the specific activities of the pentose phosphate pathway enzymes, G6PDH and

6PGDH and NAPDP-dependent isocitrate dehydrogenase in the bivalves, *Mytilus edulis, Ostrea edulis* and *Crassostrea gigas*. Comp. Biochem. Physiol. 66B, 279–284.

Gabbott, P. A. & Stephenson, R. R. 1974. A note on the relationship between the dry weight condition index and the glycogen content of adult oysters (*Ostrea edulis* L) kept in the laboratory. J. Cons. int. Explor. Mer 35, 359–361.

Gabbott, P. A. & Walker, A. J. M. 1971. Changes in the condition index and biochemical content of adult oysters (*Ostrea edulis* L.) maintained under hatchery conditions, J. Cons. int. Explor. Mer 34, 99–106.

Gabrielascu, E. 1970. The lability of lysosomes during the response of neurons to stress. Histochem. J. 2, 123–130.

Gäde, G. 1980. Biological role of octopine formation in marine molluscs. Mar. Biol. Lett. 1, 121–135.

Gahan, P. B. 1965. Reversible activation of lysosomes in rat liver. J. Histochem. Cytochem. 13, 334–338.

Gee, J. M., Maddock, L. & Davey J. T. 1977. The relationship between infestation by *Mytilicola intestinalis,* Steuer (Copepoda, Cyclopoidea) and the condition index of *Mytilus edulis* in South West England. J. Cons. int. Explor. Mer 37, 300–308.

Gee, S. J., Krieger, R. I., Lim, L. O. & Wellings, S. R. 1979. Disposition processes in mussels *Mytilus californianus*. In: Soc. Toxicol. New Orleans, Louisiana. Toxicology and applied pharmacology, Academic Press, New York, p. 61.

George, S. G., Carpene, E., Coombs, T. L., Overnell, J. & Youngson, A. 1979. Characterisation of cadmium-binding proteins from mussels, *Mytilus edulis* (L), exposed to cadmium. Biochim. biophys. Acta 580, 225–233.

George, S. G., Pirie, B. J. S. & Coombs, T. L. 1976. The kinetics of accummulation and excretion of ferric hydroxide in *Mytilus edulis* (L) and its distribution in the tissue. J. exp. mar. Biol. Ecol. 23, 71–84.

GESAMP 1980. Monitoring biological variables related to marine pollution, UNESCO, Paris, 22 pp.

Giam, C. S. 1978. Pollution effects on marine organisma, Lexington Books, D. C. Heath and Company, Lexington, Massachusetts, Toronto, 213 pp.

Gibson, J. R., Ludke, J. L. & Ferguson, D. E. 1969. Sources of error in the use of fish-brain acetylcholinesterase activity as a monitor for pollution. Bull. Environ. Contam. Toxicol. 4, 17–23.

Giesy, J. P., Duke, R., Bingham, R. & Denzer, S. 1978. Energy charges in several molluscs and crustaceans: Natural values and responses to cadmium stress. Bull. ecol. Soc. Am. 59, 66.

Gilfillan, E. S. 1975. Decrease of net flux in two species of mussels caused by extracts of crude oil. Mar. Biol. 29, 53–58.

Gilfillan, E. S., Jiang, L. C., Donovan, D., Hanson, S. & Mayo, D. W. 1976. Reduction in carbon flux in Mya arenaria caused by a spill of No. 2. fuel oil. Mar. Biol. 37, 115–123.

Gilfillan, E. S., Mayo, D. W., Page, D. S., Donovan, D. & Hanson, S. 1977. Effects of varying concentrations of petroleum hydrocarbons in sediments on carbon flux in Mya arenaria. In: Physiological responses of marine biota to pollutants, edited by F. J. Vernberg, A. Calabrese, F. P. Thurberg & W. B. Vernberg, Academic Press, New York, pp. 299–314.

Gilfillan, E. S. & Vandermeulen, J. H. 1978. Alterations in growth and physiology in chronically oiled soft-shell clams, Mya arenaria, chronically oiled with Bunker C from Chedabucto Bay, Nova Scotia, 1970–76. J. Fish. Res. Bd Can. 35, 630–636.

Gilson, W. E. 1963. Differential respirometer of simplified and improved design. Science, N.Y. 141, 531–532.

Glende, E. A. 1972. On the mechanism of carbon tetrachloride toxicity— coincidence of loss of drug-metabolizing activity with peroxidation of microsomal lipid. Biochem. Pharmac. 21, 2131–2138.

Goddard, C. K. & Martin, A. W. 1966. Carbohydrate metabolism. In: Physiology of mollusca, Vol. 2, edited by K. M. Wilbur & C. M. Yonge, Academic Press, New York, pp. 275–302.

Goldberg, E. D. 1975. The mussel watch: A first step to global marine monitoring. Mar. Poll. Bull. 6, 111.

Goldberg, E. D. 1980. Assimilative capacity of U.S. coastal waters for pollutants. National Oceanic and Atmospheric Administration, Washington, 284 pp.

Goldberg, E. D., Bowen, V. T., Farrington, J. W., Harvey, G., Martin, J. H., Parker, P. L., Risebrough, R. W., Robertson, W., Schneider, E. &

Gamble, E. 1978. The mussel watch. Environ. Conserv. 5, 101–125.

Goldman, D. E. 1970. The role of certain metals in axon excitability processes. In: Effects of metals on cells, subcellular elements and macro-molecules, edited by J. Maniloff, J. R. Coleman & M. W. Miller, Charles C Thomas, Springfield, Ill., pp. 275–282.

Gonzaleze, J. G. & Yevich, P. 1976. Responses of an estuarine population of the blue mussel *Mytilus edulis* to heated water from a steam generating plant. Mar. Biol. 34, 177–189.

Gould, E. 1979. Alteration of enzymes in winter flounder, *Pseudopleuronectes americanus*, exposed to sublethal amounts of cadmium chloride. In: Physiological responses of marine biota to pollutants, edited by F. J. Vernberg, A. Calabrese, F. P. Thurberg & W. B. Vernberg, Academic Press, New York, pp. 209–224.

Gould, E. 1980. Low-salinity stress in American lobster, *Homarus americanus* after chronic sublethal exposure to cadmium: Biochemical effects. Helgoländer wiss. Mceresunters. 33, 36–46.

Gould, E., Collier, R. S., Karolus, J. J. & Givens, S. 1976. Heart transaminase in the Rock Crab, *Cancer irroratus*, exposed to cadmium salts. Bull. Environ. Contam. Toxicol. 15, 635–643.

Gould, E. & Karolus, J. J. 1974. V. Observations on the biochemistry. In: Physiological response of the cunner *Tautogolabrus adspersus* to cadmium, NOAA Technical Report NMFS SSRF-681, U.S. Department of Commerce, Seattle, pp. 21–25.

Gray, J. S. 1979. Pollution induced changes in populations. Phil. Trans. R. Soc. Lond. B. 286, 545–556.

Gray, J. S. 1980. The measurement of the effects of pollutants on benthic communities. Rapp. P.-v. Réun. Cons. int. Explor. Mer 179, 188–193.

Gray, J. S., Boesch, D., Heip, C., Jones, A. M., Lassig, N., Vanderhorst, R. & Wolfe, D. 1980. The role of ecology in marine production monitoring. Rapp. p.-v. Réun. Cons. int. Explor. Mer 179, 237–252.

Gregory, W. D., Miller, M. W., Carstensen, E. L., Cataldo, F. L. & Reddy, M. M. 1974. Non-thermal effects of 2 MHz ultra-sound on the growth and cytology of *Vicia faba* roots. Br. J. Radiol. 47, 122–129.

Griffiths, C. L. & King, J. A. 1979. Energy expended on growth and gonad output in the ribbed mussel *Aulacomya ater*. Mar. Biol. 53, 217–222.

Grimäs, U. 1979. The biotest basis of the Fossmark nuclear power plant, Sweden. An experiment on the ecosystem level. In: Methodology for assessing imports of radioactivity on aquatic ecosystems, Technical Reports Series No. 190, IAEA, Vienna, pp. 217–226.

Gruger, E. H., Robisch, P. A. & Wekell, M. M. 1977. Effects of chlorinated biphenyls and petroleum hydrocarbons on the activity of hepatic aryl hydrocarbon hydroxylase of coho salmon (*Oncorhynus kisutch*) and chinook salmon (*O. tshawytscha*). In: Fate and effects of petroleum hydrocarbons in marine organisms and ecosystems, edited by D. A. Wolfe, Pergamon, New York, pp. 323–331.

Guarino, A. M., Janicki, R. H. & Kinter, W. B. 1971. Distribution and metabolism of ^{14}C-DDT in eel (*Anguilla rostrata*) after 6 hrs uptake from ambient water. Bull. Mt. Desert Isl. Mar. Lab. 10, 23–24.

Guillaume, J. R., Carles, D., Leveau, M., Bertrand J. C. & Gilewicz, M. 1984. Induction of cytochrome P-450 by hydrocarbons in a mollusc bivalve: *Mytilus galloprovincialis*. In: Proceedings of the 5th Congress of the European Society for Comparative Physiology and Biochemistry, Springer-Verlag, Berlin (in press).

Hammen, C. S. 1975. Succinate and lactate oxidoreductases of bivalve molluscs. Comp. Biochem. Physiol. 50B, 407–412.

Haukioja, E. & Hakala, T. 1979. Asymptotic equations in growth studies—An analysis based on *Anodonta piscinalis* (Mollusca, Unionidae). Ann. Zool. Fennici. 16, 115–122.

Hardonk, M. J. & Koudstaal, J. 1976. Enzyme histochemistry as a link between biochemistry and morphology. Prog. Histochem. Cytochem. 8, 1–68.

Harrison, F. L. & Jones, I. M. 1982. An *in vivo* sister chromatid exchange assay in the larvae of the mussel *Mytilus edulis*: Response to 3 mutagens. Mutation Res. 105, 235–242.

Haskin, H. H. 1954. Age determination in molluscs. Trans. N.Y. Acad. Sci. (Ser. III). 16, 300–304.

Hayes, W. J. 1975. Toxicology of pesticides, Williams & Wilkins, Baltimore, 580 pp.

Hazel, J. R. & Prosser, C. L. 1974. Molecular mechanisms of temperature compensation in poikilotherms. Physiol. Rev. 54, 620–627.

Heip, C. 1980. Meiobenthos as a tool in the assessment of marine environmental quality. Rapp. P.-v. Réun. Cons. int. Explor. Mer 179, 182–187.

Heitz, J. R., Lewis, L., Chambers, J. & Yarbrough, J. D. 1974. The acute effects of empire mix crude oil on enzymes in oysters, shrimp and mullet. In: Pollution and physiology of marine organisms, edited by F. J. Vernberg & W. B. Vernberg, Academic Press, New York, pp. 311–328.

Helm, M. M., Holland, D. L. & Stephenson, R. R. 1973. The effect of supplementary algal feeding of a hatchery breeding stock of Ostrea edulis L. on larval vigour. J. mar. biol. Ass. U.K. 53, 673–684.

Henderson, B. 1979. Quantitative dehydrogenase cytochemistry in the study of cellular metabolism with special reference to rheumatoid arthritis. In: Quantitative cytochemistry and its applications, edited by J. R. Pattison, L. Bitensky & J. Chayen, Academic Press, New York, pp. 83–98.

Herbert, D. W. M. 1952. Measurement of the toxicity of substances to fish. J. Inst. Sew. Purif. 1, 60–68.

Hess, B. & Brand, K. 1974. Cell and Tissue Disintegration. In: Methods of enzymatic analysis, Vol. 1, edited by H. U. Bergmeyer, Academic Press, New York, pp. 396–413.

Hildreth, D. I. & Crisp, D. J. 1976. A corrected formula for calculation of filtration rate of bivalve molluscs in an experimental flowing system. J. mar. biol. Ass. U.K. 56, 111–120.

Hodgson, E. 1976. Comparative toxicology: Cytochrome P-450 and mixed function oxidase activity in target and non-target organisms. Essays Toxicol. 7, 73–97.

Holland, D. L. 1978. Lipid reserves and energy metabolism in the larvae of benthic marine invertebrates. In: Biochemical and biophysical perspectives in marine biology, edited by D. C. Malins & J. R. Sargent, Academic Press, London, pp. 85–123.

Holland, H. T., Coppage, D. L. & Butler, P. A. 1967. Use of fish brain acetylcholinesterase to monitor pollution by organophosphorous pesticides. Bull. Environ. Contam. Toxicol. 2, 156–162.

Holtzman, E. 1969. Lysosomes in the physiology and pathology of neurons. In: Lysosomes in biology and pathology, Vol. 1, edited by J. T. Dingle

& H. B. Fell, North Holland/American Elsevier, Amsterdam, New York, pp. 192–216.

Holwerda, D. A. & De Zwaan, A. 1973. Kinetic and molecular characteristics of allosteric pyruvate kinase from muscle tissue of the sea mussel *Mytilus edulis* L. Biochim. biophys. Acta 309, 296–306.

Hook, E. B. 1982. Contribution of chromosome abnormalities to human morbidity and mortality. Cytogent. Cell Genet. 33, 101–106.

Hori, S. H. & Takahashi, T. 1974. Phenobarbital-induced increase of hexose-6-phosphate dehydrogenase activity. Biochem. biophys. Res. Commun. 61, 1064–1070.

Hughs, G. M. & Perry, S. F. 1976. Morphometric study of trout gills: A light microscope method suitable for the evaluation of pollutant action. J. exp. Biol. 64, 447–460.

Hutson, D. H. 1976. Gluthathione conjugates. In: Bound and conjugated pesticide residues, edited by R. F. Gould, American Chemical Society, Washington, D.C., pp. 103–131.

IAEA. 1979. Methodology for assessing impacts of radioactivity on aquatic ecosystems. Technical Reports Series No. 190. IAEA, Vienna, 416 pp.

I.C.E.S. 1978. On the feasibility of effects monitoring. Coop. Res. Rep. 75, International Council for the Exploration of the Sea, Charlottenlund, Denmark, 42 pp.

Imai, Y. & Sato, R. 1966. Substrate interaction with hydroxylase system in liver microsomes. Biochem. biophys. Res. Commun. 22, 620–626.

Irons, R. D. & Smith, J. C. 1976. Prevention by copper of cadmium sequestration by metallothionein in liver. Chem. Biol. Interactions. 15, 289–294.

Irving, H. & Williams, R. J. P. 1953. The stability of transition-metal complexes. J. Chem. Soc. 1953, 3192–3210.

Ivanovici, A. M. 1977. Adenylate energy charge and physiological stress in the estuarine gastropod, *Pyrazinus ebeninus*. Ph.D. thesis, University of Sidney, Australia, 225 pp.

Ivanovici, A. M. 1980a. Adenylate energy charge: An evaluation of applicability to assessment of pollution effects and directions for future research. Rapp. P.-v. Réun. Cons. int. Explor. Mer 179, 23–28.

Ivanovici, A. M. 1980b. The adenylate energy charge in the estuarine mollusc, *Pyrazinus ebeninus*. Laboratory studies of responses to salinity and temperature. Comp. Biochem. Physiol. 66A, 43–55.

Ivanovici, A. M. & Wiebe, W. J. 1981. Towards a working definition of 'Stress': A review and critique. In: Stress effects on natural ecosystems, edited by G. W. Barrett & R. Rosenberg, Wiley-Interscience, New York, pp. 13–27.

Ivlev, V. S. 1934. Eine Mikromethode zur bestimming des Kaloriengehalts von Nahrstoffen. Biochem. Z. 275, 49–55.

Ivlev, V. S. 1961. Experimental ecology of the feeding of fishes. Yale University Press, New Haven, 302 pp.

Jackim, E. 1973. Influence of lead and other metals on fish δ-aminolevulinate dehydrase activity. J. Fish. Res. Bd Can. 30, 560–562.

Jackim, E. 1974. Enzyme responses to metals in fish. In: Pollution and physiology of marine organisms, edited by F. J. Vernberg & W. B. Vernberg, Academic Press, New York, pp. 59–65.

Jackim, E., Hamlin, J. M. & Sonis, S. 1970. Effects of metal poisoning on five liver enzymes in the Killifish *(Fundulus heteroclitus)*. J. Fish. Res. Bd Can. 27, 383–390.

Jakoby, W. B. 1978. The glutathione S-transferases: A group of multifunctional detoxification proteins. In: Advances in enzymology, 46, edited by A. Meister, Wiley, New York, pp. 383–415.

Jakubowski, M., Piotowski, J. & Trojanowska, B. 1970. Binding of mercury in the rat: Studies using $^{203}HgCl_2$ and gel filtration. Toxic. appl. Pharmac. 16, 743–752.

James, M. O., Fouts, J. R. & Bend, J. R. 1977. Xenobiotic metabolizing enzymes in marine fish. In: Pesticides in the aquatic environment, edited by M. A. Khan, Plenum Press, New York, pp. 171–189.

James, M. O., Khan, M. A. Q. & Bend, J. R. 1979. Hepatic microsomal mixed-function oxidase activities in several marine species common to coastal Florida. Comp. Biochem. Physiol. 63C, 155–164.

Janicki, R. H. & Kinter, W. B. 1971. DDT: Disrupted osmoregulatory events in the intestine of the eel *Anguilla rostrata* adapted to seawater. Science, N.Y. 173, 1146–1147.

Jaworek, D., Gruber, W. & Bergmeyer, H. U. 1974. Adenosine-5'triphosphate: Determination with 3-phosphoglycerate kinase. In: Methods of enzymatic analysis, Vol. 4, edited by H. U. Bergmeyer, Academic Press, New York, pp. 2097–2101.

Jeffries, H. P. 1972. A stress syndrome in the hard clam, *Mercenaria mercenaria*. J. Invertebr. Pathol. 20, 242–287.

Jenkins, K. D., Brown, D. A., Perkins, E. M., Oshida, P. S., Palacio, J.-L.Y., Jennema, E. M. & Alfafara, J. F. 1983. Cytosolic metal distribution and histopathology of urchins and mussels from the Southern California Bight (in press).

Jennings, J. R., Rainbow, P. S. & Scott, A. G. 1979. Studies on the uptake of cadmium by the crab *Carcinus maenas* in the laboratory. II. Preliminary investigation of cadmium-binding proteins. Mar. Biol. 50, 141–149.

Jerina, D. M. & Daly, J. W. 1974. Arene oxides: A new aspect of drug metabolism. Science, N.Y. 185, 573–582.

John, B. & Lewis, K. R. 1968. The chromosome complement. Springer-Verlag, Vienna, 206 pp.

Johnson, F. G. 1977. Sublethal biological effects of petroleum hydrocarbon exposures: Bacteria, algae and invertebrates. In: Effects of petroleum on arctic and subarctic marine environments and organisms, Vol. II. Biological effects, edited by D. C. Malins, Academic Press, New York, pp. 271–318.

Johnston, R. E., Schnell, R. C. & Miga, T. S. 1974. Cadmium potentiation of drug response: Lack of change in brain sensitivity. Toxic. appl. Pharmac. 30, 90–95.

Jorgensen, C. B. 1975. On gill function in the mussel, *Mytilus edulis* L. Ophelia 13, 187–232.

Kägi, J. H. R. & Vallee, B. L. 1960. Metallothionein: A cadmium and zinc containing protein from equine renal cortex. J. biol. Chem. 235, 3460–3465.

Kägi, J. H. R. & Vallee, B. L. 1961. Metallothionein: A cadmium and zinc containing protein from equine renal cortex. II. Physicochemical properties. J. biol. Chem. 236, 2435–2442.

Kaufman, I. A., Hall, N. F., Deluca, M. A., Ingwall, J. S. & Mayer, S. E. 1977. Metabolism of adenine nucleotides in the cultured fetal mouse heart. Am. J. Physiol. 233, H282–H288.

Kaw, J. L., Beck, E. G. & Bruck, J. 1975. Studies of quartz cytotoxicity on peritoneal macrophages of guinea pigs pretreated with polyvinyl pyridine N-oxide. Environ. Res. 9, 313–320.

Keizer, P. D., Gordan, D. C. Jr. & Dale, J. 1977. Hydrocarbons in Eastern Canadian marine waters determined by fluorescence spectroscopy and gas-liquid chromatography. J. Fish. Res. Bd Can. 34, 347–353.

Kennish, M. J. 1980. Shell microgrowth analysis. In: Skeletal growth of aquatic organisms, edited by D. C. Rhoads & R. D. Lutz, Plenum Press, New York, pp. 255–294.

Khan, M. A. Q. 1970. Genetic and biochemical characteristics of cyclodiene epoxidase in the housefly. Biochem. Pharmac. 19, 903–910.

Khan, M. A. Q., Chang, J. L., Sutherland, D. J., Rosen, J. D. & Kamal, A. 1970. Housefly microsomal oxidation of some foreign compounds. J. econ. Ent. 63, 1807–1813.

Khan, M. A. Q., Coello, W., Khan, A. A. & Pinto, H. 1972a. Some characteristics of the microsomal mixed function oxidase in the freshwater crayfish, Cambarus. Life Sci. 2, 405–415.

Khan, M. A. Q., Kamal, A., Wolin, R. J. & Runnels, J. 1972b. In vivo and in vitro epoxidation of aldrin by aquatic food chain organisms. Bull. Environ. Contam. Toxicol. 8, 219–228.

Khan, M. A. Q., Stanton, R. H. & Reddy, G. 1974. Detoxification of foreign chemicals by invertebrates. In: Survival in toxic environments, edited by M. A. Q. Khan & J. P. Bederka, Academic Press, New York, pp. 177–201.

Kihlman, B. A. 1966. Actions of chemicals on dividing cells. Prentice-Hall, Englewood Cliffs, N.J., 260 pp.

Kihlman, B. A. 1977. Root tips of Vicia faba for the study of the induction of chromosomal aberrations. In: Handbook of mutogenicity test procedures, edited by B. J. Kilby, M. Legator, W. Nichols & C. Ramel, Elsevier, Amsterdam, New York, Oxford, pp. 389–400.

Kimura, K., Endou, H., Sudo, J. & Saki, F. 1979. Glucose dehydrogenase (hexose-6-phosphate dehydrogenase) and the microsomal electron transport system. J. Biochem., Tokyo 85, 319–326.

King, P. J. 1977. An assessment of the potential carcinogenic hazard of petroleum hydrocarbons in the marine environment. In: Petroleum hydrocarbons in the marine environment, edited by A. D. McIntyre &

K. J. Whittle, Rapp. P.-v, Réun. Cons. int. Explor. Mer 171, pp. 202–211.

Kinne, O. 1964. The effects of temperature and salinity on marine and brackish-water animals. I. Temperature. Oceanogr. Mar. Biol. Ann. Rev. 1, 301–340.

Kinoshita, N. & Gelboin, H. V. 1978. β-Glucuronidase catalysed hydrolysis of benzo(a)pyrene-3-glucuronide and binding to DNA. Science, N.Y. 199, 307–309.

Kinter, W. B., Merkens, L. S., Janicki, R. H. & Guarino, A. M. 1972. Studies on the mechanism of toxicity of DDT and polychlorinated biphenyls (PCBs): Disruption of osmoregulation in marine fish. Environ. Hlth. Perspec. 1, 169–173.

Kiorboe, T. & Møhlenberg, F. 1981. Particle selection in suspension-feeding bivalves. Mar. Ecol. Prog. Ser. 5, 291–296.

Kiorboe, T., Møhlenberg, F. & Nohr, O. 1980. Feeding, particle selection and carbon absorption in *Mytilus edulis* in different mixtures of algae and resuspended bottom materials. Ophelia 19, 193–205.

Kligerman, A. D. 1979. Cytogenetic methods for the detection of radiation-induced chromosome damage in aquatic organisms. In: Methodology for assessing impacts of radioactivity on aquatic ecosystems. Technical Reports Series No. 190. IAEA, Vienna, pp. 349–367.

Knight-Jones, E. W. 1951. Gregariousness and some other aspects of the setting behaviour of *Spirorbis*. J. mar. biol. Ass. U.K. 30, 201–222.

Knowles, C. J. 1977. Microbial metabolic regulation by adenine nucleotide pool. In: Microbial energetics, edited by B. A. Haddock & W. A. Hamilton, Cambridge University Press, London, pp. 241–283.

Kobayashi, N. 1971. Fertilised sea urchin eggs as an indicatory material for marine pollution bioassay, preliminary experiments. Publs. Seto mar. biol. Lab. 18, 379–406.

Kobayashi, N., Nogami, H. & Doi, K. 1972. Marine pollution bioassay by using sea urchin eggs in the inland sea of Japan (the Seto-Naikai). Publs Seto mar. biol. Lab. 19, 359–381.

Koenig, H. 1963. Intravital staining of lysosomes by basic dyes and metallic ions. J. Histochem. Cytochem. 11, 120–121.

Kohli, K. K., Siddiqui, F. A. & Venkitasubramanian, T. A. 1977. Effect of dieldrin on the stability of lysosomes in the rat liver. Bull. Environ. Contam. Toxicol. 18, 617–623.

Kojima, Y. & Kägi, J. H. R. 1978. Metallothionein. Trends biochem. Sci. 3, 90–92.

Koudstaal, J. & Hardonk, M. J. 1969. Histochemical demonstration of enzymes related to NADPH-dependant hydroxylating systems in rat liver after phenobarbital treatment. Histochemie 23, 68–77.

Koudstaal, J. & Hardonk, M. J. 1972. Relations between biochemically determined hydroxylations and some enzyme-histochemical reactions in rat liver after phenobarbital and methylcholanthrene treatment. Acta histochem. (Suppl). 12, 279–282.

Krebs, C. T. 1973. Unpublished observations after the West Falmouth oil spill. St. Marys College, St. Marys City, Maryland.

Krieger, R. I., Gee, S. J., Lim, L. O., Ross, J. H. & Wilson, A. 1979. Disposition of toxic substances in mussels (Mytilus californianus): Preliminary metabolic and histologic studies. In: Pesticide and xenobiotic metabolism in aquatic organisms, edited by M. A. Q. Khan., J. J. Lech & J. J. Menn, American Chemical Society, Washington, D.C., pp. 259–277.

Kurelec, B., Britvic, S., Rijavec, M., Müller, W. E. G. & Zahn, R. K. 1977. Benzo(a)pyrene monooxygenase induction in marine fish—Molecular response to oil pollution. Mar. Biol. 44, 211–216.

Kurelec, B., Matijasevic, Z., Rijavec, M., Alacevic, M., Britvic, S., Müller, W. E. G. & Zahn, R. K. 1979. Induction of benzo(a)pyrene monooxygenase in fish and the Salmonella Test as a tool for detecting mutagenic/carcinogenic xenobiotics in the aquatic environment. Bull. Environ. Contam. Toxicol. 21, 799–807.

Kurtz, D. A. 1977. Adsorption of PCB's and DDT's on membrane filters—A new analysis method. Bull. Environ. Contam. Toxicol. 17, 391–398.

La Cour, L. F. 1941. Acetic-orcein. Stain Technol. 16, 169–174.

Lammens, J. J. 1967. Growth and reproduction of a tidal flat population of Macoma balthica (L). Neth. J. Sea Res. 3, 315–382.

Lamprecht, W. & Trautschold, I. 1974. Adenosine-5′-triphosphate: Determination with hexokinase and glucose-6-phosphate dehydrogenase. In: Methods of enzymatic analysis, Vol. 4, edited by H. U. Bergmeyer, Academic Press, New York, pp. 2101–2110.

Lane, C. E. & Scura, E. D. 1970. Effects of dieldrin on glutamic oxaloacetic transaminase in *Poecilia latipinna.* J. Fish. Res. Bd Can. 27, 1869–1871.

Lange, R. 1972. Some recent work on osmotic, ionic and volume regulation in marine animals. Oceanogr. mar. Biol. A. Rev. 10, 97–135.

Langston, W. J. 1978. Accumulation of polychlorinated biphenyls in the cockle *Cerastoderma edule* and the Tellin *Macoma balthica.* Mar. Biol. 45, 265–272.

Langton, R. W. 1975. Synchrony in the digestive diverticula of *Mytilus edulis.* J. mar. biol. Ass. U.K. 55, 221–229.

Langton, R. W. & Gabbot, P. A. 1974. The tidal rhythm of extracellular digestion and the response to feeding in *Ostrea edulis.* Mar. Biol. 24, 181–197.

Law, R. J. 1978. Petroleum hydrocarbon analyses conducted following the wreck of the supertanker *Amoco Cadiz.* Mar. Poll. Bull. 9, 293–296.

Lawton, J. H. & Richards, J. 1970. Comparability of Cartesian diver, Gilson, Warburg and Winkler methods of measuring the respiratory rates of aquatic invertebrates in ecological studies. Oecologia 4, 319–324.

Leber, A. P. 1974. A mechanism for cadmium- and zinc-induced tolerance to cadmium toxicity: Involvement of metallothionein. Ph.D. diss. Purdue University, University Microfilms, Ann Arbor, Michigan, 72 pp.

Lee, R. F. 1975. Fate of petroleum hydrocarbons in marine zooplankton. In: Conference on prevention and control of oil spills, American Petroleum Institute, Washington, D.C., pp. 549–553.

Lee, R. F. 1981. Mixed function oxygenases (MFO) in marine invertebrates. Mar. Biol. Lett. 2, 87–105.

Lee, R. F., Davies, J. M., Freeman, H. C., Ivanovici, A., Moore, M. N., Stegeman, J. & Uthe, J. F. 1980. Biochemical techniques for monitoring biological effects of pollution in the sea. Rapp. P.-v, Réun. Cons. int. Explor. Mer 179, 48–55.

Lee, R. F., Furlong, E. & Singer, S. 1977. Metabolism of hydrocarbons in marine invertebrates: Aryl hydrocarbon hydroxylase from the tissues of the Blue Crab, *Callinectes sapidus* and the polychaete worm, *Nereis* sp. In: Pollutant effects on marine organisms, edited by C. S. Giam, Lexington Books, D. C. Heath and Company, Lexington, Massachusetts, Toronto, pp. 111–124.

Lee, R. F., Ryan, C. & Neuhauser, M. L. 1976. Fate of petroleum hydrocarbons taken up from food and water by the blue crab, *Callinectes sapidus*. Mar. Biol. 37, 363–370.

Lee, R. F., Sauerheber, R. & Benson, A. A. 1972a. Petroleum hydrocarbons: Uptake and discharge by the marine mussel *Mytilus edulis*. Science, N.Y. 177, 344–346.

Lee, R. F., Sauerheber, R. & Dobbs, G. H. 1972b. Uptake, metabolism and discharge of polycyclic aromatic hydrocarbons by marine fish. Mar. Biol. 17, 201–208.

Lee, R. F. & Singer, S. C. 1980. Detoxifying enzymes system in marine polychaetes: Increases in activity after exposure to aromatic hydrocarbons. Rapp. P.-v. Réun. Cons. int. Explor. Mer 179, 29–32.

Lee, R. F., Singer, S. C. & Page, D. S. 1981. Responses of cytochrome P-450 systems in marine crab and polychaetes to organic pollutants. Aquat. Toxicol. 1, 355–365.

Lehninger, A. L. 1975. Biochemistry. Worth Publishers, New York, 1104 pp.

Léonard, A. 1977. Tests for heritable translocations in male mammals. In: Handbook of mutagenicity test procedures, edited by B. J. Kilberg, M. Legator, W. Nichols & C. Ramel, Elsevier, Oxford, pp. 293–299.

Levan, A., Fredga, K. & Sandberg, A. V. 1964. Nomenclature for centromeric position on chromosomes. Hereditas 52, 201–220.

Levinton, J. S. & Koehn, R. K. 1976. Population genetics. In: Marine mussels: Their ecology and physiology, edited by B. L. Bayne, Cambridge University Press, Cambridge, pp. 357–384.

Lindner, E. & Beyhl, F. E. 1978. Induction of microsomal drug-metabolising enzymes caused by hexobarbital. Experientia 34, 226–227.

Livingstone, D. R. 1975. A comparison of the kinetic properties of pyruvate kinase in three populations of *Mytilus edulis* L. from different environments. In: Proc. 9th Europ. mar. biol. Symp., edited by H. Barnes, Aberdeen University Press, Aberdeen, pp. 151–164.

Livingstone, D. R. 1976. Some kinetic and regulatory propeties of the cytoplasmic L-malate dehydrogenases from the posterior adductor muscle and mantle tissues of the common mussel *Mytilus edulis*. Biochem. Soc. Trans. 4, 447–451.

Livingstone, D. R. 1980. Enzymic aspects of the seasonal control of metabolism in the common mussel *Mytilus edulis* L. and in marine invertebrates in general. In: Control processes, edited by K. A. Munday, University of Southampton, Southampton, pp. 41–42.

Livingstone, D. R. 1981. Induction of enzymes as a mechanism for the seasonal control of metabolism in marine invertebrates: Glucose-6-phosphate dehydrogenases from the mantle and hepatopancreas of the common mussel *Mytilus edulis* L. Comp. Biochem. Physiol. 69B, 147–156.

Livingstone, D. R. & Bayne, B. L. 1974. Pyruvate kinase from the mantle tissue of *Mytilus edulis* L. Comp. Biochem. Physiol. 48B, 481–497.

Livingstone, D. R. & Bayne, B. L. 1977. Responses of *Mytilus edulis* to low oxygen tension: Anaerobic metabolism of the posterior adductor muscle and mantle tissues. J. Comp. Physiol. 114, 143–155.

Livingstone, D. R. & Farrar, S. V. 1984. Tissue and subcellular distribution of enzyme activities of mixed-function oxygenase and benzo(a)pyrene metabolism in the common mussel *Mytilus edulis* L. Sci. Tot. Environ. (in press).

Livingstone, D. R., Widdows, J. & Fieth, P. 1979. Aspects of nitrogen metabolism of the common mussel *Mytilus edulis*: Adaptation to abrupt and fluctuating changes in salinity. Mar. Biol. 53, 41–55.

Löhr, G. W. & Waller, H. D. 1974. Glucose-6-phosphate dehydrogenase. In: Methods of enzymatic analysis Vol. 2, edited by H. U. Bergmeyer, Academic Press, New York, pp. 636–643.

Longwell, A. C. 1976. Chromosome mutagenesis in developing mackerel eggs sampled from the New York Bight. NOAA Technical Memorandum ERC MESA-7, 1–61.

Loomis, W. F. 1953. The cultivation of *Hydra* under controlled conditions. Science, N.Y. 117, 565–566.

Loomis, W. F. 1954. Environmental factors controlling growth in *Hydra*. J. exp. Zool. 126, 223–234.

Lowe, D. M. & Moore, M. N. 1978. Cytology and quantitative cytochemistry of a proliferative atypical hemocytic condition in *Mytilus edulis*. (Bivalvia, Mollusca). J. natn. Cancer. Inst. 60, 1455–1459.

Lowe, D. M. & Moore, M. N. 1979. The cytochemical distribution of zinc (ZnII) and iron (FeIII) in the common mussel, *Mytilus edulis*, and their relationship with lysosomes. J. mar. biol. Ass. U.K. 59, 851–858.

Lowe, D. M., Moore, M. N. & Bayne, B. L. 1982. Aspects of gametogenesis in the marine mussel *Mytilus edulis*. J. mar. biol. Ass. U.K. 62, 133–145.

Lowe, D. M., Moore, M. N. & Clarke, K. R. 1981. Effects of oil on digestive cells in mussels: Quantitative alterations in cellular and lysosomal structure. Aquat. Toxicol. 1, 213–226.

Lowry, O. H., Rosebrough, N. J., Farr, A. L. & Randall, R. J. 1951. Protein measurement with the folin phenol reagent. J. biol. Chem. 193, 265–275.

Lubet, P. 1957. Cycle sexuel de *Mytilus edulis* L. et de *Mytilus galloprovincialis* Lmk. dans le Bassin d'Arcachon (Gironde). Année biologique 33, 19–29.

Lubet, P. 1959. Recherches sur le cycle sexuel et l'emission des gametes chez les Mytilidês les Pectinidés. Revue des travaux Inst des pechês maritimes 23, 396–545.

Ludke, J. L., Gibson, J. R. & Lusk, G. I. 1972. Mixed function oxidase activity in freshwater fish: Aldrin epoxidation and parathion activation. Toxic. appl. Pharmac. 21, 89–97.

Luoma, S. N., 1977. Detection of trace contaminant effects in aquatic ecosystems. J. Fish. Res. Bd Can. 34, 436–439.

Lutz, R. D. & Rhoads, D. C. 1980. Growth patterns within the molluscan shell: An overview. In: Skeletal growth of aquatic organisms, edited by D. C. Rhoads & R. A. Lutz, Plenum Press, New York, pp. 203–254.

McGinnis, A. J. & Kasting, R. 1964. Chromic oxide indicator method for measuring food utilization in a plant feeding insect. Science 144, 1464–1465.

MacInnes, J. R., Thurberg, F. P., Greig, R. A. & Gould, E. 1977. Long-term cadmium stress in the cunner, *Tautogolabrus adspersus*. Fishery Bull. Fish Wildl. Serv. U.S. 75, 199–203.

McIntyre, A. D., Bayne, B. L., Rosenthal, N. & White, I. C. 1978. On the feasibility of effects monitoring. Cooperative Research Report No. 75. International Council for the Exploration of the Sea, Charlottenlund, 42 pp.

McIntyre, A. D. & Pearce, J. B. 1980. Biological effects of marine pollution and the problems of monitoring. Rapp. P.-v. Réun. cons. int. Explor. Mer. 179, 340–346.

Mackie, P. R., Hardy, R., Butler, E. I., Holligan, P. M. & Spooner, M. F. 1978. Early samples of oil in water and some analyses of zooplankton. Mar. Poll. Bull. 9, 294–297.

Mackie, P. R., Hardy, R. & Whittle, K. J. 1978. Preliminary assessment of the presence of oil in the ecosystem at Ekofisk after the blowout, April 22–30. J. Fish. Res. Bd Can. 35, 544–551.

McKim, J. M., Christensen, G. M. & Hunt, E. P. 1970. Changes in the blood of brook trout (*Salvelinus fontinalis*) after short-term and long-term exposure to copper. J. Fish. Res. Bd Can. 27, 1883–1889.

Maclean, F. I., Lucis, O. J., Shakh, Z. A. & Jansz, E. E. R. 1972. The uptake and subcellular distribution of Cd and Zn in micro-organisms. Proc. Fedn. Am. Socs. exp. Biol. 31, 699.

Magee, P. N. 1977. The relationship between mutagenesis, carcinogenesis and teretogenesis. In: Progess in genetic toxicology, edited by D. Scott, B. A. Bridges & F. H. Sobels, Elsevier/North Holland, Amsterdam, pp. 15–27.

Mailman, R. B. & Hodgson, E. 1972. The cytochrome P-450 substrate optical difference spectra of pesticides with mouse hepatic microsomes. Bull. Environ. Contam. Toxicol. 8, 186–192.

Makino, S. & Nishimura, I. 1952. Water-pretreatment squash technic. A new and simple practical method for the chromosome study of animals. Stain Technol. 27, 1–7.

Mantoura, R. F. C., Dickson, A. & Riley, J. P. 1978. The complexation of metals with humic materials in natural waters. Estuar. cstl. mar. Sci. 6, 387–408.

Marafante, E. 1976. Binding of mercury and zinc to cadmium-binding protein in liver and kidney of goldfish (*Carassius auratus L*). Experientia 32, 149–150.

Margoshes, M. & Vallee, B. L. 1957. A cadmium protein from equine kidney cortex. J. Am. chem. Soc. 79, 4813–4814.

Matsubura, T., Koike, M., Touchi, A., Tochino, Y. & Sugeno. K. 1976. Quantitative determination of cytochrome P-450 in rat liver homogenate. Analyt. Biochem. 75, 596–603.

Matthay, R. A., Baker, D. A., Putman, C. E., Gee, J. B. L., Smith, G. J. W. & Greenspan, R. H. 1977. Tantalum oxide and silica particles—Effects on alveolar macrophage viability and lysosomal enzyme release. Invest. Radiol. 12, 411.

Mawdesley-Thomas, L. E. 1974. Diseases of fish. MSS Information Corporation, New York, 277 pp.

Mayzaud, P. 1973. Respiration and nitrogen excretion of zooplankton. II. Studies of the metabolic characteristics of starved animals. Mar. Biol. 21, 19–28.

Mearns, A. J. & Sherwood, M. J. 1976. Ocean wastewater discharge and tumours in a southern Californian flatfish. Prog. Exp. Tumour. Res. 20, 75–85.

Meister, A. 1975. Biochemistry of glutathione. In: Metabolic pathways. Metabolism of sulphur compounds, edited by M. Greenberg, Academic Press, New York, pp. 102–188.

Mesarovic, M. D., Macko, D. & Takahara, Y. 1970. Theory of hierarchical, multilevel systems. Academic Press, New York, 321 pp.

Miovic, M. L. & Gibson, J. 1973. Nucleotide pools and adenylate energy charge in balanced and unbalanced growth of *Chromatium*. J. Bact. 114, 86–95.

Mitton, J. & Koehn, R. C. 1975. A marine fish affected by reactor effluent. Genetics 79, 97–111.

Mix, M. C. 1972. Chronic tissue degeneration in the Pacific oyster, *Crassostrea gigas*, following acute γ-irradiation. Rad. Res. 49, 176–189.

Mix, M. C. 1975. Proliferative characteristics of atypical cells in native oysters (*Ostrea lurida*) from Yaquina Bay, Oregon. J. invertebr. Pathol. 26, 289–298.

Mix, M. C. 1976. A review of the histopathological effects of ionizing radiation on the Pacific oyster, *Crassostrea gigas*. Mar. Fish. Fev. 38, 12–15.

Mix, M. C., Hawkes, J. C. & Sparks, A. K. 1979. Observations on the ultrastructure of large cells associated with putative neoplastic disorders of mussels, *Mytilus edulis*, from Yaquina Bay, Oregon. J. Invertebr. Pathol. 34, 41–56.

Mix, M. C., Schaffer, R. L. & Hemingway, S. J. 1981. Polynuclear aromatic hydrocarbons in Bay mussels (*Mytilus edulis*) from Oregon. In: Phyletic approaches to cancer, edited by C. J. Dawe, J. C. Harshbarger., S.

Kondo., T. Sugimura & S. Takayama. Japan Scientific Press, Tokyo, pp. 167–177.

Mix, M. C. & Sparks, A. K. 1970. Studies on the histopathological effects of ionizing radiation on the oyster, *Crassostrea gigas*. J. Invertebr. Pathol. 16, 14–37.

Mix, M. C. & Sparks, A. K. 1971a. Repair of digestive tubule tissue of the Pacific oyster *Crassostrea gigas* damaged by ionizing radiation. J. Invertebr. Pathol. 17, 172–177.

Mix, M. C. & Sparks, A. K. 1971b. The histopathological effects of various doses of ionizing radiation on the gonad of the oyster, *Crassostrea gigas*. Proc. Nat. Shellfish Soc. 61, 64–70.

Møhlenberg, F. & Riisgard, H. U. 1978. Efficiency of particle retention in 13 species of suspension feeding bivalves. Ophelia 17, 239–246.

Møhlenberg, F. & Riisgard, H. U. 1979. Filtration rate, using a new indirect technique, in thirteen species of suspension-feeding bivalves. Mar. Biol. 54, 143–147.

Montague, M. D. & Dawes, E. A. 1974. The survival of *Peptococcus prevotii* in relation to the adenylate energy charge. J. gen. Microbiol. 80, 291–299.

Moore, M. N. 1976. Cytochemical demonstration of latency of lysosomal hydrolases in digestive cells of the common mussel, *Mytilus edulis*, and changes induced by thermal stress. Cell Tissue Res. 175, 279–287.

Moore, M. N. 1977. Lysosomal responses to environmental chemicals in some marine invertebrates. In: Pollutant effects on marine organisms, edited by C. S. Giam, Lexington Books, D. C. Heath and Company, Lexington, Massachusetts, Toronto, pp. 143–154.

Moore, M. N. 1979. Cellular responses to polycyclic aromatic hydrocarbons and phenobarbital in *Mytilus edulis*. Mar. Environ. Res. 2, 255–263.

Moore, M. N. 1980a. Cytochemical determination of cellular responses to environmental stressors in marine organisms. Rapp. P-v, Réun. Cons. int. Explor. Mer 170, 7–15.

Moore, M. N. 1980b. A quantitative cytochemical investigation of alterations in the latency of lysosomal arylsulphatase in the marine mussel, *Mytilus edulis*, induced by copper, steroids and salinity changes. In: Abstracts of the VIth international histochemistry and cytochemistry congress

1980, edited by B. D. Lake, O. Bayliss High, S. J. Hold & P. J. Stoward, Royal Microscopical Society, Oxford, pp. 269.

Moore, M. N. 1981. Elemental accumulation in organisms and food chains. In: Analysis of marine ecosystems, edited by A. R. Longhurst, Academic Press, London, New York and San Francisco, pp. 535-569.

Moore, M. N. & Bayne, B. L. 1982. Responses of the mussel *Mytilus edulis* to environmental stress and pollution. In: Seminari internazionali sull inquinomento marino, edited by N. Della Croce, Gruppo Ricerca Oceanologica, Genova, pp. 65-73.

Moore, M. N. & Halton, D. W. 1973. Histochemical changes in the digestive gland of *Lymnea truncatula* infected with Fasciola hepatica. Z. Parasitenk 43, 11-16.

Moore, M. N. & Halton, D. W. 1977. The cytochemical localisation of lysosomal hydrolases in the digestive cells of littorinids and changes induced by larval trematode infection. Z. Parasitenk 53, 115-122.

Moore, M. N., Livingstone, D. R., Donkin, P., Bayne, B. L., Widdows, J. & Lowe, D. M. 1980. Mixed function oxygenases and xenobiotic detoxication/toxication systems in bivalve molluscs. Helgoländer wiss. Meeresunters. 33, 278-291.

Moore, M. N. & Lowe, D. M. 1977. The cytology and cytochemistry of the hemocytes of *Mytilus edulis* and their responses to experimentally injected carbon particles. J. Invertebr. Pathol. 29, 18-30.

Moore, M. N., Lowe, D. M. & Fieth, P. E. M. 1978a. Responses of lysosomes in the digestive cells of the common mussel, *Mytilus edulis* to sex steroids and cortisol. Cell Tissue Res. 188, 1-9.

Moore, M. N., Lowe, D. M. & Fieth, P. E. M. 1978b. Lysosomal responses to experimentally injected anthracene in the digestive cells of *Mytilus edulis*. Mar. Biol. 48, 297-302.

Moore, M. N., Lowe, D. M. & Gee, J. M. 1978c. Histopathological effects induced in *Mytilus edulis* by *Mytilicola intestinalis* and the histochemistry of the copepod intestinal cells. J. Cons. int. Explor. Mer. 38, 6-11.

Moore, M. N., Lowe, D. M. & Moore, S. L. 1979. Induction of lysosomal destabilisation in marine bivalve molluscs exposed to air. Mar. Biol. Letts. 1, 44-57.

Moore, M. N., Pipe, R. K. & Farrar, S. V. 1982. Lysosomal and microsomal responses to environmental factors in *Littorina littorea* from Sullom Voe. Mar. Poll. Bull. 13, 340–345.

Moore, M. N. & Stebbing, A. R. D. 1976. The quantitative cytochemical effects of three metal ions on a lysosomal hydrolase of a hydroid. J. mar. biol. Ass. U.K. 56, 995–1005.

Morris, A. W. 1984. Practical procedures for estuarine studies, edited by A. W. Morris, Natural Environment Research Council, Swindon, 261 pp.

Morton, B. S. 1971. The diurnal rhythm and tidal rhythm of feeding and digestion in *Ostrea edulis*. Biol. J. Linn. Soc. 3, 329–342.

Morton, B. S. 1977. The tidal rhythm of feeding and digestion in the Pacific oyster, *Crassostrea gigas* (Thunberg). J. exp. mar. Biol. Ecol. 26, 135–151.

Neff, J. M., Cox, B. A., Dixit, D. & Anderson, J. W. 1976. Accumulation and release of petroleum-derived aromatic hydrocarbons by four species of marine animals. Mar. Biol. 38, 279–289.

Nevo, E., Shimony, T. & Libni, M. 1977. Thermal selection of allozyme polymorphisms in barnacles. Nature, Lond. 267, 699–700.

Nevo, E., Shimony, T. & Libni, M. 1978. Pollution selection of allozyme polymorphism in barnacles. Experientia 34, 1562–1564.

Newell, R. C., 1973. Factors affecting the respiration of intertidal invertebrates. Amer. Zool. 13, 513–528.

Newell, R. C. 1979. Biology of intertidal animals, 3rd ed., Marine Ecological Surveys Ltd., Faversham, Kent, 781 pp.

Newell, R. I. E., 1977. The eco-physiology of *Cardium edule* L. Ph.D. Thesis, University of London, 215 pp.

Newsholme, E. A. & Start, C. 1973. Regulation in metabolism. Wiley, London, 349 pp.

Nichols, W. W., Miller, R. C. & Bradt, C. 1977. In vitro anaphase and metaphase preparations in mutations resting. In: Handbook of mutagenicity test procedures, edited by B. J. Kilbey, M. Legator, W. Nichols & C. Ramel, Elsevier, Oxford, pp. 225–233.

Nicholson, H. P. 1967. Pesticide pollution control. Science, N.Y. 158, 871–876.

Noël-Lambert, F. 1976. Distribution of cadmium, zinc and copper in the mussel *Mytilus edulis*. Existence of cadmium-binding proteins similar to metallothioneins. Experientia 32, 324–326.

Nordberg, G. F. 1972. Cadmium metabolism and toxicity. Experimental studies on mice with special reference to the use of biological materials as indices of retention and the possible role of metallothionein in transport and detoxification of cadmium. Environ. Physiol. Biochem. 2, 7–36.

Nordberg, G.F. & Piscator, M. 1972. Influence of long-term cadmium exposure on urinary excretion of protein and cadmium in mice. Environ. Physiol. Biochem. 2, 37–49.

Odum, H. T. 1967. Work circuits and system stress. In: Symposium on primary productivity and mineral cycling in natural ecosystems, edited by H. E. Young, University of Maine Press, Orono, pp. 81–138.

Olafson, R. W., Kearns, A. & Sim, R. G. 1979. Heavy metal induction of metallothionein synthesis in the hepatopancreas of the crab *Scylla serrata*. Comp. Biochem. Physiol. 62B, 417–424.

Olafson, R. W. & Thompson, J. A. J. 1974. Isolation of heavy metal binding proteins from marine vertebrates. Mar. Biol. 28, 83–86.

Omura, T. & Sato, R. 1964a. The carbon-monoxide binding pigment of liver microsomes: I. Evidence for its hemoprotein nature. J. biol. Chem. 239, 2370–2378.

Omura, T. & Sato, R. 1964b. The carbon-monoxide binding pigment of liver microsomes: II. Solubilization, purification and properties. J. biol. Chem. 239, 2379–2385.

Osborne, M. R. 1979. Diolepoxides—The key to hydrocarbon carcinogenesis? Trends biochem. Sci. 5, 213–215.

Osterroht, C. 1977. Dissolved PCBs and chlorinated hydrocarbon insecticides in the Baltic, determined by two different sampling procedures. Mar. Chem. 5, 113–121.

Owen, G., 1966. Digestion. In: Physiology of mollusca II, edited by K. M. Wilbur & C. M. Yonge, Academic Press, New York, London, pp. 53–88.

Owen, G. 1970. The fine structure of the digestive tubules of the marine bivalve *Cardium edule*. Phil. Trans. R. Soc. Lond. B. 258, 245–260.

Owen, G. 1972. Lysosomes, peroxisomes and bivalves. Sci. Prog. 60, 299–318.

Ozawa, K., Ida, T., Kamano, T., Garbus, J. & Cowley, R. A. 1977. Different response to hepatic energy charge and adenine nucleotide concentrations to hemorrhagic shock. Res. Exp. Med. 169, 145–153.

Paine, R. T. 1974. Intertidal community structure: Experimental studies on the relationship between a dominant competitor and its principal predator. Oecologia, Berl. 15, 92–120.

Paloheimo, J. E. & Dickie, L. M. 1965. Food and growth of fishes. I. A growth curve derived from experimental data. J. Fish. Res. Bd Can. 22, 521–542.

Paloheimo, J. E. & Dickie, L. M. 1966a. Food and growth of fishes. II. Effects of food and temperature on the relation between metabolism and body weight. J. Fish. Res. Bd Can. 23, 869–908.

Paloheimo, J. E. & Dickie, L. M. 1966b. Food and growth of fishes. III. Relations among food, body size and growth efficiency. J. Fish. Res. Bd Can. 23, 1209–1248.

Pani, P., Sanna, A., Brigaglia, M. I., Columbano, A. & Congiu, L. 1976. Early investigations on the effect of methyl mercuric chloride upon DMN— acute hepatotoxicity. Experientia 32, 1449–1451.

Parry, M. J., Tweats, D. J. & Al-Mossawi, A. J. 1976. Monitoring the marine environment for mutagens. Nature, Lond. 264, 538–540.

Pauley, G. B. 1969. A critical review of neoplasia and tumour-like lesions in mollusks. Natl. Cancer. Inst. Monogr. 31, 509–539.

Payne, J. F., 1976. Field evaluation of benzopyrene hydroxylase induction as a monitor for marine petroleum pollution. Science, N.Y. 191, 945–946.

Payne, J. F. 1977. Mixed function oxidases in marine organisms in relation to petroleum hydrocarbon metabolism and detection. Mar. Poll. Bull. 8, 112–116.

Payne, J. F., Maloney, R. & Rahimtula, A. 1979. Are petroleum hydrocarbons an important source of mutagens in the marine environment. In: Proceedings of the 1979 oil spill conference, American Petroleum Institute, Publication No. 4308, Washington, D.C., pp. 533–536.

Payne, J. F., Maloney, R., Rahimtula, A. & Martins, I. 1982. Petroleum and petroleum combustion by-products as potential sources of marine environmental mutagens. In: Carcinogenic polynuclear aromatic hydrocarbons in the marine environment, U.S. Environmental Protection Agency, Washington, D.C., pp. 102–109.

Payne, J. F. & Martins, I. 1980. Monitoring for mutagenic compounds in the marine environment. Rapp. P.-v. Réun. Cons. int. Explor. Mer 179, 292–298.

Payne, J. F., Martins, I. & Rahimtula, A. 1978. Crankcase oils: Are they a major mutagenic burden in the aquatic environment? Science, N.Y. 200, 329–330.

Payne, J. F. & May, N. 1978. Oxidative transformation of complex mixtures of pollutant aromatic hydrocarbons by fish. Chemosphere 7, 815–819.

Payne, J. F. & May, N. 1979. Further studies on the effect of petroleum hydrocarbons on mixed function oxidases in marine organisms. In: Pesticide and xenobiotic metabolism in aquatic organisms, edited by M. A. Q. Khan, J. L. Lech & J. J. Menn, American Chemical Society, Washington, D.C., pp. 339–347.

Payne, J. F. & Penrose, W. R. 1975. Induction of aryl hydrocarbon (benzo(a) pyrene) hydroxylase in fish by petroleum. Bull. Environ. Contam. Toxicol. 14, 112–116.

Pearse, A. G. E. 1972. Histochemistry, theoretical and applied, Vol. 2, Churchill Livingstone, London, 757 pp.

Pedersen, M. G., Hershberger, W. K. & Jachau, M. R. 1974. Metabolism of 3,4-benzopyrene in rainbow trout (Salmo gairdneri). Bull. Environ. Contam. Toxicol. 12, 481–486.

Pedersen, M. G., Hershberger,W. K., Zachariah, P. K. & Jachau, M. R. 1976. Hepatic biotransformation of environmental xenobiotics in six strains of rainbow trout (Salmo gairdneri). J. Fish. Res. Bd Can. 33, 666–675.

Penrose, W. R. 1978. Specific biological methods for petroleum baseline and pollution monitoring. Mar. Poll. Bull. 9, 231–234.

Pesch, G. G. & Pesch, C. E. 1980. Neanthes arenaceodentata (Polychaeta: Annelida), a preposed cytogenetic model for marine genetic toxicology. Com. J. Fish. Aquat. Sci. 37, 1225–1228.

Pesch, G. G. & Pesch, C. E. 1980. Neanthes arenaceodentata (Polychaeta: Annelida), a proposed cytogenetic model for marine genetic toxicology. Com. J. Fish. Aquat. Sci. 37, 1225–1228.

Peterson, G. L. 1979. Review of the folin phenol protein quantitation method of Lowry, Rosebrough, Farr and Randall. Analyt. Biochem. 100, 201–220.

Phillips, D. J. H. 1979. Trace metals in the common mussel, *Mytilus edulis* (L) and the alga *Fucus vesiculosus* (L) from the region of the sound (Öresund). Environ. Pollut. 18, 31–43.

Philpot, R. M., James, M. O. & Bend, J. R. 1976. Metabolism of benzo(a)-pyrene and other xenobiotics by microsomal mixed function oxidases in marine species. In: Sources, effects and sinks of petroleum in the aquatic environment, Amer. Inst. Biol. Sci. Symposium, Washington, D.C., pp. 184–199.

Pickering, A. D. 1981. Stress and fish. Academic Press, London, 367 pp.

Piotrowski, J. K., Bolanowska, W. & Sapota, A. 1973. Evaluation of metallothionein content in animal tissues. Acta. biochim. pol. 20, 207–215.

Piscator, M. 1964. On cadmium in normal human kidneys together with a report on the isolation of metallothionein from livers of cadmium-exposed rabbits. Nord. hyg. Tidskr. 45, 76–82.

Plapp, F. W., Tate, L. F. & Hodgson, E. 1976. Biochemical genetics of oxidative resistance to diazinon in the housefly. Pest. Biochem. Physiol. 6, 175–182.

Pohl, R. J., Bend, J. R., Guarino, A. M. & Fouts, J. R. 1974. Hepatic microsomal mixed function oxidase activity of several marine species from coastal Maine. Drug Metab. Dispos. 2, 545–555.

Poland, A. & Glover, E. 1977. Chlorinated biphenyl induction of aryl hydrocarbon hydroxylase activity: A study of the structure-activity relationship. Molec. Pharmacol. 13, 924–938.

Porter, H., 1974. The particulate half-cystine-rich copper protein of new-born liver. Relationship to metallothionein and subcellular localisation in non-mitochondrial particles possibly representing heavy lysosomes. Biochem. biophys. Res. Commun. 56, 661–668.

Precht, H. 1958. Concepts of temperature adaptation of unchanging reaction systems of cold-blooded animals. In: Physiological adaptation, edited by C. L. Prosser, Ronald Press, New York, pp. 50–78.

Premakumar, R., Winge, D. R., Wiley, R. D. & Rajagopalan, K. V. 1975. Copper-induced synthesis of copper-chelatin in rat liver. Archs Biochem. Biophys. 170, 267–277.

Premdas, F. H. & Anderson, J. M. 1963. Uptake and detoxification of ^{14}C-labelled DDT in Atlantic salmon, *Salmo salar*. J. Fish. Res. Bd Can. 20, 827–837.

Pritchard, J. B. & Kinter, W. B. 1970. Fate and distribution and metabolism of DDT in winter flounder. Bull. Mt. Desert Isl. Mar. Lab. 10, 64–67.

Prosser, C. L. 1958. General summary: The nature of physiological adaptation. In: Physiological adaptation, edited by C. L. Prosser, Ronald Press, New York, pp. 167–180.

Pruell, R. J. & Engelhardt, F. R. 1980. Liver cadmium uptake, catalase inhibition, and cadmium thionein production in the killifish (*Fundulus heteroclitus*) induced by experimental cadmium exposure. Mar. Environ. Res. 3, 101–111.

Pulido, P., Kägi, J. H. R. & Vallee, B. L. 1966. Isolation and some properties of human metallothionein. Biochemistry, N.Y. 5, 1768–1777.

Purich, D. L. & Fromm, H. J. 1972. Studies on factors influencing enzyme responses to adenylate energy charge. J. biol. Chem. 247, 249–255.

Purich, D. L. & Fromm, H. J. 1973. Additional factors influencing enzyme responses to the adenylate energy charge. J. biol. Chem. 248, 461–466.

Rabinowitz, J. C. 1974. Determination of adenosine-5'-triphosphate with formyltetrahydrofolate synthetase. In: Methods of enzymatic analyses, edited by H. U. Bergmeyer, Academic Press, New York, pp. 2110–2111.

Rahman, Y. E. & Lindebaum, A. 1964. Lysosome particles and subcellular distributions of polymeric tetravalent plutonium-239. Radiat. Res. 21, 575–583.

Rainer, S. F., Ivanovici, A. M. & Wadley, V. A. 1979. Effect of reduced salinity on adenylate energy charge in three estuarine molluscs. Mar. Biol. 54, 91–99.

Read, K. R. H. & Cumming, K. B. 1967. Thermal tolerance of the bivalve molluscs *Modiolus modiolus* L., *Mytilus edulis* L. and *Brachidontes demissus Dillwyn*. Comp. Biochem. Physiol. 22, 149–155.

Rees, W. J. & Russell, F. S. 1937. On rearing the hydroids of certain medusae, with an account of the methods used. J. mar. biol. Ass. U.K. 22, 61–82.

Reichenback-Klinke, H. & Elkan, E. 1965. The principle diseases of lower vertebrates. Academic Press, London, New York, 600 pp.

Renfro, J. L., Schmidt-Nielsen, B., Miller, D., Benos, D. & Allen. J. 1974. Methylmercury and inorganic mercury: Uptake, distribution and effect on osmoregulatory mechanism in fishes. In: Pollution and physiology of marine organisms, edited by F. J. Vernberg & W. B. Vernberg, Academic Press, New York, pp. 101–122.

Report of the Ad Hoc Committee of the Environmental Mutagen Society, 1972. Chromosome methodologies in mutation testing. Toxic. appl. Pharmac. 22, 269–275.

Richards, T. C. 1973. Histochemical changes in developing mouse liver after administration of phenobarbital. Am. J. Anat. 138, 449–464.

Richardson, C. A., Crisp, D. J., Runham, N. W. & Gruffydd, Ll. D. 1980. The use of tidal growth bands in the shell of Cerastoderma edule to measure seasonal growth rates under cool temperate and sub-arctic conditions. J. mar. biol. Ass. U.K. 60, 977–989.

Ridge, W. 1972. Hypoxia and the energy charge of the cerebral adenylate pool. Biochem. J. 127, 351–355.

Riisgard H. U. 1977. On measurements of the filtration rates of suspension feeding bivalves in a flow system. Ophelia, 16, 167–173.

Riley, J. P. & Taylor, D. 1968. Chelating resins for the concentrations of trace elements from seawater and their analytical use in conjunction with atomic absorption spectrophotometry. Analytica chim. Acta 40, 479–485.

Riordan, J. R. 1977. The role of metals in enzyme activity. Ann. Clin. Lab. Sci. 7, 119–129.

Risebrough, R. W., DeLappe, B. W. & Schmidt, T. T. 1976. Bioaccumulation factors of chlorinated hydrocarbons between mussels and seawater. Mar. Poll. Bull. 7, 225–228.

Roberts, D. 1976. Mussels and pollution. In: Marine mussels, their ecology and physiology, edited by B. L. Bayne, Cambridge University Press, Cambridge, pp. 67–80.

Roberts, K. S., Cryer, A., Kay, J., De, L. G., Solbie, J. F., Wharfe, J. R. & Simpson, W. R. 1979. The effects of exposure to sub-lethal concentrations of cadmium on enzyme activities and accumulation of the metal in tissues and organs of rainbow and brown trout (Salmo gairdneri, Richardson and Salmo trutta fario L). Comp Biochem. Physiol. 62C, 135–140.

Roesijadi, G. 1979. Taurine and glycine in the gills of the clam *Protothaca staminea* exposed to chlorinated seawater. Bull. Environ. Contam. Toxicol. 22, 543–547.

Roesijadi, G. 1980. Influence of copper on the clam *Protothaca staminea:* Effects on gills and occurence of copper-binding proteins. Biol. Bull. mar. biol. Lab., Woods Hole 158, 233–247.

Roesijadi, G. 1981. The significance of low molecular weight, metallothionein-like proteins in marine invertebrates: Current status. Marine. Environ. Res. 4, 167–179.

Roesijadi, G. & Anderson, J. W. 1979. Condition index and free amino acid content of *Macoma inquinata* exposed to oil-contaminated marine sediments. In: Marine pollution: Functional responses, edited by W. B. Vernberg, F. P. Thurberg, A. Calabrese & F. J. Vernberg, Academic Press, New York, pp. 69–83.

Roesijadi, G., Anderson, J. W. & Giam, C. S. 1976. Osmoregulation of the Grass Shrimp *Palaemonetes pugio* exposed to polychlorinated biphenyls (PCBs). II. Effect on free amino acids of muscle tissues. Mar. Biol. 38, 357–363.

Rugstad, H. E. & Norseth, T. 1975. Cadmium resistance and content of cadmium-binding protein in cultured human cells. Nature, Lond. 257, 136–137.

Sabbioni, E. & Marafante, E. 1975. Heavy metals in rat liver cadmium-binding protein. Environ. Physiol. Biochem. 5, 132–141.

Salemaa, H. 1979, The chromosomes of *Asellus aquaticus* (L.)—A technique for isopod karyology. Crustaceana 36, 316–318.

Sansone, G., Biondi, A. & Noviello, L. 1978. Free amino acids in fluids and tissues of *Mytilus galloprovincialis* in relation to the environment. Their behaviour as an index of normality of metabolism. Comp. Biochem. Physiol. 61A, 133–139.

Savage, J. R. K. 1975. Classification and relationships of induced chromosomal structural changes. J. Med. Genet. 12, 103–122.

Sax, K. 1938. Chromosome aberrations induced by X-rays. Genetics 23, 494–516.

Saxena, J. & Howard, P. H. 1977. Environmental transformation of alkylated and inorganic forms of certain metals. Adv. Appl. Microbiol. 21, 185–226.

Schafer, R. D. 1961. Effects of pollution on the free amino acid content of two marine invertebrates. Pacif. Sci. 15, 49–55.

Schafer, R. D. 1963. Effects of pollution on the amino acid content of *Mytilus edulis*. Pacif. Sci. 17, 246–250.

Schenkman, J. B. 1970. Studies on the nature of the Type I and Type II spectral changes in liver microsomes. Biochemistry, N.Y. 9, 2081–2091.

Schenkman, J. B., Remmer, H. & Estabrook, R. W. 1967. Spectral studies of drug interactions with hepatic microsomal cytochrome. Molec. Pharmacol. 3, 113–123.

Schenkmann, J. B. & Kupfer, D. (editors). 1982. Hepatic cytochrome P-450 monooxygenase system. In: International encyclopaedia of pharmacology and therapeutics, Section 108, Pergamon, Oxford, 841 pp.

Scheuer, P. J., Thorpe, M. E. C. & Marriott, P. 1969. A method for the demonstration of copper under the electron microscope. J. Histochem. Cytochem. 15, 300–301.

Schmid, O. J. & Mann, H. 1961. Action of a detergent (dodecylbenzenesulphonate) on the gills of the trout. Nature, Lond. 192, 675.

Schmidt-Nielsen, B., Sheline, J., Miller, D. S. & Deldonno, M. 1977. Effect of methylmercury upon osmoregulation, cellular volume, and ion regulation in winter flounder, *Pseudopleuronectes americanus*. In: Physiological responses of marine biota to pollutants, edited by F. J. Vernberg, A. Calabrese, F. P. Thurberg & V. B. Vernberg, Academic Press, New York, pp. 105–117.

Schoffeniels, E. 1976. Adaptations with respect to salinity. In: Biochemical adaptation to environmental change, edited by R. M. S. Smellie & J. F. Pennock, The Biochemical Society, London, pp. 179–204.

Schoffeniels, E. & Gilles, R. 1972. Ionoregulation and osmoregulation in Mollusca. In: Chemical zoology, Vol. VII, edited by M. Florkin & B. T. Scheer, Academic Press, New York, London, pp. 393–420.

Schonbrod, R. D., Philleo, W. W. & Terriere, L. C. 1965. Hydroxylation as a factor in resistance in house flies and blowflies. J. econ. Ent. 53, 71–77.

Scott, D., Bridges, B. A. & Sobels, F. H. 1977. Progress in genetic toxicology. Elsevier/North Holland, Amsterdam, 335 pp.

Selye, H. 1950. Stress. Acta Inc., Montreal, 638 pp.

Shafee, M. S. 1979. Ecological energy requirements of the green mussel, *Perna viridis* L. from Ennore estuary. Madras. Oceanologica Acta. 2, 69–74.

Shaikh, Z. Z. & Lucis, O. J. 1971. Isolation of cadmium-binding proteins. Experientia 27, 1024–1025.

Sharma, A. K. & Sharma, A. 1980. Chromosome techniques, theory and practice, 3rd edn., Butterworths, England 724 pp.

Shaw, B. L. & Battle, H. I. 1957. The gross and microscopic anatomy of the digestive tract of the oyster *Crassostrea virginica* Gmelin. Can. J. Zool. 35, 325–347.

Shaw, W. H. R. 1961. Cation toxicity and the stability of transition-metal complexes. Nature, Lond. 192, 754–755.

Shaw, W. N., Tubiash, H. S. & Baker, A. M. 1967. Freeze-drying for determining total solids in shellfish. J. Fish. Res. Bd Can. 24, 1413–1417.

Sheridan, P. F. 1975. Uptake, metabolism and distribution of DDT in organs of the blue crab, *Callinectes sapidus*. Chesapeake Science, 16, 20–26.

Shumway, S. E., Gabbott, P. A. & Youngson, A. 1977. The effect of fluctuating salinity on the concentrations of free amino acids and ninhydrin-positive substances in the adductor muscles of eight species of bivalve molluscs. J. exp. mar. Biol. Ecol. 29, 131–150.

Shumway, S. E. & Youngson, A. 1979. The effects of fluctuating salinity on the physiology of *Modiolus demissus* (Dillwyn). J. exp. mar. Biol. Ecol. 40, 167–181.

Siegel, S. 1956. Nonparametric statistics for the behavioral sciences, McGraw-Hill, New York, 312 pp.

Simmonds, J. A. & Dumbroff, E. B. 1974. High energy charge as a requirement for axis elongation in response to gibberelic acid and kinetin during stratification of *Acer saccharum* seeds. Pl. Physiol. Lancaster, 53, 91–95.

Simpson, R. D. 1979. Uptake and loss of zinc and lead by mussel (*Mytilus edulis*) and relationships with body weight and reproductive cycle. Mar. Poll. Bull. 10, 74–78.

Sinderman, C. J. 1970. Principle diseases of marine fish and shellfish. Academic Press, New York, London, 369 pp.

Singer, S. C. & Lee, R. F. 1977. Mixed function oxidase activity in blue crab, *Callinectes sapidus* tissue distribution and correlation with changes during molting and development. Biol. Bull. 153, 377–386.

Sivarajah, K., Franklin, C. S. & Williams, W. P. 1978. The effects of polychlorinated biphenyls on plasma steroid levels and hepatic microsomal enzymes in fish. J. Fish Biol. 13, 401–409.

Skidmore, J. F. & Tovell, P. W. 1972. Toxic effects of zinc sulphate on the gills of rainbow trout. Water Res. 6, 217–230.

Skjoldal, H. R. & Bakke, T. 1978. Relationship between ATP and energy charge during lethal metabolic stress of the marine isopod, *Cirolana borealis*. J. biol. Chem. 253, 3355–3356.

Skjoldal, H. R. & Bamstedt. U. 1976. Studies on the deep-water pelagic community of Korsfjorden, Western Norway. Adenosine phosphates and nucleic acids in *Meganyctiphanes norvegica* (Euphausiacea) in relation to the life cycle. Sarsia 61, 1–14.

Slater, T. F. 1969. Lysosomes and experimentally induced tissue injury. In: Lysosomes in biology and pathology, Vol. 1, edited by J. T. Dingle & H. B. Fell, North Holland/American Elsevier, Amsterdam, pp. 467–492.

Slater, T. F. 1979. Mechanisms of protection. In: Biochemical mechanism of liver injury, edited by T. F. Slater, Academic Press, New York, pp. 745–801.

Slobodkin, L. B. & Richman, S. 1961. Calories/gm in species of animals. Nature, Lond. 191, 299.

Smyth, J. D. 1966. The physiology of trematodes. Oliver and Boyd, Edinburgh, London, 256 pp.

Snedecor, G. W. & Cochran, W. G. 1967. Statistical methods, 6th ed., Iowa State University Press, 593 pp.

Solorzano, L. 1969. Determination of ammonia in natural waters by the phenolhypochlorite method. Limnol. Oceanogr. 14, 799–801.

Sparks, A. K. 1972. Invertebrate pathology, noncommunicable diseases. Academic Press, New York, London, 387 pp.

Squibb, K. S. & Cousins, R. J. 1974. Control of cadmium-binding protein synthesis in rat liver. Environ. Physiol. Biochem. 4, 24–30.

Stanton, R. H. & Khan, M. A. Q. 1973. Mixed function oxidase activity towards cyclodiene insecticides in bass and bluegill sunfish. Pest. Biochem. Physiol. 3, 351–357.

Stebbing, A. R. D. 1971. Growth of *Flustra foliacea* (Bryozoa). Mar. Biol. 9, 267–272.

Stebbing, A. R. D. 1976. The effects of low metal levels on a clonal hydroid. J. mar. biol. Ass. U.K. 56, 977–994.

Stebbing, A. R. D. 1979. An experimental approach to the determinants of biological water quality. Phil. Trans. R. Soc. Lond. B. 286, 465–481.

Stebbing, A. R. D. 1980a. The biological measurement of water quality. Rapp. P.-v. Réun. Cons. int. Explor. Mer 179, 310–314.

Stebbing, A. R. D. 1980b. Increase in gonozooid frequency as an adaptive response to stress in *Campanularia flexuosa*. In: Developmental and cellular biology of coelenterates, edited by P. Tardent & R. Tardent, Elsevier/North Holland, Amsterdam, pp. 27–32.

Stebbing, A. R. D. 1981a. The kinetics of growth control in a colonial hydroid. J. mar. biol. Ass. U.K. 61, 35–63.

Stebbing, A. R. D. 1981b. The effects of reduced salinity on colonial growth and membership in a hydroid. J. exp. mar. Biol. Ecol. 55, 233–241.

Stebbing, A. R. D. 1981c. Hormesis—Stimulation of colony growth in *Campanularia flexuosa* (Hydrozoa) by copper, cadmium and other toxicants. Aquat. Toxicol. 1, 227–238.

Stebbing, A. R. D. 1981d. Stress, health and homeostasis. Mar. Poll. Bull. 12, 326–329.

Stebbing, A. R. D. 1982. Hormesis—The stimulation of growth by low levels of inhibitors. Sci. Tot. Environ. 22, 213–234.

Stebbing, A. R. D., Akesson, B., Calabrese, A., Gentile, J. H., Jensen, A. & Lloyd, R. 1980. The role of bioassays in marine pollution monitoring. Rapp. P.-v. Réun. Cons. int. Explor. Mer 179, 322–332.

Stebbing, A. R. D., Cleary, J. J., Brinsley, M., Goodchild, C. & Santiago-Fandino V. 1983. Responses of a hydroid to surface water samples from the River Tamar and Plymouth Sound in relation to metal concentrations. J. mar. biol. Ass. U.K. 63, 695–711.

Stebbing, A. R. D. & Pomroy, A. J. 1978. A sublethal technique for assessing the effects of contaminants using *Hydra littoralis*. Water Res. 12, 631–635.

Stegeman, J. J. 1974. Hydrocarbons in shellfish chronically exposed to low levels of fuel oil. In: Pollution and physiology of marine organisms, edited by F. J. Vernberg & W. B. Vernberg, Academic Press, New York, pp. 329–347.

Stegeman, J. J. 1978. Influence of environmental contamination on cytochrome P-450 mixed-function oxygenases in fish: Implications for recovery in the Wild Harbor Marsh. J. Fish. Res. Bd Can. 35, 668–674.

Stegeman, J. J. 1980. Mixed-function oxygenase studies in monitoring for effects of organic pollution. Rapp, P.-v. Réun. Cons. int. Explor. Mer 179, 33–38.

Stegeman, J. J. 1981a. Polynuclear aromatic hydrocarbons and their metabolism in the marine environment. In: Polycyclic hydrocarbons and cancer, Vol. 3, edited by H. V. Gelboin & P. O. P. Ts'O, Academic Press, New York, pp. 1–60.

Stegeman, J. J. 1981b. Metabolism of aromatic hydrocarbons by the bivalve mollusc *Mytilus edulis*. In: 1980–81 Annual sea grant report, Woods Hole Oceanographic Institution, 15 pp.

Stegeman, J. J. & Klotz, A. V. 1979. A possible role for microsomal hexose-6-phosphate dehydrogenase in microsomal electron transport and mixed-function oxygenase activity. Biochem. biophys. Res. Commun. 87, 410–415.

Stegeman, J. J. & Sabo, D. J. 1976. Aspects of the effects of petroleum hydrocarbons on intermediary metabolism and xenobiotic metabolism in marine fish. In: Sources, effects and sinks of hydrocarbons in the aquatic environment. American Institute of Biological Science, pp. 424–436.

Stegeman, J. J. & Teal, J. M. 1973. Accumulation, release and retention of petroleum hydrocarbons by the oyster *Crassostrea virginica*. Mar. Biol. 22, 37–44.

Sternlieb, I. & Goldfischer, S. 1976. Heavy metals and lysosomes. In: Lysosomes in biology and pathology, Vol. 5, edited by J. T. Dingle & R. T. Dean, North Holland/American Elsevier, Amsterdam, pp. 185–202.

Stewart, H. L. 1976. Some observations on comparative vertebrate and invertebrate pathology: A summary discussion of the workshop. Mar. Fish. Rev. 38, 46–48.

Stickle, W. B. & Sabourin, T. D. 1979. Effects of salinity on the respiration and heart rate of the common mussel, *Mytilus edulis* L., and the black chiton, Katherina tunicata (Wood). J. exp. mar. Biol. Ecol. 41, 257–268.

Strehler, B. L. 1974. Adenosine-5'-triphosphate and creatine phosphate: Determination with luciferase. In: Methods of enzymatic analysis, Vol. 4, edited by H. U. Bergmeyer, Academic Press, New York, pp. 2112–2121.

Strickland, J. D. H. & Parsons, T. R. 1972. A practical handbook of seawater analysis, rev. ed. Bull. Fish. Res. Bd Can. 167, 1–311.

Sugawara, C. & Sugawara. N. 1975. The inductive effect of cadmium on protein synthesis of rat intestine. Bull. Environ. Contam. Toxicol. 14, 159–162.

Summer, A. T. 1969. The distribution of some hydrolytic enzymes in the cells of the digestive gland of certain lamellibranchs and gastropods. J. Zool. (Lond). 158, 277–291.

Sutton, H. E. & Harris, M. I. 1972. Mutagenic effects of environmental contaminants (Papers Conf. Bethesdal), Academic Press, New York, London, 195 pp.

Swanson, C. P. 1957. Cytology and cytogenetics, Prentice-Hall, Englewood Cliffs, N.J., 536 pp.

Sweeney, M. J., Ashmore, J., Morris, H. P. & Weber, G. 1963. Comparative biochemistry of hepatomas IV. Isotope investigation of carbohydrate metabolism in liver tumors of different growth rates. Cancer Res. 23, 995–1002.

Talbot, V. & Mageo, R. J. 1978. Naturally-occurring heavy metal binding proteins in invertebrates. Arch. Environ. Contam. Toxicol. 7, 73–81.

Tardent, P. 1963. Regeneration in the hydrozoa. Biol. Rev. 38, 293–333.

Thillart, G., Kisbeke F. & Waarde, A. 1976. Influence of anoxia on the energy metabolism of goldfish *Carassius auratus* (L). Comp. Biochem. Physiol. 55A, 329–336.

Thompson, R. J. 1972. Feeding and metabolism in the mussel, *Mytilus edulis*. Ph.D. thesis, University of Leicester, 176 pp.

Thompson, R. J. 1979. Fecundity and reproductive effort in the blue mussel (*Mytilus edulis*), the sea urchin (*Strongylocentratus droebachiensis*) and the snow crab (*Chionoecetes opilio*) from populations in Nova Scotia and Newfoundland. J. Fish. Res. Bd Can. 36, 955–964.

Thompson, R. J. & Bayne, B. L. 1972. Active metabolism associated with feeding in the mussel *Mytilus edulis*. J. exp. mar. Biol. Ecol. 9, 111–124.

Thompson, R. J. & Bayne, B. L. 1974. Some relationships between growth, metabolism and food in the mussel, *Mytilus edulis*. Mar. Biol. 27, 317–326.

Thompson, R. J., Bayne, C. J., Moore, M. N. & Carefoot, T. H. 1978. Haemolymph volume, change in the biochemical composition of the blood and cytochemical responses of the digestive cells in *Mytilus californianus* Conrad, induced by nutritional, thermal and exposure stress. J. Comp. Physiol. 127, 287–298.

Thompson, R. J., Ratcliffe, N. A. & Bayne, B. L. 1974. Effects of starvation on the structure and function in the digestive gland of the mussel (*Mytilus edulis*). J. mar. biol. Ass. U.K. 54, 699–712.

Thurberg, F. P., Calabrese, A., Gould, E., Greig, R. A., Dawson, M. A. & Tucker, R. K. 1977. Response of the lobster, *Homarus americanus,* to sublethal levels of cadmium and mercury. In: Physiological responses of marine biota to pollutants, edited by F. J. Vernberg, A. Calabrese, F. P. Thurberg & V. B. Vernberg, Academic Press, New York, pp. 185–197.

Tiffon, Y. 1971. Detection cytochemique d'hydrolases lysosomiales dans les doisons septales steriles de *Cerianthus lloydi.* (Coelentere Anthozoaire). C.R. Acad. Sci. Paris 273, 1953–1956.

Topping, G. 1977. Mesurement and effects of sub-lethal levels of some heavy metals on marine life in simulated marine ecosystems. Proc. Analyt. Div. chem. Soc. 14, 222–224.

Trautman, T. D., Gee, S. J., Krieger, R. I. & Thongsinthusak, T. 1979. Sensitive radioassay of microsomal o-demethylations of $^{14}CH_3O$- or C^3H_3O-p-nitroanisole for comparative studies. Comp. Biochem. Physiol. 63C, 333–339.

Trenholm, S. R. & Mix, M.C. 1978. Regeneration of radiation-damaged digestive tissues in juvenile Pacific oysters (*Crassostrea gigas*). J. Invertebr. Pathol. 32, 249–257.

Tsytsugina, V. G. 1979. Methods of demonstrating cytogenetic radiation damage to aquatic organisms in vivo or in systems of tissue cultures. In: Methodology for assessing impacts of radioactivity on aquatic ecosystems. Technical Reports Series No. 190, IAEA, Vienna, pp. 369–380.

Tucker, R. K. 1979. Effects of *in vivo* cadmium exposure on ATPases in gill of the lobster, *Homarus americanus*. Bull. Environ. Contam. Toxicol. 23, 33–35.

Ulanowicz, R. E. 1978. Modelling environmental stress. In: Energy and environmental stress in aquatic systems, edited by J. H. Thorpe & J. W. Gibbons, Technical Information Center, U.S. Dept. of Energy, Virginia, pp. 1–18.

Uncles, R. J. 1982. Computed and observed residual currents in the Bristol Channel. Oceanologica Acta 5, 11–20.

Uthe, J. F., Freeman, H. C., Mounib, S. & Lockhart, W. L. 1980. Selection of biochemical techniques for detection of environmentally induced sublethal effects in organisms. Rapp. P.-v. Réun. Cons. int. Explor. Mer 179, 39–47.

Vaes, G. 1969. Lysosomes and the cellular physiology of bone resorption. In: Lysosomes in biology and pathology, Vol. 1, edited by J. T. Dingle & H. B. Fell, North Holland/American Elsevier, Amsterdam, pp. 217–253.

Vahl, O. 1972. Efficiency of particle retention in *Mytilus edulis* L. of different sizes. Ophelia 12, 45–52.

Vance, R. R. 1973. On reproductive strategies in marine benthic invertebrates. Amer. Natur. 107, 339–361.

Vandermeulen, J. H. & Penrose, W. R. 1978. Absence of aryl hydrocarbon hydroxylase (AHH) in three marine bivalves. J. Fish. Res. Bd Can. 35, 643–647.

Van Duijn, C. 1967. Diseases of fishes. Iliffe Books Ltd., London, 309 pp.

Van Weel, P. B. 1961. The comparative physiology of digestion in molluscs. Am. Zool. 1, 245–252.

Vaughan, J., Bleaney, B. & Williamson, M. 1967. The uptake of plutonium in bone marrow: A possible leukaemic risk. Br. J. Haemat. 13, 492–502.

Verity, M. A. & Reith, A. 1967. Effect of mercurial compounds on structure-linked latency of lysosomal hydrolases. Biochem. J. 105, 685–690.

Viarengo, A., Pertica, M., Mancinelli, G., Palmero, S. & Orunesu, M. 1980. Rapid induction of copper-binding proteins in the gills of metal exposed mussels. Comp. Biochem. Physiol. 67C, 215–218.

Viarengo, A., Pertica, M., Mancinelli, G., Palmero, S., Zanicchi, G. & Orunesu, M. 1982. Evaluation of general and specific stress indices in mussels collected from populations subjected to different levels of heavy metal pollution. Mar. Environ. Res. 6, 235–243.

Viarengo, A., Pertica, M., Mancinelli, G., Zanicchi, G., Palmero, S. & Orunesu M. Sintesi di proteine capaci di legare il Cu^{++} in diversi tessuti di Mitili esposti al metallo. In: Atti del Congresso della Societa Italiana di Fisiologia L'Aqvila, 27–29 Settembre, No. 127.

Villareale, M., Gould, L. V., Wasserman, R. H., Barr, A., Chiroff, R. T. & Bergstrom, W. H. 1974. Diphenylhydantoin: Effects on calcium metabolism in the chick. Science, N.Y. 183, 671–673.

Vink, G. J. 1975. Uptake of dieldrin and dieldrin-induced changes in the activities of microsomal liver enzymes of the marine flat fish, *Pleuronectes platessa*. L. In: Sublethal effects of toxic chemicals in aquatic animals, edited by J. H. Koeman and J. Strik, Elsevier, Amsterdam, pp. 145–157.

Voogt, P. A. 1972. Lipid and sterol components and metabolism in mollusca. In: Chemical zoology Vol. VII, edited by M. Florkin & B. T. Scheer, Academic Press, New York, London. pp. 245–300.

Wallis, R. L. 1975. Thermal tolerance of *Mytilus edulis* in Eastern Australia. Mar. Biol. 30, 183–191.

Walne, P. R. 1970. The seasonal variation of meat and glycogen content of seven populations of oysters *Ostrea edulis* L. and a review of the literature. Fishery Invest., Lond., Ser. 2, 26, 35 pp.

Walters, J. M., Cain, R. B., Higgins, I. J. & Corner, E. D. S. 1979. Cell-free benzo(a)pyrene hydroxylase activity in marine zooplankton. J. mar. biol. Ass. U.K. 59, 553–563.

Walton, D. G., Penrose, W. R. & Green, J. M. 1978. The petroleum-inducible mixed-function oxidase of cunner (*Tautogolabrus adspersus* Walbaum 1972): Some characteristics relevant to hydrocarbon monitoring. J. Fish. Res. Bd Can. 35, 1547–1552.

Warren, G. E. & Davis, G. E. 1967. Laboratory studies on the feeding, bioenergetics and growth of fish. In: The biological basis of freshwater fish production, edited by S. D. Gerking, Blackwell Scientific Publications, Oxford, pp. 175–214.

Webb, M. 1972. Binding of cadmium by rat liver and kidney. Biochem. Pharmac. 21, 2751–2765.

Weber, G. 1963. Behaviour and regulation of enzyme systems in normal liver and in hepatomas of different growth rates. In: Advances in enzyme regulation, 1, edited by G. Weber, Pergamon, Oxford, pp. 321–340.

Weibel, E. R. 1969. Stereological principles for morphometry in electron microscope cytology. Int. Rev. Cytol. 26, 235–302.

Weibel, E. R. & Elias, H. 1967. Quantitative methods in morphology, Springer-Verlag, Berlin, Heidelberg, New York, 267 pp.

Weiss, C. M. 1958. The determination of cholinesterase in the brain tissue of three species of fresh water fish and its inactivation *in vivo*. Ecology 39, 194–199.

Weiss, C. M. 1959. Stream pollution. Responses of fish to sublethal exposures of organic phosphorus insecticides. Sewage Ind. Wastes 31, 580–593.

Weiss, C. M. 1961. Physiological effect of organic phosphorus insecticides on several species of fish. Trans. Am. Fish. Soc. 90, 143–152.

Weiss, C. M. 1965. Use of fish to detect organic insecticides in water. J. Wat. Pollut. Control Fed. 37, 647–658.

Wellings, S. R., McCain, B. B. & Miller, B. S. 1976. Epidermal papillomas in pleuronectidae of Puget Sound, Washington. Prog. Exp. Turmour. Res. 20, 55–74.

Wells, H. W. & Gray, I. E. 1960. The seasonal occurrence of *Mytilus edulis* on the Carolina coast as a result of transport around Cape Hatteras. Biol. Bull. mar. biol. Lab., Woods Hole 119, 550–559.

Whittle, K. J., Hardy, R., Holden, A. V., Johnston, R. & Pentreath, R. J. 1977. Occurence and fate of organic and inorganic contaminants in marine animals. Ann. N.Y. Acad. Sci. 298, 47–79.

Wickens, J. F. 1972. The food value of brine shrimp, *Artemia salina* L. to larvae of the prawn, *Palaemon serratus* Pennant. J. exp. mar. Biol. Ecol. 10, 151–170.

Widdows, J. 1972. Thermal acclimation by *Mytilus edulis*. Ph.D. thesis, University of Leicester, Leicester, 131 pp.

Widdows, J. 1976. Physiological adaptation of *Mytilus edulis* to cyclic temperatures. J. Comp. Physiol. 105, 115–128.

Widdows, J. 1978a. Combined effects of body size, food concentration, and season on the physiology of *Mytilus edulis*. J. mar. biol. Ass. U.K. 58, 109–124.

Widdows, J. 1978b. Physiological indices of stress in *Mytilus edulis*. J. mar. biol. Ass. U.K. 58, 125–142.

Widdows, J., Bakke, T., Bayne, B. L., Donkin, P., Livingstone, D. R., Lowe, D. M., Moore, M. N., Evans, S. V. & Moore, S. L. 1982. Responses of *Mytilus edulis* L. on exposure to the water accomodated fraction of North Sea Oil. Mar. Biol. 67, 15–31.

Widdows, J. & Bayne, B. L. 1971. Temperature acclimation of *Mytilus edulis* with reference to its energy budget. J. mar. biol. Ass. U.K. 51, 827–843.

Widdows, J., Bayne, B. L., Donkin, P., Livingstone, D. R., Lowe, D. M., Moore, M. N. & Salkeld, P. N. 1981a. Measurement of the responses of mussels to environmental stress and pollution in Sullom Voe: A baseline study. Proc. Roy. Soc. Edin. B. 80, 323–338.

Widdows, J., Bayne, B. L., Livingstone, D. R., Newell, R. I. E. & Donkin, P. 1979a. Physiological and biochemical responses of bivalve molluscs to exposure to air. Comp. Biochem. Physiol. 62A, 301–308.

Widdows, J., Fieth, P. & Worrall, C. M. 1979b. Relationships between seston, available food and feeding activity in the common mussel *Mytilus edulis*. Mar. Biol. 50, 195–207.

Widdows, J., Phelps, D. K. & Galloway, W. 1981b. Measurement of physiological condition of mussels transplanted along a pollution gradient in Narragansett Bay. Mar. Environ. Res. 4, 181–194.

Wiebe, W. J. & Bancroft, K. 1975. Use of the adenylate energy charge ratio to measure growth state of natural microbial communities. Proc. natn. Acad. Sci. U.S.A. 72, 2112–2115.

Wijsman, T. C. M. 1976. Adenosine phosphates and energy charge in different tissues of *Mytilus edulis* under aerobic and anaerobic conditions. J. Comp. Physiol. 107, 129–140.

Williams, R. J. 1970. Freezing tolerance in *Mytilus edulis*. Comp. Biochem. Physiol. 35, 145–161.

Wilson, D. P. 1951. A biological difference between natural waters. J. mar. biol. Ass. U.K. 30, 1–21.

Wilson, D.P. & Armstrong, F. A. T. 1961. Biological differences between sea waters: Experiments in 1960. J. mar. biol. Ass. U.K. 41, 663–681.

Winberg, G. G. 1960. Rate of metabolism and food requirements of fishes. Fish. Res. Bd Can. Transl. Ser. 194, 1–253.

Winberg, G. G. 1971. Methods for the estimation of production of aquatic animals. Academic Press, London, 175 pp.

Winge, A., Handler, P. & Smith, E. L. 1973. Cadmium accumulation in rat liver: Correlation between bound metal and pathology. In: Trace element metabolism Vol. 2, edited by W. G. Hoekstra., J. W. Suttie., H. E. Ganther & W. Mertz, University Park Press, Baltimore, pp. 500–501.

Winge, D. R., Premakumar, R. & Rajagopalan, K. V. 1975. Metal-induced formation of metallothionein in rat liver. Arch. Biochem. Biophys. 170, 242–252.

Woelke, C. E. 1967. Measurement of water quality with the Pacific oyster embryo bioassay. Water Quality Criteria 416, 112–120.

Woelke, C. E. 1968. Application of shellfish bioassay results to the Puget Sound pulp mill pollution problem. N.W. Sci. 42, 125–133.

Woelke, C. E. 1972. Development of a receiving water quality bioassay criterion based on the 48 hour Pacific oyster (*Crassostrea gigas*) embryo. Washington Department of Fisheries, Technical Report 9, 1–93.

Woodger, J. H. 1930. The 'concept of organism' and the relation between embryology and genetics. Part II. Q. Rev. Biol. 5, 438–463.

Yang, S. K., McCourt, D. W., Leutz, J. C. & Gelboin, H. V. 1977. Benzo(a)pyrene diol epoxides: Mechanism of enzymatic formation and optically active intermediates. Science, N.Y. 196, 1199–1201.

Yap, H. H., Desaiah, D., Cutkomp, L. K. & Koch, R. B. 1971. Sensitivity of fish ATPases to polychlorinated biphenyls. Nature, Lond. 233, 61.

Yoshida, T., Ito, Y. & Suzuki, Y. 1976. Inhibition of hepatic drug metabolizing enzyme by cadmium in mice. Bull. Environ. Contam. Toxicol. 15, 402–405.

Zaba, B. N., De Zwaan, A. & de Bont, A. M. T. 1978. Preparation and properties of mitochondria from tissues of the sea mussel, *Mytilus edulis*. Int. J. Biochem. 9, 191–197.

Zammitt, V. A. & Newsholme, E. A. 1976. The maximum activities of hexokinase, phosphorylase, phosphofructokinase, glycerol phosphate dehydrogenases, lactate dehydrogenase, octopine dehydrogenase, phosphoenolpyruvate carboxykinase, nucleoside diphosphatekinase, glutamate-oxaloacetate transaminase and arginine kinase in relation to carbohydrate utilization in muscles from marine invertebrates. Biochem. J. 160, 447–462.

Zurburg, W. & De Zwaan, A. 1981. The role of amino acids in anaerobiosis and osmoregulation in bivalves. J. exp. Zool. 215, 315–325.

Zurburg, W., Kluytmans, J. H., Pieters, H. & Zandee, D. I. 1979. The influence of seasonal changes on energy metabolism in *Mytilus edulis* L. II. Organ specificity. In: Proc. 13th Europ. mar. biol. symp, edited by E. Naylor & R. G. Hartnoll, Pergamon, Oxford, New York, pp. 293–300.

Index

bioassay, 133–140
    approach, rationale for, 133–134
    techniques, 135–137
    of water samples, 288–293
biological effects monitoring, application of AEC to, 100–107
biosynthesis, inhibition of, 303
Bishop, S. H., 86, 91
Bitensky, L., 64, 65, 189, 190, 191, 192
Blackstock, J. D., 115, 216
body component index, 44–45
body condition index, 1, 39–44
    calculation of, 178
    definition of, 39–41
    factors affecting, 41–44
Boehm, P. D., 121
Bostock, C. J., 78
Bouquegneau, J. M., 126, 130, 259
Brand, A. R., 15
Brand, K., 220, 221
Braverman, M., 267
Bremner, I., 126
Bresnick, E., 124
Brett, J. R., 12
Briarty, J. R., 185
Bronowski, J., 306
Brown, D. A., 126, 127, 128, 129, 130, 132, 258, 259, 262, 263, 264, 265, 266
Brown, V. M., 268
Bruce, W. R., 208
Brun, A., 65
Brunk, U., 65
Bryan, G. W., 133, 134, 312
Bubel, A., 54
Buhler, D. R., 252, 255, 257
Burns, J. J., 71
Burns, K. A., 118, 119, 120, 251, 252, 255, 257, 258
Butcher, R. G., 203
byphenyl, polychlorinated, 122
cadmium, 66, 101, 112, 127, 128, 132, 266
Cairns, J., 310
Calanus hyperboreus, 8, 32
Caldwell, R. S., 112
Calow, P., 16, 17, 155
Campanuluria flexuosa, 65, 66, 137, 268–297, 302
Campbell, J. W., 86
Canzonier, W. J., 47
Capitella capitata, 119
carbohydrate, depletion of, 84
carbon tetrachloride, 65
carcinogens, 71, 75, 120, 122

Cardium edule, 59
Carlson, G. P., 119, 252, 255, 257
Carter, C. O., 77
cell
    daughter, 76
    mutation, somatic, 77
    quantitative analysis of, 185–189
Cerastoderma edule, 7, 147
Chan, T. M., 252
Chapman, A. G., 100, 101
Chatel, K. W., 128, 258, 263, 265, 266
Chayen, J., 71, 204
Chevion, M., 258
Chipman, W. A., 75
Chipperfield, P. N. J., 57
chromosomal
    mutations, 77–79
    structural aberrations, 212, 213
chromosome, 77
    banding technique, 79
    prevention of overcondensation of, 213
Clarke, K. R., 80, 214
clearance rate, 14–15
    measurement of, 165–168
Cochran, W. G., 233
Coleman, N., 48
Colombatti, A., 75
Conney, A. H., 118
Conney, A. K., 71
Connor, P. M., 135
Conover, R. J., 17, 18, 36, 169
Conover ratio, 17–19, 169
contaminants, biologically significant, identification of, 294
Cook, L. M., 77
copper, 51, 65, 66, 127, 128, 266, 275, 286, 295
Corbicula fluminea, 101
Corner, E. D. S., 36, 251, 252, 268
Coughlan, J., 15
Cousins, R. J., 127
Cowey, C. B., 36
Crabtree, B., 114
Crangon crangon, 30
Crassostrea
    gigas, 52, 59
    virginica, 7, 54, 58–59, 119
Creaven, P. J., 252, 255, 257
Crisp, D. J., 12, 13, 136, 157, 166, 167
Cumming, K. B., 48
cysteine, 126, 266
cytochemical measurements, and response to stress, 46–74

376

cytochrome P-450, 71, 116, 121, 250,
253-255
cytological measurements, and
response to stress, 46-74
cytology, preparation of tissue
sections for, 179-185
cytoplasmic changes, 49-50
cytoplasmic pool, concentration of
metals in, 264-266
Daly, J. W., 118
Dare, P. J., 43
Darlington, C. D., 211
Darrow, D. C., 251
Davey, E. W., 295
Davies, N. T., 126
Davies, P. Spencer-, 12
Davis, G. E., 5, 6
Davis, H. C., 136
Davison, W., 18
Dawes, E. A., 100
Dayton, P. K., 142
DDT, 107
DePierre, J. W., 115, 116, 117, 118,
119
destabilisation of lysosomes, 63-70
DesVoigne, D. M., 54, 92, 106, 107,
112, 114
detoxication, rates of, in fish,
120-121
Dewaide, J. H., 255, 257
De Wilde, P. A. W. J., 148
De Zwaan, A., 11, 86, 93, 112, 113,
114, 216
Dickie, L. M., 12, 34, 145, 146
digestion
in bivalves, 58-62
efficiency of, 16-17
measurement of, 14-19
digestive gland index, 45
digestive tubules
loss of synchrony in, 58-62
quantitative analysis of, 186-188
Dingle, J. T., 63, 65
DiSalvo, L. H., 47, 121
Dixon, D. R., 77, 80, 214, 312
DNA, 51, 52, 85
damage to, 75, 76
Donax vittatus, 38
Drake, J. W., 77
Dumbroff, E. B., 100
Dvorchik, B. H., 251
Ebberink, R. H. M., 112, 114
Edwards, D. B., 43
Edwards, R. R. C., 30
effluent
cooling-water, 153

industrial, 133
pulp mill, 138
egg quality, 155-157
Eigener, U., 101
Elcombe, C. R., 118, 122
Elias, H., 185
Elliott, J. M., 18
Elmamlouk, T. H., 119, 252, 254,
255, 257
embryos
analphase analysis of, 213
in bioassay, 210
metaphase analysis of, 210-213
Emmerson, B. K., 85
Emmerson, J., 85
endocytosis, 64
energy charge, adenylate, 97-100,
220-239
energy equation
balanced, 5
physiological components of,
6-19
Engel, D. W., 112, 127
Engelhardt, F. R., 127
environment
assimilative capacity of, 307,
310-311
chronically polluted, 70
environmental contamination, and
temporal sequence of effects in
organisms, 305
environmental mutagenesis, test
system for, 205-214
environmental quality, strategy for
monitoring of, 311-314
environmental stress, and body condition index, 43-44
enzyme
as indicator of metabolic stress,
114
NADPH-producing, 71, 121, 124-
125, 247-250
enzyme activities, 107-115
maximal, 239-246
enzyme cytochemistry, preparation of
tissue sections for, 189
Ericsson, J. L. E., 63, 64
Ernster, L., 115, 116, 117, 118, 119
Evans, H. J., 78, 79, 212
extracellular regulation, anisosmotic,
93
Farley, C. A., 48, 52, 74, 123-124
Farrar, S. V., 119
Farrington, J. W., 121
fecundity, 148-153
feeding, measurement of, 14-19

mussels, as indicators of environmental
    pollution, 47–48
Mya arenaria, 6, 30, 32
Mytilicola intestinalis, 56
Mytilus
    edulis, 6, 9, 14–45, 48, 50, 52, 54,
        55, 59, 65, 66, 71, 72, 74, 80,
        86, 90, 93, 94, 95, 101, 107, 113,
        114, 119, 122, 123, 125, 129,
        142–157, 167, 170, 185–189,
        194, 204, 215–226, 239–250,
        256, 257, 302, 312
    galloprovincialus, 121, 129
    californianus, 62, 119
N-acetyl-β-hexosaminidase, 190–191
NADPH, 117, 226–227
NADPH-neotetrazolium reductase,
    50–51, 121
    microsomal, 70–74
    stimulation of, 203–204
naphthalene, 251
natural environmental stressors, effect
    of, on scope for growth, 20–27
nauplii, 268, 270–271, 273
Neanthes arenaceodentata, 80, 91
Neff, J. M., 121
neoplasia, 47, 77
neoplasms, haemopoietic, 52
net growth efficiency, calculation of,
    177
Nevo, E., 75
Newell, R. C., 12
Newsholme, E. A., 114, 220, 225, 238
Nichols, W. W., 79, 212, 213
nickel, 65
Nishimura, I., 211
nitrogen, excretion of, 19
Noël-Lambert, F., 126, 129, 130,
    259, 262
Nordberg, G. F., 126, 259
Norseth, T., 126
nucleotides
    adenine, extraction of, 221–225
    efficiency of extraction of, 238
nucleotide concentrations, calculation
    of, 232–233
nucleotide ratios, calculation of,
    233
nucleus, as indicator of cell condition,
    49
Olafson, R. W., 126, 130, 258, 262
Omura, T., 253
O:N ratio, 1, 4, 36–38
    calculation of, 177–178
    and response to stress, 36–39

oocytes, 208–209, 210
organism, hierarchical organisation of
    and impact of toxicant on, 303–
    305
O'Riordan, M. L., 212
Osborne, M. R., 118
Osterroht, C., 295
Ostrea
    edulis, 45, 59, 156
    lurida, 52
oxygen consumption
    calculation of rate of, 171
    measurement of, 11–13
    relationship of to body size,
        163–164
Owen, G., 59, 60, 63
Ozawa, K., 100
Paine, R. T., 142
Palaemonetes pugio, 91
Paloheimo, J. E., 34
Pani, P., 121
parasitic infections, screening for, 188
parasitic infestation, 56
parasitology, 47
Parophrys vetulus, 132
Parry, M. J., 75
Parsons, T. R., 126, 127, 168, 258,
    259, 263, 265
particulate organic matter (POM), 16,
    168, 175
Pauley, G. B., 52
Payne, J. F., 71, 75, 118, 119, 120–
    121, 122, 124, 252, 255, 258
PCBs, 107, 112
Pearce, J. B., 306, 309
Pearse, A. G. E., 51
Pedersen, M. G., 118, 252, 255, 257,
    258
Penrose, W. R., 82, 118, 119, 121,
    122, 123, 252, 255, 258
PEP, 226–267
Perna viridis, 7
Perry, S. F., 47
Pesch, C. E., 80
pesticides, 70, 118
Phaeodactylum tricornutum, 162, 165
Phillips, D. J. H., 47
Philpot, R. M., 255
phosphagens, 106
phosphate groups, high-energy, 98
phosphofructokinase, 114
phosphorylation potential, 99
physiological stress
    experimental approaches to
        measurement of, 161

381